Study Guide

Clinical Procedures
for Medical Assistants

Study Guide

Clinical Procedures
for Medical Assistants

Ninth Edition

Kathy Bonewit-West, BS, MEd
Coordinator and Instructor
Medical Assistant Technology
Hocking College
Nelsonville, Ohio

Former Member, Curriculum Review Board of the
American Association of Medical Assistants

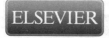

3251 Riverport Lane
St. Louis, Missouri 63043

STUDY GUIDE FOR
CLINICAL PROCEDURES FOR MEDICAL ASSISTANTS

ISBN: 978-1-4557-4835-8

Executive Content Strategist: Jennifer Janson
Senior Content Development Specialist: Jennifer Bertucci
Publishing Services Manager: Hemamalini Rajendrababu
Project Manager: Saravanan Thavamani
Design Direction: Karen Pauls

Printed in the United States

Last digit is the print number: 9 8 7 6 5 4 3 2 1

Working together to grow libraries in developing countries

www.elsevier.com • www.bookaid.org

Contents

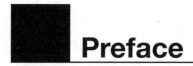

Preface

Outcome-based education prepares individuals to perform the prespecified tasks of an occupation under real-world conditions at a level of accuracy and speed required of the entry-level practitioner of that profession. Outcome-based education plays an important role in medical assisting programs in preparing qualified individuals for careers in medical offices, clinics, and related health care facilities. The *Study Guide for Clinical Procedures for Medical Assistants* has been developed using a thorough outcome-based approach. It meets the criteria stipulated by the Commission on Accreditation of Allied Health Education (CAAHEP)* Standards and Guidelines for the Medical Assisting Educational Programs and the Accrediting Bureau of Health Education Schools (ABHES) Programmatic Evaluation Standards for Medical Assisting. Instructors should find this Study Guide a valuable teaching aid for training students who are able to think critically and to perform competently in the clinical setting.

Each study guide chapter is organized into the following sections:

1. *ASSIGNMENT SHEETS*: The textbook and Study Guide Assignment Sheets indicate the assignments required for each chapter, along with a space provided for the student to document the following: the date each assignment is due, completion of the assignment, and points earned for each assignment. The Laboratory Assignment Sheet indicates the procedures required for each chapter, along with the textbook and Study Guide reference pages, the number of practices required to attain competency, and a space for documenting the score earned on the Performance Evaluation Checklist.

2. *PRETEST AND POSTTEST*: These tests have been included for each chapter using true/false questions that allow the student to test his or her acquisition of knowledge for each chapter before and after completing the chapter. These tests can be used as a study guide to prepare for chapter tests.

3. *KEY TERM ASSESSMENT*: This section provides the student with an assessment of his or her knowledge of the medical terms covered in each chapter. This section also includes an assessment of the word parts of the medical terms (prefixes, suffixes, and combining forms) to evaluate the student's knowledge of the meaning of the medical term through its word parts.

4. *EVALUATION OF LEARNING*: These questions help the student evaluate his or her progress throughout each chapter. After the student has completed these questions and checked them for accuracy, they provide an ongoing review of the textbook material. Individuals preparing for a certification examination will find the completed Evaluation of Learning sections useful study aids for the clinical aspect of the examination.

5. *CRITICAL THINKING ACTIVITIES*: In this section, the student performs activities that enhance his or her ability to think critically. Some situations require the student to become involved in a game or play a role; others require the student to use independent study to answer questions posed by a patient. Independent study helps the student become familiar with resources available to acquire additional knowledge and skills outside the classroom. By learning techniques of self-development, the medical assisting student may become aware of the necessity for continuing education after graduation and entrance into the medical assisting profession.

6. *VIDEO EVALUATION*: The video evaluation sheets assess the student's knowledge of key points in the clinical skills presented in the procedural videos presented on the Evolve site (http://evolve.elsevier.com/Bonewit).

7. *PRACTICE FOR COMPETENCY*: This section consists of worksheets that provide the student with a guide for the practice of each clinical skill presented in the textbook.

---

*The CAAHEP competencies used for the Evaluation of Competency sheets were used with permission from the American Association of Medical Assistants, Chicago, Illinois, and the Commission on Accreditation of Allied Health Education Programs, Clearwater, Florida.

8. *EVALUATION OF COMPETENCY*: This section has two parts. The first part is the Performance Objective, which provides an exact description of what the learner must be able to demonstrate to attain competency and has been developed to correspond to the procedures presented in the textbook. A performance objective consists of the (1) outcome, (2) conditions, and (3) standards. The second part is the Performance Evaluation Checklist, which provides quality control by comparing the student's performance against an established set of performance standards.

9. *SUPPLEMENTAL EDUCATION*: Several medical assisting content areas are more difficult than others for the student to comprehend and perform. Because students have special difficulty in taking patients' symptoms and in calculating drug dosage, two supplemental education sections have been incorporated into this manual. The section "Taking Patients' Symptoms" provides supplemental education for Chapter 1 (The Medical Record) in the textbook; the section "Drug Dosage Calculation" provides supplemental education for Chapter 11 (Administration of Medication). In these two sections, a step-by-step, self-directed approach has been used, beginning with basic concepts and advancing to more difficult ones. The student should find that this type of approach facilitates the process of becoming proficient in these areas.

10. *EVOLVE SITE*: The Evolve site (http://evolve.elsevier.com/Bonewit) offers many opportunities for students to apply the theory and skills learned throughout the textbook. Organized by chapter, the Evolve site includes several games (e.g., Quiz Show, Road to Recovery) to provide entertainment while the student is learning important concepts related to selected chapters, matching exercises, labeling exercises, identification exercises, and other helpful activities. Of particular importance on the Evolve site are the following:
   a. *Apply Your Knowledge*: These multiple-choice questions allow the student to test his or her acquisition of practical knowledge for each chapter. These test questions can be used as a study guide to prepare for chapter tests and for a national certification examination.
   b. *Practicum Activity worksheets*: Practicum Activity worksheets are completed by the student at his or her practicum site. These worksheets assist the student in relating classroom knowledge to the real-world setting of the medical office.
   c. *Procedural Videos*: These step-by-step procedural videos directly correlate to procedures found in the textbook. They give students a visual representation of the reading material and reinforce how to perform correct clinical procedures.
   d. *Nutrition Nuggets*: These documents are provided with every chapter and provide students with supplemental nutritional coverage related to each chapter's content. After students read the relevant supplemental material, they can answer questions related to the topic at hand.

I want to thank the staff at Elsevier for their assistance and support in preparing this Study Guide. I would also like to express my appreciation to the following individuals who provided encouragement and friendship throughout this endeavor: Dave Brennan, Marlene Donovan, Dawn Shingler, Deborah Murray, Rob Bonewit, Hollie Bonewit-Cron, Tristen West, and Caitlin Brennan.

Kathy Bonewit-West, BS, MEd

Message to the Student

This Study Guide has been designed to facilitate the attainment of competency in the clinical theory and procedures in your textbook. Each chapter of the manual has been organized into the eight components outlined below. By completing each component, it is hoped that your ability to assimilate the theory and perform the clinical skills will be greatly enhanced.

1. **TEXTBOOK AND STUDY GUIDE ASSIGNMENT SHEETS**
   A. Each time your instructor makes an assignment from the textbook, Study Guide, or Evolve site, document the date due in the appropriate space on the Textbook or Study Guide Assignment Sheet.
   B. Complete each assignment by the due date. Place a checkmark in the appropriate space on the Textbook or Study Guide Assignment Sheet after completing each assignment.
   C. Grade the assignment according to the directions stipulated by your instructor.
   D. Record your points earned in the appropriate space on the Textbook or Study Guide Assignment sheet.

2. **LABORATORY ASSIGNMENT SHEET**
   A. Your instructor will assign the procedures to be completed for each laboratory practice session. Check the assigned procedures in the appropriate space on the Laboratory Assignment Sheet.
   B. Refer to the page numbers on the Laboratory Assignment Sheet for the Practice for Competency and Evaluation of Competency worksheets required for each procedure your instructor assigned.
   C. Locate and tear out the worksheets required for each procedure to be performed, and bring them to your laboratory practice session.
   D. Record the score you earned on the Evaluation of Competency Performance Evaluation Checklist in the appropriate space on the Laboratory Assignment Sheet. This will provide you with a record of your progress on clinical procedures.

3. **PRETEST AND POSTTEST**
   A. Complete the Pretest before beginning a study of each chapter. Complete the Posttest after completing the study of the chapter. Place a checkmark in the appropriate space on the Study Guide Assignment Sheet after completing each test.
   B. Check your work for accuracy against the textbook, and correct any errors.
   C. Grade the tests according to the directions stipulated by your instructor.
   D. Record the points you earned in the appropriate space on the Study Guide Assignment Sheet.
   E. Review the Pretest and Posttest before taking your chapter test.

4. **KEY TERM ASSESSMENT**
   A. Study the Terminology Review section located at the end of each chapter in the textbook.
   B. Match the medical terms with the definitions and complete the word parts table. Place a checkmark in the appropriate space on the Study Guide Assignment Sheet after completing the exercise.
   C. Check your work for accuracy against the textbook, and correct any errors.
   D. Grade the exercise according to the directions stipulated by your instructor.
   E. Record the points you earned in the appropriate space on the Study Guide Assignment Sheet.
   F. Review the Key Term Assessment before taking your chapter test.

5. **EVALUATION OF LEARNING QUESTIONS**
   A. Read the textbook chapter.
   B. Complete the Evaluation of Learning questions. Place a checkmark in the appropriate space on the Study Guide Assignment Sheet after completing the questions.
   C. Check your work for accuracy against the textbook, and correct any errors.
   D. Grade the questions according to the directions stipulated by your instructor.
   E. Record the points you earned in the appropriate space on the Textbook Assignment Sheet.
   F. Review the Evaluation of Learning questions before taking your chapter test.

6. **CRITICAL THINKING ACTIVITIES**
    A. Review the information required to complete the Critical Thinking Activities.
    B. Obtain any additional materials or resources required.
    C. Complete each Critical Thinking Activity. Place a checkmark in the appropriate space on the Study Guide Assignment Sheet after completing each assigned activity.
    D. Grade each Critical Thinking Activity according to the directions stipulated by your instructor.
    E. Record the points you earned in the appropriate space on the Textbook Assignment Sheet.

7. **EVOLVE SITE ACTIVITIES**
    A. Complete each Evolve site activity listed on the Study Guide Assignment Sheet. Place a checkmark in the appropriate space on the Assignment Sheet after completing each assigned activity.
    B. Record the points you earned in the appropriate space on the Assignment Sheet.

8. **APPLY YOUR KNOWLEDGE**
    A. Complete the Apply Your Knowledge questions on the Evolve site after studying the chapter. Place a checkmark in the appropriate space on the Study Guide Assignment Sheet after completing the questions.
    B. Record the points you earned in the appropriate space on the Study Guide Assignment Sheet.
    C. Review the Apply Your Knowledge questions before taking your chapter test.

9. **VIDEO EVALUATION**
    A. View the procedural videos assigned by your instructor (available on the Evolve site).
    B. Complete the video evaluation questions, and place a checkmark in the appropriate space on the Study Guide Assignment Sheet.
    C. Check your work for accuracy, and correct any errors.
    D. Grade the questions according to the directions stipulated by your instructor.
    E. Record the points you earned in the appropriate space on the Study Guide Assignment Sheet.
    F. Review the Video Evaluation questions before being evaluated on each clinical skill by your instructor.

10. **PRACTICE FOR COMPETENCY**
    A. Your instructor will assign procedures to be completed for each laboratory practice session. For each procedure assigned, place a checkmark in the appropriate space on the Laboratory Assignment Sheet.
    B. Refer to the page numbers on the Laboratory Assignment Sheet for the Practice for Competency and Evaluation of Competency sheets required for each procedure your instructor assigned. Locate and tear out the sheets required for each procedure to be performed, and bring them to your laboratory practice session.
    C. Practice each assigned procedure the required number of times indicated on the Laboratory Assignment Sheet or as designated by your instructor. Use the following guidelines when practicing the procedure to attain competency over each procedure:
        1. Information indicated on the Practice for Competency sheet
            a. Record your practices in the chart provided.
        2. Procedure as presented in your textbook
        3. Video of the procedure (on the Evolve site)
            a. View each procedure several times to make sure you understand the correct technique and theory.
        4. Evaluation of Competency Performance Checklist
            a. Ensure you can perform each procedure according to the criteria stipulated under conditions and standards.
        5. Peer evaluation
            a. If directed by your instructor, obtain a peer evaluation using the Evaluation of Competency Performance Evaluation Checklist.
    D. Bring the completed Practice for Competency sheet to your laboratory testing session, and present it to your instructor for his or her review before testing on the procedure.

11. **EVALUATION OF COMPETENCY PERFORMANCE CHECKLIST**
    A. Write your name and date in the space indicated on the Evaluation of Competency Performance Evaluation Checklist.
        1. Do not chart the procedure (in advance) on the Evaluation of Competency sheet. You do this after you have been tested on the procedure.
    B. For each procedure being evaluated, bring the following to your laboratory testing session, and present them to your instructor:
        1. Completed Practice for Competency sheet
        2. Evaluation of Competency Performance Checklist
        3. Outcome Assessment Record

C. Demonstrate the proper procedure for performing the clinical skill for your instructor.

D. Record results (if required) in the chart provided on the Evaluation of Competency Checklist.

E. Obtain your instructor's initials on your Outcome Assessment Record indicating you have performed the procedure with competency.

F. Record the score you earned in the appropriate space on your Laboratory Assignment Sheet.

After you have completed each chapter in this Study Guide, place the perforated sheet into a three-ring notebook. This will provide an ongoing record of your academic progress. The notebook provides a classroom reference and a certification examination review resource.

I hope that this Study Guide will assist your attainment of competency in clinical medical assisting procedures and will facilitate your transition from the classroom to the workplace.

Kathy Bonewit-West, BS, MEd

Outcome Assessment Record

This list of outcomes is used to maintain an ongoing record of classroom and practicum outcome assessment. Your instructor should initial each outcome when you have performed it with competency in the classroom. When you have performed the outcome with competency at your externship facility, it should be initialled by your practicum supervisor. Space is provided for three externship experiences in the event that you extern at more than one practicum site.

Name_____	Classroom Performance	Practicum	Practicum	Practicum
THE MEDICAL RECORD				
Complete a consent form for treatment.				
Assist a patient in completion of a consent form for release of medical information.				
Release information according to a completed form for release of medical information.				
Prepare a medical record for a new patient.				
Complete or assist the patient in completing a health history form.				
Obtain and record a patient's symptoms.				
MEDICAL ASEPSIS AND THE OSHA STANDARD				
Wash hands.				
Apply an alcohol-based hand rub.				
Apply and remove clean disposable gloves.				
Adhere to the OSHA Standard.				
STERILIZATION AND DISINFECTION				
Sanitize instruments.				
Chemically disinfect contaminated articles.				
Wrap an instrument for autoclaving.				
Sterilize articles in the autoclave.				
VITAL SIGNS				
Measure oral body temperature.				
Measure axillary body temperature.				

Name_____	Classroom Performance	Practicum	Practicum	Practicum
Measure rectal body temperature.				
Measure aural body temperature.				
Measure temporal artery body temperature.				
Measure radial pulse and respiration.				
Measure apical pulse.				
Perform pulse oximetry.				
Measure blood pressure.				
THE PHYSICAL EXAMINATION				
Measure weight and height.				
Demonstrate proper body mechanics.				
Position and drape an individual.				
Transfer a patient from and to a wheelchair.				
Prepare the examining room.				
Prepare a patient for a physical examination.				
Assist the physician with a physical examination.				
EYE AND EAR PROCEDURES				
Assess distance visual acuity.				
Assess color vision.				
Perform an eye irrigation.				
Perform an eye instillation.				
Perform an ear irrigation.				
Perform an ear instillation.				
PHYSICAL AGENTS TO PROMOTE TISSUE HEALING				
Apply a heating pad.				
Apply a hot soak.				
Apply a hot compress.				
Apply an ice bag.				
Apply a cold compress.				

Name_____	Classroom Performance	Practicum	Practicum	Practicum
Apply a chemical cold and hot pack.				
Assist with the application and removal of a cast.				
Instruct a patient in proper cast care.				
Apply a splint.				
Apply a brace.				
Measure an individual for axillary crutches.				
Instruct an individual in mastering crutch gaits.				
Instruct an individual in the use of a cane.				
Instruct an individual in the use of a walker.				
THE GYNECOLOGIC EXAMINATION AND PRENATAL CARE				
Provide instructions for a breast self-examination.				
Prepare the patient for a gynecologic examination.				
Assist with a gynecologic examination.				
Complete a cytology requisition form.				
Prepare the patient for a prenatal examination.				
Assist with a prenatal examination.				
THE PEDIATRIC EXAMINATION				
Carry an infant in the following positions: cradle and upright.				
Measure the weight and length of an infant.				
Measure the head circumference of an infant.				
Measure the chest circumference of an infant.				
Plot pediatric measurements on a growth chart.				

Name_____	Classroom Performance	Practicum	Practicum	Practicum
Apply a pediatric urine collector.				
Collect a specimen for a newborn screening test.				
MINOR OFFICE SURGERY				
Apply and remove sterile gloves.				
Open a sterile package.				
Add an article to a sterile field from a peel-apart package.				
Pour a sterile solution into a container on a sterile field.				
Change a sterile dressing.				
Remove sutures.				
Remove staples.				
Apply and remove adhesive skin closures.				
Set up a tray for minor office surgery.				
Assist the physician with minor office surgery.				
Apply the following bandage turns: circular, spiral, spiral-reverse, figure-eight, and recurrent.				
Apply a tubular gauze bandage.				
ADMINISTRATION OF MEDICATION				
Complete a medication record form.				
Prepare and administer oral medication.				
Prepare an injection from a vial.				
Prepare an injection from an ampule.				
Reconstitute a powdered drug.				
Administer a subcutaneous injection.				
Locate the following intramuscular injection sites: dorsogluteal, deltoid, vastus lateralis, and ventrogluteal.				
Administer an intramuscular injection.				

Name_____	Classroom Performance	Practicum	Practicum	Practicum
Administer an injection using the Z-track method.				
Administer an intradermal injection.				
Administer a tuberculin skin test and read the test results.				
CARDIOPULMONARY PROCEDURES				
Record a 12-lead, three-channel electrocardiogram (ECG).				
Instruct a patient in the guidelines for wearing a Holter monitor.				
Apply a Holter monitor.				
Perform a spirometry test.				
Measure peak flow rate.				
COLON PROCEDURES				
Instruct a patient for a fecal occult blood test.				
Develop a fecal occult blood test.				
Instruct a patient in the preparation for a sigmoidoscopy.				
Assist the physician with a sigmoidoscopy.				
Instruct a patient in the preparation for a colonoscopy.				
Provide instructions for a testicular self-examination.				
RADIOLOGY AND DIAGNOSTIC IMAGING				
Instruct a patient in the proper preparation required for each of the following x-ray examinations: mammogram, bone density scan, upper gastrointestinal (GI), lower GI, and intravenous pyelogram.				
Instruct a patient in the proper preparation required for each of the following: ultrasonography, computed tomography, magnetic resonance imaging, and nuclear medicine study.				

Name_____	Classroom Performance	Practicum	Practicum	Practicum
INTRODUCTION TO THE CLINICAL LABORATORY				
Use a laboratory directory.				
Complete a laboratory request form.				
Instruct the patient in advance preparation requirements for a laboratory test.				
Collect a specimen.				
Properly handle and store a specimen.				
Review a laboratory report.				
URINALYSIS				
Instruct a patient in clean-catch midstream urine specimen collection.				
Instruct a patient in 24-hour urine specimen collection.				
Assess the color and appearance of a urine specimen.				
Perform a chemical assessment of a urine specimen.				
Prepare a urine specimen for microscopic analysis.				
Perform a rapid urine culture test.				
Perform a urine pregnancy test.				
PHLEBOTOMY				
Perform a venipuncture using the vacuum tube method.				
Perform a venipuncture using the butterfly method.				
Separate serum from a blood specimen.				
Perform a skin puncture with a disposable semiautomatic lancet device.				
Perform a skin puncture with a reusable semiautomatic lancet device.				
HEMATOLOGY				
Perform a hemoglobin determination.				

Outcome Assessment Record

Name_____	Classroom Performance	Practicum	Practicum	Practicum
Perform a hematocrit determination.				
Prepare a blood smear.				
Perform a prothrombin time (PT) and international normalized ratio (INR) test.				
BLOOD CHEMISTRY AND IMMUNOLOGY				
Perform a fasting blood glucose test using a glucose monitor.				
Perform blood chemistry testing.				
Perform a rapid mononucleosis test.				
MICROBIOLOGY				
Use a microscope.				
Collect a throat specimen.				
Obtain a specimen using a collection and transport system.				
Perform a rapid strep test.				
Prepare a wet-mount slide.				
Prepare a microbiologic smear.				
ADDITIONAL OUTCOMES (List)				

1 The Medical Record

√ After Completing	Date Due	Textbook Pages	TEXTBOOK ASSIGNMENTS	Possible Points	Points You Earned
		1–49	Read Chapter 1: The Medical Record		
		5 46	Read Case Study 1 Case Study 1 questions	5	
		27 46	Read Case Study 2 Case Study 2 questions	5	
		33 46	Read Case Study 3 Case Study 3 questions	5	
			Total points		

√ After Completing	Date Due	Study Guide Pages	STUDY GUIDE ASSIGNMENTS (CTA = Critical Thinking Activity)	Possible Points	Points You Earned
		5	Pretest	10	
		6	Term Key Term Assessment	20	
		6–12	Evaluation of Learning questions	53	
		13	CTA A: Medication Administration Record	4	
		13	CTA B: Consultation Report	4	
		13	CTA C: Radiology Report	3	
		13	CTA D: Diagnostic Imaging Report	4	
		14	CTA E: Discharge Summary Report	5	
		14	CTA F: Release of Medical Information	4	
		14–15	CTA G: Chief Complaint	6	
		15	CTA H: Crossword Puzzle	23	
			Evolve Site: Road to Recovery: Medical Abbreviations (Record points earned)		

√ After Completing	Date Due	Study Guide Pages	STUDY GUIDE ASSIGNMENTS (CTA = Critical Thinking Activity)	Possible Points	Points You Earned
		40–46	Taking Patient Symptoms: Supplemental Education for Chapter 1 (10 points for each problem)	60	
			e Evolve Site: Chapter 1 Nutrition Nugget: Nutrition Basics	10	
			e Evolve Site: Apply Your Knowledge questions	10	
		17	*e* Video Evaluation	12	
		5	Posttest	10	
			ADDITIONAL ASSIGNMENTS		
			Total points		

√ When Assigned by Your Instructor	Study Guide Pages	Practices Required	LABORATORY ASSIGNMENTS (Procedure Number and Name)	Score*
	19–21	1	Practice for Competency Health History Form Textbook reference: pp. 34–36	
	22	1	Practice for Competency 1-1: Completion of a Consent to Treatment Form Textbook reference: p. 22	
	25–27		Evaluation of Competency 1-1: Completion of a Consent to Treatment Form	*
	23	1	Practice for Competency 1-2: Release of Medical Information Textbook reference: p. 23	
	29–32		Evaluation of Competency 1-2: Release of Medical Information	*
	23	2	Practice for Competency 1-3: Preparing a Medical Record Textbook reference: pp. 30–31	
	33–35		Evaluation of Competency 1-3: Preparing a Medical Record	*
	23	5	Practice for Competency 1-4: Obtaining and Recording Patient Symptoms Textbook reference: pp. 44–45	
	37–39		Evaluation of Competency 1-4: Obtaining and Recording Patient Symptoms	*
			ADDITIONAL ASSIGNMENTS	

Notes

Name _____ Date _____

86010

True or False

___T___ 1. The medical record serves as a legal document.

___T___ 2. The purpose of progress notes is to update the medical record with new information.

___F___ 3. The patient registration record consists of a list of the problems associated with the patient's illness.

___T___ 4. All OTC medications taken by the patient should be charted on the medication record form.

___T___ 5. A consultation report is a narrative report of a clinical opinion about a patient's condition by a practitioner other than the primary physician.

___F___ 6. A report of the analysis of body specimens is known as a diagnostic report.

___T___ 7. Medical impressions are conclusions drawn from an interpretation of data.

___F___ 8. A consent to treatment form is required for tuberculin skin testing.

___T___ 9. Diabetes mellitus is an example of a familial disease.

___T___ 10. Pain is an example of an objective symptom.

📄 **POSTTEST**

76000

True or False

___True___ 1. The purpose of HIPAA is to provide patients with more control over the use and disclosure of their health information.

___True___ 2. The health history provides subjective data about a patient to assist the physician in arriving at a diagnosis.

___True___ 3. Physical therapy helps a patient with a disability learn new skills to perform the activities of daily living.

___True___ 4. A copy of the patient's emergency room report is sent to the patient's family physician.

___True___ 5. When a medical assistant witnesses a patient's signature on a form, it means that the medical assistant is verifying that the patient understands the information on the form.

___True___ 6. SOAP is the acronym for the format used to organize POR progress notes.

___True___ 7. The chief complaint is the symptom causing the patient the most trouble.

___True___ 8. The social history includes information on the patient's lifestyle, such as health habits and living environment.

___True___ 9. The patient's name must be included at the beginning of each entry charted in the patient's medical record.

___False___ 10. A decrease in the amount of water in the body is known as edema.

Term **KEY TERM ASSESSMENT**

Directions: Match each medical term (numbers) with its definition (letters).

Q _____ 1. Attending physician

E _____ 2. Charting

B _____ 3. Consultation report

N _____ 4. Diagnosis

R _____ 5. Diagnostic procedure

J _____ 6. Discharge summary report

I _____ 7. Electronic medical record

P _____ 8. Familial

A _____ 9. Health history report

F _____ 10. Informed consent

S _____ 11. Inpatient

H _____ 12. Medical impressions

K _____ 13. Medical record

L _____ 14. Objective symptom

T _____ 15. Patient

O _____ 16. Physical examination report

C _____ 17. Problem

M _____ 18. Prognosis

D _____ 19. Subjective symptom

G _____ 20. Symptom

A. A collection of subjective data about a patient

B. A narrative report of an opinion about a patient's condition by a practitioner other than the attending physician

C. Any condition that requires further observation, diagnosis, management, or patient education

D. A symptom felt by the patient but not observed by an examiner

E. The process of documenting information about a patient in the medical record

F. The consent given by a patient for a medical procedure after being informed of the procedure

G. Any change in the body or its functioning that indicates the presence of disease

H. Conclusions drawn by the physician from an interpretation of data

I. A medical record that is stored on a computer

J. A brief summary of the significant events of a patient's hospitalization

K. A written record of the important information regarding a patient

L. A symptom that can be observed by an examiner

M. The probable course and outcome of a disease and the prospects for recovery

N. The scientific method of determining and identifying a patient's condition

O. A report of the objective findings from the physician's assessment of each body system

P. Occurring or affecting members of a family more frequently than would be expected by chance

Q. The physician responsible for the care of a hospitalized patient

R. A procedure performed to assist in the diagnosis, management, or treatment of a patient's condition

S. A patient who has been admitted to the hospital for at least one overnight stay

T. An individual receiving medical care

EVALUATION OF LEARNING

Directions: Fill in each blank with the correct answer.

1. List three functions of the medical record.

_____

_____

_____

2. What is the meaning of the acronym HIPAA?

_____

6

Chapter 1 **The Medical Record**

3. What is the purpose of the HIPAA Privacy Rule?

_____

_____

4. Who must comply with HIPAA?

_____

5. What is a Notice of Privacy Practices?

_____

_____

6. List examples of when HIPAA does not require written consent for the use or disclosure of a patient's health information in the following categories:

   a. Treatment: _____

   b. Payment: _____

   c. Health care operations: _____

7. What two general categories of information are included on a patient registration record?

_____

8. List three uses of the health history.

_____

_____

_____

9. What is the purpose of the physical examination?

_____

_____

10. What is the purpose of progress notes?

_____

_____

11. List three categories of medication that may be included in a medication record.

_____

_____

12. What is the purpose of home health care?

_____

_____

13. List five examples of home health services.

_____

_____

_____

_____

_____

14. What is the purpose of a laboratory report?

_____

_____

15. List five examples of diagnostic procedure reports.

_____

_____

16. What is the purpose of a therapeutic service report?

_____

_____

17. What is the difference between physical therapy and occupational therapy?

_____

_____

_____

18. List examples of physical agents used in physical therapy.

_____

_____

19. What is speech therapy?

_____

_____

20. What is the purpose of an operative report?

_____

_____

21. What is the purpose of the discharge summary report?

_____

_____

22. What is included in a pathology report?

_____

_____

23. Why is a copy of the emergency room report sent to the patient's family physician?

_____

_____

24. When is a consent to treatment form required?

_____

_____

25. What is the purpose of a consent to treatment form?

_____

_____

26. What information must the patient receive before signing a consent to treatment form?

_____

_____

27. What does *witnessing a signature* mean? What does it not mean?

_____

_____

_____

28. When must a patient complete a release of medical information form?

_____

_____

29. When does a release of medical information form not have to be completed?

_____

_____

30. What is the difference between a PPR and an EMR?

_____

_____

31. What functions are performed by an EMR software program?

_____

_____

32. What are the advantages of the electronic medical record?

_____

_____

_____

_____

33. How are paper documents entered into a patient's electronic medical record?

_____

_____

34. What procedures typically are performed by a medical assistant using an EMR?

_____

_____

_____

_____

35. How are documents organized in a source-oriented medical record?

_____

_____

36. What is reverse chronological order?

_____

37. How are documents organized in a problem-oriented medical record (POR)?

_____

_____

38. List and describe the four parts of a POR.

_____

_____

_____

_____

39. List and describe the format used to organize progress notes in a POR.

_____

_____

40. How can a health history be entered into the EMR?

_____

_____

_____

41. What are the seven parts of the health history?

_____

_____

_____

_____

_____

_____

_____

42. What is a chief complaint?

_____

43. What guidelines should be followed in recording the chief complaint?

_____

_____

_____

44. What is the current illness, and how is this information obtained?

_____

_____

45. List five examples of information included in the past medical history.

_____

_____

_____

_____

_____

46. List three examples of familial diseases.

_____

_____

_____

47. Explain the importance of the social history.

_____

_____

48. What is the purpose of the review of systems (ROS)?

_____

_____

49. List the guidelines that should be followed to ensure accurate and concise charting.

_____

_____

_____

_____

50. List three examples of subjective symptoms.

_____

_____

_____

51. List three examples of objective symptoms.

_____

_____

_____

52. What is the difference between a productive and a nonproductive cough?

_____

_____

53. Why should the following be charted in the patient's medical record?

a. Procedures performed on the patient

_____

_____

b. Specimens collected from the patient

_____

_____

c. Laboratory tests ordered for the patient

_____

_____

d. Instructions given to the patient regarding medical care

_____

_____

CRITICAL THINKING ACTIVITIES

A. Medication Administration Record

Refer to the medication administration record (see Fig. 1-2) in your textbook, and answer the following questions.

1. Does Kristen Antle have any allergies?

_____

2. How much Rocephin was administered to Kristen?

_____

3. What was the route of administration of the Rocephin injection, and where was it administered?

_____

4. What is the name of the company that manufactures Rocephin?

_____

B. Consultation Report

Refer to the consultation report (see Fig. 1-3) in your textbook, and identify the following information using the corresponding letter (A, B, C, or D).

1. Documentation that the consultant reviewed the patient's health history

2. Documentation that the consultant examined the patient

3. A report of the consultant's impressions

4. A report of the consultant's recommendations

C. Radiology Report

Refer to the radiology report (see Fig. 1-5) in your textbook, and answer the following questions.

1. What type of radiological examination was performed on Rose Baker?

_____

2. Were the lungs clear? _____

3. Were any abnormal masses noted in the abdomen? _____

D. Diagnostic Imaging Report

Refer to the diagnostic imaging report (see Fig. 1-6) in your textbook, and answer the following questions.

1. What type of diagnostic imaging procedure was performed on Vera Ruth?

_____

2. Which vertebrae of the spine were scanned?

_____

3. What problem may affect L4-5?

_____

4. What additional tests might be scheduled for Vera Ruth?

_____

E. Discharge Summary Report

Refer to the discharge summary report (see Fig. 1-10) in your textbook, and answer the following questions.

1. How long was Susan Brennan hospitalized?

   _____

2. What was her hemoglobin level at admission?

   _____

3. What was the reason for the hospitalization?

   _____

4. Was Susan pregnant?

   _____

5. What was her discharge diagnosis?

   _____

F. Release of Medical Information

Refer to the release of medical information form (see Fig. 1-14) in your textbook, and answer the following questions.

1. What medical information is protected by law and cannot be released unless specifically authorized by the patient?

   _____

   _____

2. List three reasons why a patient may authorize the release of his or her medical information.

   _____

   _____

   _____

3. After this form is completed and signed, how long is it valid before it expires?

   _____

4. What must the patient do if he or she wants to revoke the authorization?

   _____

   _____

G. Chief Complaint

Indicate whether each of the following statements is an incorrect (I) or correct (C) example of recording a chief complaint (CC). If the example is incorrect, explain which recording guideline is not being followed.

_____ 1. CC: Low back pain _____

_____ 2. CC: Sore throat and fever for the past 2 days _____

_____ 3. CC: Dyspnea, paleness, and fatigue, similar to that associated with anemia, that have lasted for
2 weeks _____

_____ 4. CC: Poor health for the past several months _____

_____ 5. CC: Weakness and fatigue related to poor eating habits and lack of exercise

_____

_____ 6. CC: Heart palpitations occurring after drinking coffee in the morning before work

_____

_____

H. Crossword Puzzle: Symptoms

Directions: Complete the crossword puzzle using the terms provided.

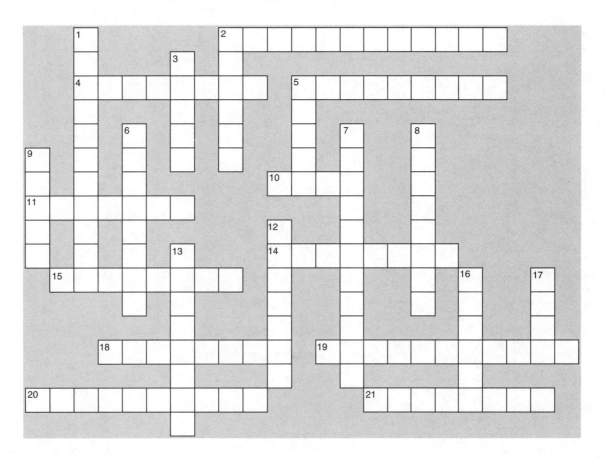

Across
- **2** Stool is hard and dry
- **4** Blue skin from lack of O_2
- **5** Nosebleed
- **10** Skin eruption
- **11** Dizziness
- **14** No appetite
- **15** Yellow skin
- **18** Severe itching
- **19** Involuntary contractions of muscles
- **20** Gas
- **21** Head pain

Down
- **1** Fast pulse rate
- **2** Shivering
- **3** May be productive or nonproductive
- **5** Fluid retention
- **6** Ejection of stomach contents
- **7** Decreased H_2O levels in the body
- **8** Red face
- **9** Elevated temp
- **12** Bad all over
- **13** Loose, watery stools
- **16** Sensation of stomach discomfort
- **17** Feeling of distress or suffering

Notes

Name: _____

Directions:

a. Watch the videos indicated.
b. Mark each true statement with a T and each false statement with an F. For each false statement, change the wording of the question so that it becomes a true statement.

Video: Procedure 1-2: Release of Medical Information

_____ 1. The information in a patient's medical record can be read by anyone who is employed by the medical office.

_____ 2. The patient must sign a consent form to release information from his or her medical record.

_____ 3. The medical assistant witnesses the patient's signature by signing the form in the appropriate space on the form.

_____ 4. The medical assistant should release only the information indicated on the release of information form.

_____ 5. The medical assistant must document the information that is being released in the appropriate space on the release form.

_____ 6. The release of information form provides legal documentation that the patient gave permission for the release of his or her medical information.

Video: Procedure 1-3: Preparing the Medical Record

_____ 1. A medical record is a written document of the important information regarding a patient.

_____ 2. The medical record includes the patient's health history, treatment, and progress.

_____ 3. Each patient must sign a Notice of Privacy Practices acknowledgement form.

_____ 4. A copy of the patient's insurance card is required for proper identification of the patient.

_____ 5. The medical assistant must enter the data on the patient registration form into the computer.

_____ 6. The patient's registration form should be placed in front of the medical record.

Notes

PRACTICE FOR COMPETENCY

Health History Form. Complete the health history form (pages 19 to 21) using yourself as the patient.

PATIENT HEALTH HISTORY

A IDENTIFICATION DATA   Please print the following information.

Today's date _____

Name _____   ___ Male ___ Female

Address _____   ___ Married ___ Separated ___ Divorced ___ Widowed ___ Single

Date of Birth _____

_____

Telephone _____
            Home number   Work number

B PAST HISTORY

Have you ever had the following: (Circle "no" or "yes", leave blank if uncertain)

Measles_____	no yes	Heart Disease_____	no yes	Diabetes_____	no yes	Hemorrhoids_____	no yes
Mumps_____	no yes	Arthritis _____	no yes	Cancer_____	no yes	Asthma _____	no yes
Chickenpox_____	no yes	Sexually Transmitted Disease	no yes	Polio_____	no yes	Allergies_____	no yes
Whooping Cough___	no yes	Anemia_____	no yes	Glaucoma_____	no yes	Eczema_____	no yes
Scarlet Fever_____	no yes	Bladder Infections___	no yes	Hernia _____	no yes	AIDS or HIV+_____	no yes
Diphtheria_____	no yes	Epilepsy_____	no yes	Blood or Plasma_____ Transfusions	no yes	Infectious Mono_____	no yes
Pneumonia_____	no yes	Migraine Headaches_	no yes	Back Trouble_____	no yes	Bronchitis_____	no yes
Rheumatic Fever___	no yes	Tuberculosis_____	no yes	High Blood Pressure _____	no yes	Mitral Valve Prolapse	no yes
Stroke_____	no yes	Ulcer_____	no yes	Thyroid Disease ___	no yes	Any other disease___	no yes
Hepatitis_____	no yes	Kidney Disease_____	no yes	Bleeding Tendency_	no yes	Please list: _____	
						_____	

MAJOR HOSPITALIZATIONS: If you have ever been hospitalized for any major medical illness or operation, write in your most recent hospitalizations below.

Hospitalizations	Year	Operation or illness	Name of hospital	City and state
1st Hospitalization				
2nd Hospitalization				
3rd Hospitalization				
4th Hospitalization				

TESTS AND IMMUNIZATIONS: Mark an X next to those that you have had.

Tests: Immunizations:

☐ TB Test   ☐ Electrocardiogram   ☐ Influenza

☐ Rectal/Hemoccult   ☐ Chest X-ray   ☐ Hepatitis B

☐ Sigmoidoscopy   ☐ Mammogram   ☐ Tetanus

☐ Colonoscopy   ☐ Pap Test   ☐ MMR

                                                 ☐ Polio

ALLERGIES: List all allergies (foods, drugs, environment). ☐ None

_____

_____

_____

_____

CURRENT MEDICATIONS: List the following that you are currently taking: Prescription medications, over-the-counter (OTC) medications, vitamin supplements, and herbal supplements.   ☐ None

Medication   Frequency

_____

_____

_____

ACCIDENTS/INJURIES: Describe all serious accidents, severe injuries, head injury, or fractures. Include the date each occurred. ☐ None

Accident/Injury: Date:

_____

_____

_____

(Continued)

C FAMILY HISTORY

For each member of your family, follow the purple or blue line across the page and check boxes for:
1. Their present state of health
2. Any illnesses they have had

	Good Health	Poor Health	Deceased	If deceased, write in age and cause of death.	Allergies or Asthma	Diabetes	Heart Disease	Stroke	Cancer	High Blood Pressure	Glaucoma	Arthritis	Ulcer	Kidney Disease	Mental Health Problems	Alcohol/Drug Abuse	Obesity	High Cholesterol	Thyroid Disease
Father:																			
Mother:																			
Brothers/Sisters:																			

D SOCIAL HISTORY

EDUCATION _____ High school _____ College _____ Post graduate

Occupation _____ Years _____

Previous occupations _____ Years _____

_____ Years _____

Have you ever been exposed to any of the following in your environment?

☐ Excess dust (coal, lime, rock)   ☐ Cleaning fluids/solvents   ☐ Radiation   ☐ Other toxic materials

☐ Sand   ☐ Hair spray   ☐ Insecticides

☐ Chemicals   ☐ Smoke or auto exhaust fumes   ☐ Paints

Please answer the follwing questions by placing an X in the box in front of the word Yes or No, except where you are asked for specific information. This information is obviously highly confidential and will be released to other health professionals or insurance carriers ONLY with your consent.

DIET:

Do you eat a good breakfast? ☐ Yes ☐ No

Do you snack between meals (soft drinks, chips, candy bars)? ☐ Yes ☐ No

Do you eat fresh fruits and vegetables each day? ☐ Yes ☐ No

Do you eat whole grain breads and cereals? ☐ Yes ☐ No

Is your diet high in fat content? ☐ Yes ☐ No

Is your diet high in cholesterol content? ☐ Yes ☐ No

Is your diet high in salt content? ☐ Yes ☐ No

Are you allergic to any foods? ☐ Yes ☐ No

How many glasses of water do you drink each day? _____

How would you describe your overall eating habits? ☐ Excellent ☐ Good ☐ Fair ☐ Poor

PERSONAL HISTORY:

Do you find it hard to make decisions? ☐ Yes ☐ No

Do you find it hard to concentrate or remember? ☐ Yes ☐ No

Do you feel depressed? ☐ Yes ☐ No

Do you have difficulty relaxing? ☐ Yes ☐ No

Do you have a tendency to worry a lot? ☐ Yes ☐ No

Have you gained or lost much weight recently? ☐ Yes ☐ No

Do you lose your temper often? ☐ Yes ☐ No

Are you disturbed by any work or family problems? ☐ Yes ☐ No

Are you having sexual difficulties? ☐ Yes ☐ No

Have you ever considered committing suicide? ☐ Yes ☐ No

Have you ever desired or sought psychiatric help? ☐ Yes ☐ No

EXERCISE:

Do you exercise on a regular basis? ☐ Yes ☐ No

Does your job require strenuous, sustained physical work? ☐ Yes ☐ No

SLEEP PATTERNS:

Do you seem to feel exhausted or fatigued most of the time? ☐ Yes ☐ No

Do you have difficulty either falling asleep or staying asleep? ☐ Yes ☐ No

USE OF TOBACCO/ALCOHOL/CAFFEINE/DRUGS: Amt:

How much do you smoke per day? ☐ Cigarettes ___

☐ Don't smoke   ☐ Cigars/pipes ___

Do you take two or more alcoholic drinks per day? ☐ Yes ☐ No

Do you drink six or more cups of coffee or tea per day? ☐ Yes ☐ No

Are you a regular user of sleeping pills, marijuana, tranquilizers, painkillers, etc.? ☐ Yes ☐ No

Have you ever used heroin, cocaine, LSD, PCP, etc.? ☐ Yes ☐ No

List any country outside the United States you have visited in the past six months. _____

When did you have your last physical examination? _____

(Continued)

Patient's Name _____

E | REVIEW OF SYSTEMS

HEAD AND NECK
_____ Frequent headaches
_____ Neck pain
_____ Neck lumps or swelling

EYES
_____ Wears glasses
_____ Blurry vision
_____ Eyesight worsening
_____ Sees double
_____ Sees halo
_____ Eye pain or itching
_____ Watering eyes
_____ Eye trouble

EARS
_____ Hearing difficulties
_____ Earaches
_____ Running ears
_____ Buzzing in ears
_____ Motion sickness

MOUTH
_____ Dental problems
_____ Swellings on gums or jaws
_____ Sore tongue
_____ Taste changes

NOSE AND THROAT
_____ Congested nose
_____ Running nose
_____ Sneezing spells
_____ Head colds
_____ Nose bleeds
_____ Sore throat
_____ Enlarged tonsils
_____ Hoarse voice

RESPIRATORY
_____ Wheezes or gasps
_____ Coughing spells
_____ Coughs up phlegm
_____ Coughed up blood
_____ Chest colds
_____ Excessive sweating,
      night sweats

CARDIOVASCULAR
_____ High blood pressure
_____ Racing heart
_____ Chest pains
_____ Dizzy spells
_____ Shortness of breath
_____ Shortness of breath at night
_____ More pillows to breathe
_____ Swollen feet or ankles
_____ Leg cramps
_____ Heart murmur

DIGESTIVE
_____ Heartburn
_____ Bloated stomach
_____ Belching
_____ Stomach pains
_____ Nausea
_____ Vomited blood
_____ Difficulty swallowing
_____ Constipation
_____ Loose bowels
_____ Black stools
_____ Gray stools
_____ Pain in rectum
_____ Rectal bleeding

URINARY
_____ Night frequency
_____ Day frequency
_____ Wets pants or bed
_____ Burning on urination
_____ Brown, black, or bloody urine
_____ Difficulty starting urine
_____ Urgency

MALE GENITAL
_____ Weak urine stream
_____ Prostate trouble
_____ Burning or discharge
_____ Lumps on testicles
_____ Painful testicles

FEMALE GENITAL
__/__/__ Last menstrual period
__/__/__ Last Pap test
_____ Postmenopausal or hysterectomy
_____ Noticed vaginal bleeding
_____ Abnormal LMP
_____ Heavy bleeding during periods
_____ Bleeding between periods
_____ Bleeding after intercourse
_____ Recent vaginal itching/discharge
_____ No monthly breast exam
_____ Lump or pain in breasts
_____ Complications with birth control

OBSTETRIC HISTORY
_____ Gravida
_____ Para
_____ Preterm
_____ Miscarriages
_____ Stillbirths
_____ Has had an abortion

MUSCULOSKELETAL
_____ Aching muscles
_____ Swollen joints
_____ Back or shoulder pains
_____ Painful feet
_____ Disability

SKIN
_____ Skin problems
_____ Itching or burning skin
_____ Bleeds easily
_____ Bruises easily

NEUROLOGICAL
_____ Faintness
_____ Numbness
_____ Convulsions
_____ Change in handwriting
_____ Trembles

F | PROGRESS NOTES

Date	

Procedure 1-1: Consent to Treatment. Complete the consent to treatment form using a classmate as the patient.

(attach label or complete blanks)

First name: _____ Last name: _____

Date of Birth: _____ Month _____ Day _____ Year

Account Number: _____

Procedure Consent Form

I, _____, hereby consent to have

Dr. _____, perform _____.

I have been fully informed of the following by my physician:

1. The nature of my condition.
2. The nature and purpose of the procedure.
3. An explanation of risks involved with the procedure.
4. Alternative treatments or procedures available.
5. The likely results of the procedure.
6. The risks involved with declining or delaying the procedure.

My physician has offered to answer all questions concerning the proposed procedure.

I am aware that the practice of medicine and surgery is not an exact science, and I acknowledge that no guarantees have been made to me about the results of the procedure.

Patient _____ Date _____
      (or guardian and relationship)

Witnessed _____ Date _____

Procedure 1-2: Release of Medical Information. Complete the release of medical information form using a classmate as the patient.

RELEASE OF MEDICAL INFORMATION

All information contained in the medical record is confidential and the release of information is closely controlled. A properly completed and signed authorization is required for the release of the following information.

PATIENT INFORMATION

Patient Name _____

Address _____   Social Security # _____

City _____ State _____ ZIP _____   Birth Date _____ / _____ / _____

Phone (Home) _____ Work _____

RELEASE FROM: RELEASE TO:

Name _____   Name _____

Address _____   Address _____

City _____ State _____ ZIP_____   City _____ State _____ ZIP_____

INFORMATION TO BE RELEASED:

1. GENERAL RELEASE:

____Entire Medical Record (excluding protected information)

____Hospital Records only (specify)_____

____Lab Results only (specify) _____

____X-ray Reports only (specify) _____

____Other Records (specify) _____

2. INFORMATION PROTECTED BY STATE/FEDERAL LAW:
If indicated below, I hereby authorize the disclosure and release of information regarding:

____Drug Abuse Diagnosis/Treatment

____Alcoholism Diagnosis/Treatment

____Mental Health Diagnosis/Treatment

____Sexually Transmitted Disease

PURPOSE/NEED FOR INFORMATION:

____Taking records to another doctor

____Moving

____Legal purposes

____Insurance purposes

____Workman's Compensation

____Other/Explain:_____

METHOD OF RELEASE:

____ US Mail

____ Fax

____ Telephone

____ To Patient

PATIENT AUTHORIZATION TO RELEASE INFORMATION:

Authorization is valid for 60 days only from the date of my signature. I reserve the right to revoke this authorization at any time prior to 60 days (except for action that has already been taken) by notifying the medical office in writing.

I understand that my records are protected under HIPAA (Health Insurance Portability and Accountability Act) Standards for Privacy of Individually Identifiable Information (45 CFR Parts 160 and 164) unless otherwise permitted by federal law. Any information released or received shall not be further relayed to any other facility or person without my written authorization. I also understand that such information will not be given, sold, transferred, or in any way relayed to any other person or party not specified above without my further written authorization.

I hereby grant authorization to release the information listed above. I certify that this request has been made voluntarily and that the information given above is accurate to the best of my knowledge.

_____   _____
Signature of Patient/Legally Responsible Party   Date

_____   _____
Witness Signature   Date

OFFICE USE ONLY

Information indicated above released on _____
                                                    Date

Explanation of information released: _____

_____

Signature and credentials of individual releasing information: _____

Procedure 1-3: Preparing a Medical Record. Prepare a medical record.

Procedure 1-4: Obtaining and Recording Patient Symptoms. Practice obtaining patient symptoms, by completing Taking Patient Symptoms: Supplemental Education for Chapter 1 (pages 40 to 46 in this study guide).

Notes

📋 **EVALUATION OF COMPETENCY**

Procedure 1-1: Completion of a Consent to Treatment Form

Name: _____ Date: _____

Evaluated by: _____ Score: _____

Performance Objective

Outcome:	Complete a consent to treatment form.
Conditions:	Given a consent to treatment form.
Standards:	Time: 10 minutes. Student completed procedure in _____ minutes.
	Accuracy: Satisfactory score on the Performance Evaluation Checklist.

Performance Evaluation Checklist

Trial 1	Trial 2	Point Value	Performance Standards
		•	Typed or printed required information on the consent to treatment form.
		•	Confirmed that the physician discussed the procedure with the patient.
		▷	Explained why the procedure should be discussed with the patient before the form is signed.
		•	Greeted the patient and introduced yourself.
		•	Identified the patient by full name and date of birth.
		•	Explained the purpose of the form to the patient.
		•	Gave the consent form to the patient to read.
		•	Asked whether the patient had any questions.
		•	Asked the patient to sign the form.
		•	Witnessed the patient's signature and dated the form.
		▷	Explained what *witnessing a signature* means.
		•	Provided the patient with a copy of the completed form.
		✶	Filed the original form in the patient's medical record.
		▷	Explained why the form must be filed in the medical record.
		✶	Completed the procedure within 10 minutes.
			Totals

Evaluation of Student Performance

EVALUATION CRITERIA			COMMENTS
Symbol	**Category**	**Point Value**	
✶	Critical Step	16 points	
•	Essential Step	6 points	
▷	Theory Question	2 points	

Score calculation: 100 points

        − _____ points missed

            ____ Score

Satisfactory score: 85 or above

CAAHEP Competencies Achieved

Psychomotor (Skills)

☑ IV. 2. Report relevant information to others succinctly and accurately.

☑ IX. 7. Document accurately in the patient record.

Affective (Behavior)

☑ IV. 2. Apply active listening skills.

☑ IV. 7. Demonstrate recognition of the patient's level of understanding in communications.

☑ IV. 8. Analyze communications in providing appropriate responses or feedback.

ABHES Competencies Achieved

☑ 4. a. Document accurately.

☑ 8. aa. Are attentive, listen, and learn.

☑ 8. cc. Communicate on the recipient's level of comprehension.

☑ 8. dd. Serve as liaison between physician and others.

(attach label or complete blanks)

First name: _____ Last name: _____

Date of Birth: _____ Month _____ Day _____ Year

Account Number: _____

Procedure Consent Form

I, _____, hereby consent to have

Dr. _____, perform _____ .

I have been fully informed of the following by my physician:

1. The nature of my condition.
2. The nature and purpose of the procedure.
3. An explanation of risks involved with the procedure.
4. Alternative treatments or procedures available.
5. The likely results of the procedure.
6. The risks involved with declining or delaying the procedure.

My physician has offered to answer all questions concerning the proposed procedure.

I am aware that the practice of medicine and surgery is not an exact science, and I acknowledge that no guarantees have been made to me about the results of the procedure.

Patient _____ Date _____
           (or guardian and relationship)

Witnessed _____ Date _____

Notes

EVALUATION OF COMPETENCY

e Procedure 1-2: Release of Medical Information

Name: _____   Date: _____

Evaluated by: _____   Score: _____

Performance Objective

Outcome:	1. Assist a patient in the completion of a release of medical information form.
	2. Release information according to a completed release of medical information form.
Conditions:	Given a release of medical information form and the patient's medical record.
Standards:	Time: 15 minutes. Student completed procedure in _____ minutes.
	Accuracy: Satisfactory score on the Performance Evaluation Checklist.

Performance Evaluation Checklist

Trial 1	Trial 2	Point Value	Performance Standards
			Completion of a Release of Information form
		•	Greeted the patient and introduced yourself.
		•	Identified the patient by full name and date of birth.
		▷	Explained the procedure to follow if you do not recognize the patient.
		•	Explained the purpose of the form to the patient.
		•	Provided the patient with a release of medical information form.
		•	Asked the patient to complete the form.
		•	Provided assistance if needed.
		•	Checked to make sure all information was completed.
		•	Asked the patient to sign the form.
		•	Witnessed the patient's signature and dated the form.
		•	Provided the patient with a copy of the completed form.
		•	Copied the medical information requested on the form.
		✶	Released only the information requested.
		•	Included a copy of the completed form with the medical information.
		•	Documented what information was released along with the date of release.
		•	Signed the release form with your name and credentials verifying you were the individual releasing the information.
		✶	Filed the original document and the release form in the patient's medical record.
			Explained the reason for filing the form.
		•	Sent the medical information according to the medical office policy.

Trial 1	Trial 2	Point Value	Performance Standards
			Mailed or faxed requests
		•	Checked the expiration date on the release of medical information form.
		▷	Explained the procedure to follow if the form is expired.
		•	Verified the signature on the form.
		▷	Stated what to do if in doubt regarding the authenticity of the signature.
		•	Copied the information requested on the form.
		✶	Released only the information requested.
		•	Documented what information was released along with the date of release.
		•	Signed the document with your name and credentials.
		•	Filed the original document and the release form in the patient's medical record.
		•	Sent the medical information according to the medical office policy.
		✶	Completed the procedure within 15 minutes.
			Totals

Evaluation of Student Performance

EVALUATION CRITERIA			COMMENTS
Symbol	**Category**	**Point Value**	
✶	Critical Step	16 points	
•	Essential Step	6 points	
▷	Theory Question	2 points	

Score calculation: 100 points

− _____ points missed

_____ Score

Satisfactory score: 85 or above

CAAHEP Competencies Achieved

Psychomotor (Skills)

☑ IV. 2. Report relevant information to others succinctly and accurately.

☑ IV. 4. Explain general office policies.

☑ IX. 1. Respond to issues of confidentiality.

☑ IX. 2. Perform within scope of practice.

☑ IX. 3. Apply HIPAA rules in regard to privacy/release of information.

☑ IX. 7. Document accurately in the patient record.

☑ IX. 8. Apply local, state, and federal health care legislation and regulation appropriate to the medical assisting practice setting.

Affective (Behavior)

☑ IX. 1. Demonstrate sensitivity to patient rights.

☑ 3. Recognize the importance of local, state, and federal legislation and regulations in the practice setting.

ABHES Competencies Achieved
☑ 4. a. Document accurately.
☑ 4. b. Institute federal and state guidelines when releasing medical records or information.
☑ 4. f. Comply with federal, state, and local health laws and regulations.
☑ 8. dd. Serve as liaison between physician and others.
☑ 8. hh. Receive, organize, prioritize, and transmit information expediently.
☑ 9. p. Advise patients of office policies and procedures.

RELEASE OF MEDICAL INFORMATION

All information contained in the medical record is confidential and the release of information is closely controlled. A properly completed and signed authorization is required for the release of the following information.

PATIENT INFORMATION

Patient Name _____

Address _____   Social Security #_____

City _____ State _____ ZIP _____   Birth Date _____/_____/_____

Phone (Home) _____ Work _____

RELEASE FROM: RELEASE TO:

Name _____   Name _____

Address _____   Address _____

City _____ State _____ ZIP_____   City _____ State _____ ZIP_____

INFORMATION TO BE RELEASED:

1. GENERAL RELEASE:

____Entire Medical Record (excluding protected information)
____Hospital Records only (specify)_____
____Lab Results only (specify) _____
____X-ray Reports only (specify) _____
____Other Records (specify) _____

2. INFORMATION PROTECTED BY STATE/FEDERAL LAW:
If indicated below, I hereby authorize the disclosure and release of information regarding:

____Drug Abuse Diagnosis/Treatment
____Alcoholism Diagnosis/Treatment
____Mental Health Diagnosis/Treatment
____Sexually Transmitted Disease

PURPOSE/NEED FOR INFORMATION: METHOD OF RELEASE:

____Taking records to another doctor
____Moving
____Legal purposes
____Insurance purposes
____Workman's Compensation
____Other/Explain:_____

____ US Mail

____ Fax

____ Telephone

____ To Patient

PATIENT AUTHORIZATION TO RELEASE INFORMATION:

Authorization is valid for 60 days only from the date of my signature. I reserve the right to revoke this authorization at any time prior to 60 days (except for action that has already been taken) by notifying the medical office in writing.

I understand that my records are protected under HIPAA (Health Insurance Portability and Accountability Act) Standards for Privacy of Individually Identifiable Information (45 CFR Parts 160 and 164) unless otherwise permitted by federal law. Any information released or received shall not be further relayed to any other facility or person without my written authorization. I also understand that such information will not be given, sold, transferred, or in any way relayed to any other person or party not specified above without my further written authorization.

I hereby grant authorization to release the information listed above. I certify that this request has been made voluntarily and that the information given above is accurate to the best of my knowledge.

_____   _____
Signature of Patient/Legally Responsible Party   Date

_____   _____
Witness Signature   Date

OFFICE USE ONLY

Information indicated above released on _____
                                              Date

Explanation of information released: _____

_____

Signature and credentials of individual releasing information: _____

Procedure 1-3: Preparing a Medical Record

Name: _____   Date: _____

Evaluated by: _____   Score: _____

Performance Objective

Outcome:	Prepare a medical record for a new patient.
Conditions:	Given the following: patient registration form, Notice of Privacy Practices and acknowledgment form, file folder, metal fasteners, name labels, alphabetic labels, miscellaneous chart labels, chart dividers, preprinted forms, and a two-hole punch.
Standards:	Time: 10 minutes. Student completed procedure in _____ minutes.
	Accuracy: Satisfactory score on the Performance Evaluation Checklist.

Performance Evaluation Checklist

Trial 1	Trial 2	Point Value	Performance Standards
		•	Greeted the patient and introduced yourself.
		•	Identified the patient and verified that the patient was a new patient.
		•	Asked the patient to complete a patient registration form, read an NPP, and sign an acknowledgment form.
		•	Offered to answer questions.
		•	Checked the registration form for accuracy and legibility.
		•	Copied the patient's insurance card.
		▷	Stated the purpose of copying the card.
		•	Entered the data on the completed registration form into the computer.
		•	Assembled supplies needed to prepare the medical record.
			Typed the patient's full name on the name label.
		•	The patient's name was in transposed order.
		•	The name was typed using correct spacing.
		•	The patient's name was spelled correctly.
		•	Attached appropriate color-coded labels to the side tab.
		•	Attached the labels using the indentations on the tab.
		•	Attached the name label immediately above the alphabetical label.
		•	Attached additional labels to the folder as required.

Trial 1	Trial 2	Point Value	Performance Standards
		•	Inserted chart dividers onto the metal fasteners.
		•	Placed the original registration form in front of the medical record.
		•	Placed the signed NPP acknowledgment form in the record.
		•	Placed the insurance card (copy) in the appropriate section of the record.
		•	Labeled preprinted forms with required information.
		▷	Stated examples of preprinted forms included in the medical record.
		•	Punched holes into the forms if required.
		•	Inserted each form under its proper chart divider.
		•	Checked the medical record to make sure it was prepared properly.
		✳	Completed the procedure within 10 minutes.
			Totals

Evaluation of Student Performance

EVALUATION CRITERIA			COMMENTS
Symbol	**Category**	**Point Value**	
✳	Critical Step	16 points	
•	Essential Step	6 points	
▷	Theory Question	2 points	

Score calculation: 100 points

− _____ points missed

_____ Score

Satisfactory score: 85 or above

CAAHEP Competencies Achieved

Psychomotor (Skills)

☑ IV. 2. Report relevant information to others succinctly and accurately.

☑ IV. 4. Explain general office policies.

☑ V. 3. Organize a patient's medical record.

☑ V. 5. Execute data management using electronic health care records such as the EMR.

☑ V. 6. Use office hardware and software to maintain office systems.

☑ V. 8. Maintain organization by filing.

☑ IX. 3. Apply HIPAA rules in regard to privacy/release of information.

☑ IX. 8. Apply local, state, and federal health care legislation and regulation appropriate to the medical assisting practice setting.

Affective (Behavior)

☑ IV. 2. Apply active listening skills.

☑ IV. 8. Analyze communications in providing appropriate responses or feedback.

☑ IV. 9. Recognize and protect personal boundaries in communicating with others.

☑ IX. 3. Recognize the importance of local, state, and federal legislation and regulations in the practice setting.

ABHES Competencies Achieved

☑ 4. a. Document accurately.

☑ 4. b. Institute federal and state guidelines when releasing medical records or information.

☑ 4. c. Follow established policies when initiating or terminating medical treatment.

☑ 4. f. Comply with federal, state, and local health laws and regulations.

☑ 8. b. Prepare and maintain medical records.

☑ 8. aa. Are attentive, listen, and learn.

☑ 8. ll. Apply electronic technology.

Notes

EVALUATION OF COMPETENCY

Procedure 1-4: Obtaining and Recording Patient Symptoms

Name: _____   Date: _____

Evaluated by: _____   Score: _____

Performance Objective

Outcome:	Obtain and record patient symptoms.
Conditions:	Given the following: medical record of the patient to be interviewed and a black ink pen.
Standards:	Time: 10 minutes. Student completed procedure in _____ minutes.
	Accuracy: Satisfactory score on the Performance Evaluation Checklist.

Performance Evaluation Checklist

Trial 1	Trial 2	Point Value	Performance Standards
		•	Assembled equipment.
		•	Made sure the correct patient record was obtained.
		•	Went to the waiting room and asked the patient to come back.
		•	Escorted the patient to a quiet room.
		•	In a calm and friendly manner, greeted the patient and introduced yourself.
		•	Identified the patient by full name and date of birth.
		•	Asked the patient to be seated.
		•	Seated yourself facing the patient at a distance of 3 to 4 feet.
		▷	Explained the purpose of this seating arrangement.
			Used good communication skills.
		•	Used the patient's name of choice.
		•	Demonstrated genuine interest and concern for the patient.
		•	Maintained appropriate eye contact.
		•	Used terminology the patient could understand.
		•	Listened carefully and attentively to the patient.
		•	Paid attention to the patient's nonverbal messages.
		•	Avoided judgmental comments.
		•	Avoided rushing the patient.
		•	Located the progress note sheet in the medical record.

Trial 1	Trial 2	Point Value	Performance Standards
		•	Charted the date, time, and CC abbreviation.
		•	Used an open-ended question to obtain the chief complaint.
		▷	Explained why an open-ended question should be used.
			Charted the chief complaint.
		•	Limited the CC to one or two symptoms.
		•	Referred to a specific rather than a vague symptom.
		•	Charted concisely and briefly.
		•	Used the patient's own words as much as possible.
		•	Included the duration of the symptom.
		•	Avoided using names of diseases.
		•	Obtained additional information regarding the chief complaint using what, when, and where questions.
		•	Thanked the patient and proceeded to the next step in the patient workup.
		•	Informed the patient that the physician will be in soon.
		•	Placed the medical record in the appropriate location for review by the physician.
		✶	Completed the procedure within 10 minutes.
			Totals

CHART	
Date	

Evaluation of Student Performance

EVALUATION CRITERIA			COMMENTS
Symbol	**Category**	**Point Value**	
✶	Critical Step	16 points	
•	Essential Step	6 points	
▷	Theory Question	2 points	

Score calculation: 100 points

− _____ points missed

_____ Score

Satisfactory score: 85 or above

CAAHEP Competencies Achieved

Psychomotor (Skills)

☑ IV. 1. Use reflection, restatement, and clarification techniques to obtain a patient history.

☑ IV. 3. Use medical terminology, pronouncing medical terms correctly, to communicate information, patient history, data, and observations.

☑ IV. 7. Demonstrate telephone techniques.

☑ IV. 11. Respond to nonverbal communication.

☑ IX. 7. Document accurately in the patient record.

☑ X. 2. Develop a plan for separation of personal and professional ethics.

Affective (Behavior)

☑ IV. 2. Apply active listening skills.

☑ IV. 3. Use appropriate body language and other nonverbal skills in communicating with parents, family, and staff.

☑ IV. 4. Demonstrate awareness of the territorial boundaries of the person with whom you are communicating.

☑ IV. 9. Recognize and protect personal boundaries in communicating with others.

☑ IV. 10. Demonstrate respect for individual diversity, incorporating awareness of one's own biases in areas including gender, race, religion, age, and economic status.

ABHES Competencies Achieved

☑ 3. d. Recognize and identify acceptable medical abbreviations.

☑ 4. a. Document accurately.

☑ 5. b. Identify and respond appropriately when working/caring for patients with special needs.

☑ 8. aa. Are attentive, listen, and learn.

☑ 8. bb. Are impartial and show empathy when dealing with patients.

☑ 8. cc. Communicate on the recipient's level of comprehension.

☑ 8. ee. Use proper telephone techniques.

☑ 8. ff. Interview effectively.

☑ 8. gg. Use pertinent medical terminology.

☑ 8. ii. Recognize and respond to verbal and nonverbal communication.

☑ 8. jj. Perform fundamental writing skills including correct grammar, spelling, and formatting techniques when writing prescriptions, documenting medical records, etc.

☑ 8. kk. Adapt to individualized needs.

☑ 9. a. Obtain chief complaint, recording patient history.

TAKING PATIENT SYMPTOMS: SUPPLEMENTAL EDUCATION FOR CHAPTER 1

Taking a patient's symptoms is a frequent and important responsibility of the medical assistant, who must have a thorough knowledge of symptoms and related terminology. A **symptom** is defined as any change in the body or its functioning that indicates the presence of disease. The medical assistant can observe **objective symptoms** presented by the patient, such as coughing, rash, and swelling. The medical assistant must rely on information relayed by the patient to obtain data on **subjective symptoms**. Examples of subjective symptoms include pain, pruritus, and vertigo.

This section is designed as supplemental education for Chapter 1 (The Medical Record) in your textbook. Completion of the exercises in this section can assist you in recording a patient's symptoms effectively and thoroughly, which is essential to an accurate diagnosis by the physician.

Learning Objectives

After completing this chapter, you should be able to do the following:
1. Explain the purpose of analyzing a symptom.
2. State the seven basic types of information that must be obtained to analyze a symptom.
3. Analyze a symptom by using direct questions.

Analysis of a Symptom

Before a symptom can be analyzed, the **chief complaint** (CC) must first be identified. The chief complaint is the patient's reason for seeking care or the symptom causing the patient the most trouble. An open-ended question should be used to elicit the chief complaint from the patient, and it should be charted following the charting guidelines presented in your textbook (pages 37 and 44). The next step is to analyze the chief complaint in detail from the time of its onset. The purpose of this is to provide a complete description of the current status of the chief complaint.

Analyzing the chief complaint requires a combination of good listening and writing skills. The medical assistant must know what information should be recorded for each symptom and the questions to ask the patient to obtain this information. A list of symptoms, explanation of the information required for each symptom, and examples of questions to ask the patient are provided.

Type of Information Required

The following information is needed for each symptom to provide a full description of the current status of the chief complaint:

1. Location of the symptom. This refers to the specific area of the body where the symptom is located. Locating the symptom is the first step in determining the cause of the patient's disease. The patient may refer to the location in general terms, such as the head, arm, stomach, or back. The medical assistant must be more specific than this and determine the exact location using descriptions, such as "occurs in the lower back" or "occurs under the sternum." Several questions can assist in accomplishing this.
   - Where exactly does it hurt?
   - Can you show me where it hurts?
   - Do you feel it anywhere else?

2. Quality of the symptom. The quality of the symptom includes a complete and concise description of the symptom. The medical assistant should use informative terms to describe the character of each symptom. For example, if the patient complains of pain, the character of the pain must be included. Several terms can be used to describe pain.
   - Burning
   - Aching
   - Sharp
   - Dull
   - Throbbing
   - Cramplike
   - Squeezing

   If the patient has vomited, the medical assistant should indicate the color, odor, and consistency of the vomitus. If the patient has a cough, the medical assistant should indicate whether it is productive or nonproductive and whether blood is present. Refer to the table of terms on pages 45 and 46 of this manual, which can assist in describing symptoms. Specific examples of questions that are helpful in determining the quality of the symptom are as follows:
   - Describe it (the symptom) to me as fully as possible.
   - What is it (the symptom) like?

3. Severity of the symptom. Severity refers to the quantitative aspect of the symptom. It includes the following:
   - Intensity of the symptom (e.g., mild, moderate, severe)
   - Number (e.g., of convulsions, of nosebleeds)
   - Volume (e.g., of vomitus, of blood, of mucus)
   - Size or extent (e.g., of the rash, edema, lumps, or masses)

   This information assists the physician in determining the extensiveness or seriousness of the illness. Questions to determine severity are often specific to that symptom. For example, if the patient has a productive cough, the medical assistant should determine how much phlegm is being coughed up (e.g., teaspoon, half of a cup). At first, this area may appear difficult, but as you practice taking symptoms, you will learn what questions to ask the patient, and it eventually will become automatic. The examples at the end of this section and the student practice problems provide guidance in developing skill in this area. Some examples of general questions that can be used to determine the severity of a symptom are as follows:
   - How bad is it (the symptom)?
   - Does it (the symptom) limit your normal activities?

4. Chronology and timing of the symptom. Chronology and timing include a sequential account of the symptom up to the time the patient came to the medical office for treatment. This information is important in determining the duration of the symptom and change in it since it first occurred. Chronology and timing include the following four areas:
   a. Date of onset: The date of onset of the symptom should be indicated, if possible, as a calendar date and clock time. The patient may need some time to recall this information. Examples of questions that help obtain this information are as follows:
      - When did you experience this (the symptom) for the first time?
      - Exactly when did this begin?
   b. Duration: The duration of the symptom refers to how long the symptom lasts after it occurs, for example: 10 minutes, 2 hours, continuously. Examples of questions to obtain this information are as follows:
      - How long does it last after occurring?
      - For what length of time do you experience this symptom?
   c. Frequency: The frequency of the symptom refers to how often the symptom occurs, such as twice daily or a single attack every 2 weeks. Examples of questions to obtain this information are as follows:
      - How often does it occur?
      - How often has the symptom recurred?
   d. Change over time: This area refers to any change in the symptom since it first occurred. A change in a symptom reflects the nature of the underlying disease, which assists the physician in making a diagnosis. Examples of questions to obtain this information are as follows:
      - Has the symptom changed since it first occurred?
      - Is it (the symptom) getting better, worse, or staying the same?

5. Manner of onset. The manner of onset refers to what the patient was doing when the symptom first occurred and exactly what was experienced by the patient when the symptom began. These data help provide information on the pathologic process responsible for the symptom. For example, the patient may have been lifting a heavy object before experiencing low back pain. This information helps the physician in making an accurate diagnosis. Examples of questions that are helpful in determining the manner of onset are as follows:
   - What exactly did you experience when it (the symptom) first occurred?
   - What was the first thing you noticed?
   - Did it (the symptom) come on suddenly or gradually?
   - What were you doing when it (the symptom) began?
   - Where were you when this happened?
   - How were you feeling before it (the symptom) began?

6. Modifying factors. Symptoms are often influenced by activities or physiological processes such as physical exercise, change in weather, bodily functions (e.g., bowel movements, eating, coughing), pregnancy, emotional states, and fatigue. Some activities may aggravate the symptom while others may alleviate it. These influences may help to determine what is causing the problem. For example, pain that becomes worse after the patient eats but is relieved after taking an antacid assists the physician in focusing on gastrointestinal disorders. Questions to assist in determining modifying factors are as follows:
   - Does anything make it (the symptom) better?
   - Does anything make it worse?
   - What have you done to make it better?
   - What did you do to help it?
   - Are you taking any medication for it? Did it help?

7. Associated symptoms. There is usually more than one symptom associated with a disease process. Determining these additional symptoms gives the physician a complete picture of the illness. Examples of questions that help to identify the presence of additional symptoms are as follows:
   - Are you having any other symptoms?
   - What other problems have you noticed since you became ill?

Examples

The following examples illustrate how to analyze a symptom. The chief complaint is listed first, followed by questions to ask the patient from the seven basic categories of information.

Example: Chief complaint: Headaches that began 2 months ago.

1. Using your finger, point to the location of the headache.
2. Describe the pain. Is it sharp, dull, throbbing?
3. Are you able to carry on normal activities when you have a headache?
4. Is it sometimes more severe than usual?
5. When exactly did your headaches begin?
6. How long does your headache last when it occurs?
7. How often do you get a headache?
8. Since your headaches began, have they gotten better or worse, or have they stayed the same?
9. What were you doing the first time you experienced a headache?
10. What was your health status before your headaches began?
11. Do you get a headache before, during, or after a particular activity, such as reading or watching TV?
12. Does anything make your headache better?
13. Are you taking any medication for your headache? Does it help?
14. Have you had any other problems since your headaches began, such as nausea, vomiting, dizziness, or problems with vision?

Example: Chief complaint: The patient has been coughing for the past 3 days.

1. Does it hurt when you cough? Where? Show me with one of your fingers.
2. What is the cough like?
3. Can you cough for me?
4. Do you bring up any phlegm when you cough? What color is it? Is blood present?
5. Describe the pain. Is it sharp, dull, squeezing?
6. Do you become exhausted when you cough?
7. How much phlegm do you bring up? A teaspoon? Half a cup?
8. How much blood is present in the phlegm?
9. When did your cough first begin?
10. Does it seem like an attack? How long does the attack last?
11. How often do you get a coughing attack?
12. Does your cough seem to be getting better or worse?
13. What was the first thing you noticed when you became ill?
14. How were you feeling before your symptoms began?
15. Is there anything that makes your cough better?
16. Is there anything that makes your cough worse?
17. Do you cough more at night or during the day?
18. Are you taking any medication for it? Does it help?
19. Are you having any other problems?

Practice Problems

In the space provided, indicate examples of direct questions to ask the patient to obtain the necessary information for the symptoms presented in the chief complaint.

Problem 1

> *Chief complaint: Earache and fever for the past 2 days.*

Questions:

_____

_____

_____

_____

_____

_____

_____

_____

_____

Problem 2

> *Chief complaint: Rash with itching that began 3 days ago.*

Questions:

_____

_____

_____

_____

_____

_____

_____

_____

_____

_____

_____

Problem 3

> *Chief complaint: Pain during urination that began yesterday.*

Questions:

_____

_____

_____

_____

_____
_____
_____
_____
_____

Problem 4

Chief complaint: Low back pain for the past 3 months.

Questions:

_____
_____
_____
_____
_____
_____
_____
_____
_____

Problem 5

Chief complaint: Sore throat and fever for the past 24 hours.

Questions:

_____
_____
_____
_____
_____
_____
_____
_____

Problem 6

Chief complaint: Chest pain that occurred this morning.

Questions:

_____
_____
_____

_____

_____

_____

_____

_____

_____

_____

Terms for Describing Symptoms

Pain

    Burning, aching, sharp, dull, throbbing, cramping, squeezing

    Radiating, transient, constant

    Localized, superficial, deep

Respirations

    Rapid, irregular, shallow, deep, labored, gasping, noisy, wheezing

    Apnea, dyspnea, orthopnea

    Discomfort, pain, cyanosis, cough

Cough

    Nonproductive, productive

    Persistent, dry, hacking, barking, spasmodic

    Phlegm: color, consistency, presence or absence of blood

    Exhausting or painful

Cardiovascular system

    Pain, palpitations

    Sharp, radiating

    Dyspnea, orthopnea

    Cyanosis

Gastrointestinal system

    Abdomen: flaccid, rigid, distended

    Appetite: anorexia, intolerance to foods

    Heartburn, pain after eating, belching, nausea, vomiting, flatulence, change in bowel habits, constipation, diarrhea, black stools

Urine or Stool

    Abnormality: color, odor, consistency, frequency

    Contents: sediment, mucus, blood

    Elimination: urgency, nocturia, pain, burning

Skin

    Rash: pruritus, red, swelling, distribution

    Lesions: color, character, distribution

Pallor: flushing, jaundice, warm, dry, cold, clammy

Ecchymosis, petechiae, cyanosis, edema

Pruritus, sweating, change in color, bruises easily

Ears

Pain, loss of hearing, tinnitus, vertigo

Discharge, infection

Eyes

Itching, burning, blurry vision, seeing double, photophobia

Discharge, watering, infection

2 Medical Asepsis and the OSHA Standard

CHAPTER ASSIGNMENTS

√ After Completing	Date Due	Textbook Pages	TEXTBOOK ASSIGNMENTS	Possible Points	Points You Earned
		50–83	Read Chapter 2: Medical Asepsis and the OSHA Standard		
		62 80	Read Case Study 1 / Case Study 1 questions	5	
		68 80	Read Case Study 2 / Case Study 2 questions	5	
		71 80	Read Case Study 3 / Case Study 3 questions	5	
			Total points		

√ After Completing	Date Due	Study Guide Pages	STUDY GUIDE ASSIGNMENTS (CTA = Critical Thinking Activity)	Possible Points	Points You Earned
		51	Pretest	10	
		52 53	Term Key Term Assessment A. Definitions B. Word Parts (Add 1 point for each medical term)	23 15	
		53–58	Evaluation of Learning questions	47	
		59	CTA A: Infection Process Cycle	5	
		59–60	CTA B: Handwashing	8	
		60	CTA C: Personal Protective Equipment: Gloves	8	
		60–61	CTA D: Personal Protective Equipment	30	
		61–64	CTA E: OSHA Standard	26	
		65	CTA F: Discarding Medical Waste	20	
			Evolve Site: Chapter 2 Discard It! (Record points earned)		

√ After Completing	Date Due	Study Guide Pages	STUDY GUIDE ASSIGNMENTS (CTA = Critical Thinking Activity)	Possible Points	Points You Earned
		66	CTA G: Dear Gabby	10	
		67	CTA H: Crossword Puzzle	25	
			Evolve Site: Chapter 2 Quiz Show (Record points earned)		
			Evolve Site: Chapter 2 Nutrition Nugget: MyPlate	10	
			Evolve Site: Chapter 2 Apply Your Knowledge questions	10	
		69–71	Video Evaluation	56	
		51	Posttest	10	
			ADDITIONAL ASSIGNMENTS		
			Total points		

√ When Assigned by Your Instructor	Study Guide Pages	Practices Required	LABORATORY ASSIGNMENTS (Procedure Number and Name)	Score*
	73	5	Practice for Competency 2-1: Handwashing Textbook reference: pp. 55–57	
	75–76		Evaluation of Competency 2-1: Handwashing	*
	73	4	Practice for Competency 2-2: Applying an Alcohol-Based Hand Rub Textbook reference: pp. 57–58	
	77–78		Evaluation of Competency 2-2: Applying an Alcohol-Based Hand Rub	*
	73	5	Practice for Competency 2-3: Application and Removal of Clean Disposable Gloves Textbook reference: pp. 58–60	
	79–80		Evaluation of Competency 2-3: Application and Removal of Clean Disposable Gloves	*
			ADDITIONAL ASSIGNMENTS	

Notes

Name _____ 100% _____ Date _____

True or False

True   1. A microorganism is a tiny living plant or animal that cannot be seen with the naked eye.

False   2. A disease-producing microorganism is known as a nonpathogen.

false   3. Microorganisms grow best in an acidic environment.

True   4. Coughing and sneezing help to force pathogens from the body.

false   5. An alcohol-based hand rub should be used to sanitize hands that are visibly soiled. ✓

True   6. OSHA stands for Occupational Safety and Health Administration.

True   7. A biohazard warning label must be fluorescent orange or an orange-red color.

False   8. Prescription eyeglasses are acceptable eye protection when handling blood.

True   9. Hepatitis B is an infection of the liver caused by a virus.

True   10. Many people do not develop symptoms when they first become infected with HIV.

?☰ POSTTEST

True or False

True   1. Bacteria and viruses are examples of microorganisms.

false   2. An anaerobe can exist only in the presence of oxygen.

True   3. The optimum growth temperature is the temperature at which a microorganism grows the best.

True   4. Medical asepsis is a practice that helps keep an area free from infection.

false   5. Resident florae are picked up in the course of daily activities and are usually pathogenic.

false   6. The purpose of the OSHA Standard is to prevent exposure of employees to bloodborne pathogens.

True   7. OSHA requires the Exposure Control Plan to be updated annually.

True   8. Engineering controls include all measures and devices that isolate or remove the bloodborne pathogens hazard from the workplace.

false   9. A reagent strip that has been used to test urine is an example of regulated medical waste.

false   10. The most common means of transmitting hepatitis C is through sexual intercourse.

Term KEY TERM ASSESSMENT

A. Definitions

Directions: Match each medical term (numbers) with its definition (letters).

_C_ 1. Aerobe
_Q_ 2. Anaerobe
_U_ 3. Antiseptic
_E_ 4. Asepsis
_K_ 5. Bloodborne pathogens
_N_ 6. Cilia
_R_ 7. Contaminate
_J_ 8. Exposure incident
_V_ 9. Hand hygiene
_L_ 10. Infection
_P_ 11. Microorganism
_G_ 12. Nonintact skin
_O_ 13. Nonpathogen
_D_ 14. Occupational exposure
_T_ 15. Opportunistic infection
_H_ 16. Optimal growth temperature
_A_ 17. Pathogen
_I_ 18. pH
_W_ 19. Postexposure prophylaxis
_M_ 20. Regulated medical waste
_S_ 21. Reservoir host
_F_ 22. Susceptible
_B_ 23. Transient flora

A. A disease-producing microorganism
B. Microorganisms that reside on the superficial skin layers and are picked up in the course of daily activities
C. A microorganism that needs oxygen in order to live and grow
D. Reasonably anticipated skin, eye, mucous membrane, or parenteral contact with bloodborne pathogens or other potentially infectious materials that may result from the performance of an employee's duties
E. Free from infection or pathogens
F. Easily affected; lacking resistance
G. Skin that has a break in the surface
H. The temperature at which an organism grows best
I. The degree to which a solution is acidic or basic
J. A specific eye, mouth, other mucous membrane, nonintact skin, or parenteral contact with blood or other potentially infectious materials that results from an employee's duties
K. Pathogenic microorganisms capable of causing disease that are present in human blood
L. The condition in which the body, or part of it, is invaded by a pathogen
M. Any waste containing infectious material that may pose a threat to health and safety
N. Slender, hairlike processes that constantly beat toward the outside to remove microorganisms from the body
O. A microorganism that does not normally produce disease
P. A microscopic plant or animal
Q. A microorganism that grows best in the absence of oxygen
R. To soil or to make impure
S. The organism that becomes infected by a pathogen and also serves as a source of transfer of pathogens to others
T. An infection resulting from a defective immune system that cannot defend the body from pathogens normally found in the environment
U. An agent that inhibits the growth of or kills microorganisms
V. The process of cleaning or sanitizing the hands
W. Treatment administered to an individual after exposure to an infectious disease to prevent the disease

B. Word Parts

Directions: Indicate the meaning of each word part in the space provided. List as many medical terms as possible that incorporate the word part in the space provided.

Word Part	Meaning of Word Part	Medical Terms That Incorporate Word Part
1. aer/o	Oxygen	ex Aerobe
2. an-	Without	ex Anaerobe
3. anti-	Against	ex Anti-inflammatory
4. septic	Related to Sepsis	ex Septic shock
5. a-	Without	ex Asexual
6. micro-	Small	ex Microbiology
7. non-	Not	ex Non-intact skin
8. path/o	Relating to disease	ex Pathology
9. -gen	To Produce	ex Pathogen
10. para-	Near; beside	ex Parathyroid
11. enteron	Relating to digestive tract	ex N/A
12. -al	Pertaining to	ex Duadenal
13. peri-	Around	ex Peristalsis
14. natal	Relating to birth	ex Neonatal
15. post-	After; behind	ex Postpartum depression

EVALUATION OF LEARNING

Directions: Fill in each blank with the correct answer.

1. List four examples of types of microorganisms.

   Bacteria, Virus, Protozoa, Fungi, Parasites

2. Define medical asepsis.

   A object or area is clean and Free from infection

3. What type of microorganisms may remain on an object that is considered medically aseptic?

   Non-pathogens

4. What is the name given to the organism that uses organic or living substances for food?

   HEterotrophs

Chapter 2 Medical Asepsis and the OSHA Standard

5. Why do most microorganisms prefer a neutral pH?

   If the enviorment is too basic or too acidic they die

6. List five examples of how microorganisms can enter the body.

   Mouth, Nose, throat, Ears, Eyes.

7. List three examples of how a microorganism can be transmitted from one person to another.

   Direct contact with the infected person or discharge
   Indirect transfer includes transmission by droplets
   Contaminated hands and equipment

8. List four examples of factors that would make a host more susceptible to the entrance of a pathogen.

   Poor Health, Poor Hygiene, Poor nutrition, Stress

9. List five protective devices of the body that prevent the entrance of microorganisms.

   Skin, Mucous membranes, Mucus and cilia, Coughing and sneezing
   Tears and Sweat

10. What is the difference between resident flora and transient flora?

    Resident flora - normally resides and grows in epidermis and
    deep layer of the skin. Generally harmless and nonpathogenic.
    Transient flora - lives and grows on superficial layer of skin, Picked up by
    daily activities is often pathogenic.

11. List three examples of when handwashing should be performed in the medical office.

    when hands are visibly dirty, before eating, after using the
    restroom

12. How does antiseptic handwashing sanitize the hands?

    Hand washing with antimicrobial soap, an agent that functions to
    kill or inhibit growth of microorganisms.
    leaves antibacterial film on hands to discourage bacterial growth.

13. List three examples of when an alcohol-based hand rub may be used to sanitize the hands.

Advantage More accessible, Don't require rinsing, Faster, less damage to skin. Disadvantage Expensive, stings when applied to broke

14. What are the advantages and disadvantages of alcohol-based hand rubs?

Advantage- More accessible, Don't require rinsing, Faster, less damage to skin, Disadvantage Expensive, STING when applied to broken skin.

15. List six medical aseptic practices the medical assistant should follow in the medical office.

Keep office free from dirt and dust, Ensure ventilation, keeps rooms bright and airy, Eliminate insects, Carefully dispose of wastes, Don't let soiled items touch clothing, Don't wear a ton of jewelry,

16. What are the advantages of latex gloves?

Stretch to fit more comfortably, Thin, allowing better feel and dexterity, lower cost, Proven barrier capability.

17. What guidelines should be followed when working with gloves?

Keep fingernails trimmed, Wear correct size glove, Don't use oil-based hand lotion, Don't store gloves in temperature varying locations

18. What does the acronym OSHA stand for, and what is the purpose of OSHA?

Occupational health and Safety administration, Assist employers in providing a safe and Healthy working enviorment for their employee

19. What is the purpose of the OSHA Occupational Exposure to Bloodborne Pathogens Standard?

Designed to reduce risk of exposure to infectious disease

20. Who must follow the OSHA Standard? List examples.

Must be followed by all employees with Occupational exposure to pathogens regardless of place of employment. Ex physicians, nurses, dentist, dental Hygienists, medical laboratory, personel, emergency technicians.
personnel,

Chapter 2 Medical Asepsis and the OSHA Standard

21. What is the purpose of the Needlestick Safety and Prevention Act?

To reduce needle sticks and other sharps injuries among health care workers

22. List five examples of other potentially infectious materials (OPIMs).

Semen and vaginal secretions, Cerebrospinal, synovial, pleural, pericardial and amniotic fluids. Any body fluid that is visibly contaminated fluid with blood, Saliva, Any unfixed human tissue, ~~Any tissue~~

23. List examples of nonintact skin.

Skin with dermatitis, abrasions, cuts, Burns, Hangnails, Chapping, Acne

24. What is the purpose of the exposure control plan (ECP)?

Stipulates protective measures that must be followed in that medical office to eliminate or minimize employee exposure to bloodborne pathogen and other potentially infectious material

25. List three examples of items to which a biohazard warning label must be attached.

Containers of regulated waste, Refrigerators and freezers used to store blood and other potentially infectious materials. Containers and bags used to store, transport, or ship blood or other potentially infectious materials

26. What is the purpose of a Sharps Injury Log? What types of offices must maintain this log?

Meant to help employers and employees keep track of all the needle stick injuries, Offices with 10 or more employees at risk for Occupational exposure are required to maintain this log

27. Define an engineering control, and list three examples of engineering controls.

Engineering controls are any device or measure that isolates or removes the bloodborne pathogens hazard from the work place Ex readily accessible hand washing facilities, Safer medical devices Biohazard Sharps containers and biohazards bags Autoclaves

28. What is a safer medical device?

A medical Device that, based on reasonable, judgment, would make an exposure incident involving a contaminated sharps less likely

29. What should be done before and after gloves are applied?

Sanitize your hands

30. List six guidelines that must be followed when using personal protective equipment.

1 Must not allow blood or other potentially infectious materials to pass through or reach the skin, 2 Employer must be provided for employees who are allergic to latex, 3 Employer must provide appropriate protective equipment to you, 4 if gloves become contaminated torn, or punctured replace them as soon as possible 5 all eye-protection devices must have solid eye shields

6 Utility gloves may be decontaminated and reuse unless they no longer provide barrier

31. List four guidelines that must be followed with respect to biohazard sharps containers.

Use sharps containers closest to area of use to avoid transporting contaminated needle as much as possible, Maintain sharp container in upright position, Don't reach into sharps container, Replace sharps container on regular basis, don't allow to over fill.

32. What procedure should be followed when a sharps container located in an examining room becomes full? Explain the reason for your answer.

Replace the sharps container with a new one and store the used sharps container until waste removal service can dispose of it properly

33. Explain how to prepare regulated medical waste for pickup by a medical waste service.

Place biohazard bags and sharps containers into a receptacle provided by the service, Store biohazard boxes in locked room inside facility or in locked collection container outside, Track when is picked up by service

34. How should regulated medical waste be stored while waiting for pickup by the medical waste service? Explain why.

Away from the general public and in locked container, Aim to prevent unauthorized access to items such as needles and syringes

35. What information is included on a regulated medical waste tracking form?

Quantity of waste and where it is being sent

36. What is the most likely means of contracting hepatitis B in the health care setting?

Blood and blood components via needlestick

37. What side effects may occur after the administration of a hepatitis B vaccine?

Soreness at injection site Serious reactions are extremely rare the administration of a passive and active immunizing agent

38. What postexposure prophylaxis (PEP) is recommended for an unvaccinated individual who has been exposed to hepatitis B?

The administration of a passive and active immunizing agent

Chapter 2 Medical Asepsis and the OSHA Standard

39. What are the symptoms of acute viral hepatitis B in individuals who have symptoms?

Increased risk of liver damage, increase risk of cirrhosis
Increased risk of liver cancer

40. Why is chronic viral hepatitis B considered such a serious condition?

They become carriers of the disease and can transmit hepatitis B
to others

41. Why is chronic hepatitis C known as "an epidemic that occurred in the past"?

Symptoms may not becomes serious until to 30 years after
time of infection.

42. What are the symptoms of acute HIV infection?

loss of appetite, Diarrhea
Flu like illness, fever, Sweats, fatigue, Sweats,
Pharyngitis, Myalgia, Arthralgia, adenopathy.

43. Explain what occurs during the asymptomatic period and the symptomatic period of the AIDS infection cycle.

Asymptomatic period, long incubation period, lasting months to years
Antibodies are produced, but otherwise, individual feels normal, Sympotamatic
period, Serres of lesser symptoms caused by weakened immune system, lack of energy, weight loss

44. What are the characteristics of full-blown AIDS?

Characterized by the presence of oppertunistic infections and unusual
cancers.

45. How is HIV transmitted? How is it not transmitted?

Transmitted through Sexual contact, sharing drug needles, Not Spread throug
every day contact like sharing facilities or equipment, through the air
coughing and sneezing.

46. List five AIDS-defining conditions.

Infections that don't usually cause infections in individuals with healthy
immune systems.

47. What is the CDC's definition of AIDS?

Disorder of the immune system that eventually destroys the body
ability to figh infection

CRITICAL THINKING ACTIVITIES

A. Infection Process Cycle

Carefully review the infection process cycle and the requirements for growth needed by microorganisms. Create an environment in a medical office that would function to interrupt the infection process cycle and discourage the growth of pathogens.

_____

_____

_____

_____

B. Handwashing

Using the principles outlined in the handwashing procedure, explain what may happen under the following circumstances:

1. The medical assistant's uniform touches the sink during the handwashing procedure.

_____

_____

_____

2. The hands are not held lower than the elbows during the handwashing procedure.

_____

_____

_____

3. Friction is not used to wash the hands.

_____

_____

_____

4. Water is splashed on the medical assistant's uniform during the handwashing procedure.

_____

_____

_____

5. The medical assistant continually uses water that is too cold to wash hands.

_____

_____

_____

6. The medical assistant turns off the running water with his or her bare hands.

_____

_____

_____

7. The medical assistant does not clean his or her fingernails daily.

_____

_____

_____

8. The medical assistant's skin becomes chapped.

_____

_____

_____

C. Personal Protective Equipment: Gloves

In which of the following situations does OSHA require the use of clean disposable gloves?

_____ 1. Performing a urinalysis on a urine specimen that contains blood

_____ 2. Sanitizing operating scissors for sterilization

_____ 3. Performing a finger puncture

_____ 4. Performing a vision screening test on a school-aged child

_____ 5. Cleaning up a blood spill on a laboratory work table

_____ 6. Drawing blood from an elderly patient

_____ 7. Measuring the weight of a college student

_____ 8. Testing a blood specimen for glucose

D. Personal Protective Equipment

Create a collage of items or articles that can and cannot be used as PPE following these guidelines:

1. Using items cut from a magazine, colored pencils, or markers, create a collage of items that are designated as PPE by OSHA.

2. On the reverse side of the sheet, create a collage of items or articles that are not permitted to be used as PPE.

3. In the classroom, choose a partner and trade sheets. For each PPE item, provide examples of the procedures or tasks that may require its use. For each item that is not PPE, explain why it should not be used as PPE.

Examples of PPE:

_____

_____

_____

_____

Mikil Cherx   1/18/17   95%
                                                100% 🙂

Not examples of PPE:

_____

_____

_____

_____

E. OSHA Standard

The following situations may occur in the medical office. For each situation, indicate an appropriate **action** to take that complies with the OSHA Bloodborne Pathogens Standard.

1. **Situation:** You just gave an injection to a patient, and after withdrawing the needle, you notice that there is no sharps container in the room.
   Action:
   Make sure its covered somehow and then go get a sharp container
   _____

2. **Situation:** You are getting ready to apply gloves and notice that you have a cut on your finger.
   Action:
   You are supposed to put a bandaide on the cut then put on the gloves.
   _____

3. **Situation:** You accidentally get some blood on your bare hands while removing your gloves.
   Action:
   Wash hands immediately
   _____
   _____

4. **Situation:** A part-time clinical MA was just hired. She is not immunized against hepatitis B.
   Action:
   She should be offered the vaccine, and the risk of not being immunized explained
   _____

5. **Situation:** A clinical medical assistant who has worked at the office for 5 years changes her mind and decides she wants the hepatitis B vaccine.
   Action:
   Inform physician so she can get immunized free of charge
   _____

6. **Situation:** You are wearing a protective laboratory coat over your scrubs. While performing a laboratory test, some blood splashes onto your lab coat, but it does not penetrate through to your scrubs.
   Action:

   Change the lab coat

7. **Situation:** You go into an examining room and notice that the biohazard sharps container in that room is completely full.
   Action:

   Close the cap if possible, then store and replace with new sharps' container

8. **Situation:** You are performing laboratory testing. You accidentally drop a blood tube, and it breaks.
   Action:

   Sweep up glass, spray disinfectant, let sit, then wipe up while wearing gloves

9. **Situation:** You are wearing a protective lab coat over your scrubs, and you are getting ready to leave for the day.
   Action:

   The lab coat can't leave the office

10. **Situation:** You remove your gloves after giving an injection to a patient and accidentally discard them into the biohazard sharps container.
    Action:

    Do not dig into container just leave them there

11. **Situation:** You are separating serum from whole blood, and you accidentally spill some of the serum on the countertop.
    Action:

    Same procedure as cleaning up whole blood. Spray disinfectant let sit, then wipe up while wearing glove

12. **Situation:** By mistake, you throw a tourniquet into the sharps container after drawing a patient's blood.
    Action:

    leave it in there

Chapter **2** **Medical Asepsis and the OSHA Standard**

13. **Situation:** A new clinical medical assistant has been hired in the medical office, and she is allergic to latex gloves.
    Action: Law requires nitrile gloves to be available to her

14. **Situation:** You have just drawn blood from a patient, and you accidentally stick yourself with the needle.
    Action: ~~You cannot put your food with blood~~ Report needle stick immediately

15. **Situation:** Your office only has one refrigerator, and blood tubes need to be stored in it, but the staff would like to put their lunches in it.
    Action: You cannot ~~put~~ store your food with blood another refrigerator is needed

16. **Situation:** During an office meeting, a coworker suggests an idea to save money by emptying full sharps containers into a biohazard bag so that the containers can be reused.
    Action: It is against the law to transfer sharps

17. **Situation:** A new employee wants to know where she should eat her lunch.
    Action: In a seperate location away from where testing and procedures happen

18. **Situation:** You are applying a pair of disposable gloves, and one of the gloves tears while you are pulling it on.
    Action: Replace with a new glove

19. **Situation:** You are removing a stopper from a tube of blood so that you can transfer the serum to another tube. A small amount of serum accidentally spatters into your eye.
    Action: Eye wash immediately, for at least 15 minutes

20. **Situation:** You have just been assigned the responsibility of performing all venipunctures required in your office. You notice that the sharps container is located on the opposite side of the room from the blood drawing chair.
Action:

~~More~~ p Move it closer to your prep area

21. **Situation:** A technician is coming to your office today to repair your blood chemistry analyzer.
Action:

Decontaminate the analyzer before they get there

22. **Situation:** A new employee has been hired who has already had the hepatitis B vaccination series.
Action:

You can offer for t

23. **Situation:** Utility gloves are used and reused in your office for the sanitization of surgical instruments.
Action:

They are made to be reused

24. **Situation:** Your office has run out of biohazard bags used to transport specimens to the laboratory, and you notice that an employee is using plastic bags as a substitute.
Action:

Plastic is not acceptable, order more biohazard bag as soon as possible, you can call the lab for more in the meantime

25. **Situation:** A medical assisting practicum student does not wear gloves to recap a needle after drawing medication into a syringe to give an injection to a patient.
Action:

~~Gloves aren't necessary for drawing medication~~
Any interaction where patients receive an Injection gloves are a good Idea

26. **Situation:** You accidentally close and lock in place the lid of a sharps container that is only one-half full.
Action:

leave it, just get a new sharps container

F. Discarding Medical Waste

Using these acronyms, indicate where each of the following (used) items should be discarded:

RWC: regular waste container

BSC: biohazard sharps container

BB: biohazard bag waste container

RWC   1. Urine testing strip

BSC   2. Lancet

BB   3. Gloves with blood on them

BSC   4. Blood tube

RWC   5. Tongue depressor

BSC   6. Razor blade

BSC   7. Capillary pipet

BB   8. Dressing saturated with blood

RWC   9. Patient drape

RWC   10. An empty urine container

BB   11. Sutures caked with blood

RWC   12. Thermometer probe cover

RWC   13. Patient gown

RWC   14. Disposable diaper

BB   15. Dressing saturated with a purulent discharge

RWC   16. Clean disposable gloves

BB   17. Disposable vaginal speculum

BSC   18. An outdated vaccine

BSC   19. Syringe and needle

RWC   20. Examining-table paper

G. Dear Gabby

Gabby is away on vacation and wants you to fill in for her. In the space provided, respond to the following letter by using the knowledge you have acquired in this chapter.

Dear Gabby:

I am writing to you because I am very concerned about my younger sister "Tuesday." For the past 2 weeks, Tuesday has been extremely tired and does not feel like eating. She also vomits several times each day and says that her joints ache. Tuesday is 26 years old and a single mother with two small children. Tuesday has been dating "Alex" for the past 4 months. It is well known around town that Alex sometimes injects himself with illegal drugs, and I think there's a chance that Tuesday is also using drugs.

I told Tuesday that she needs to see her doctor right away, but she will not listen to me. She says that it seems like a prolonged case of the flu and it will probably go away soon. I did an Internet search of her symptoms, and I think she has hepatitis C.

Gabby, am I just being overprotective of my sister, or should I insist that she see her doctor?

Wanting to Know in Wyoming

Yes I think you schoold should see a doctor for your sister and I think you should see her a doctor as soon as possible she might be very ill without knowing it she may need to take a blood test.

H. Crossword Puzzle: Medical Asepsis and the OSHA Standard

Directions: Complete the crossword puzzle using the clues provided.

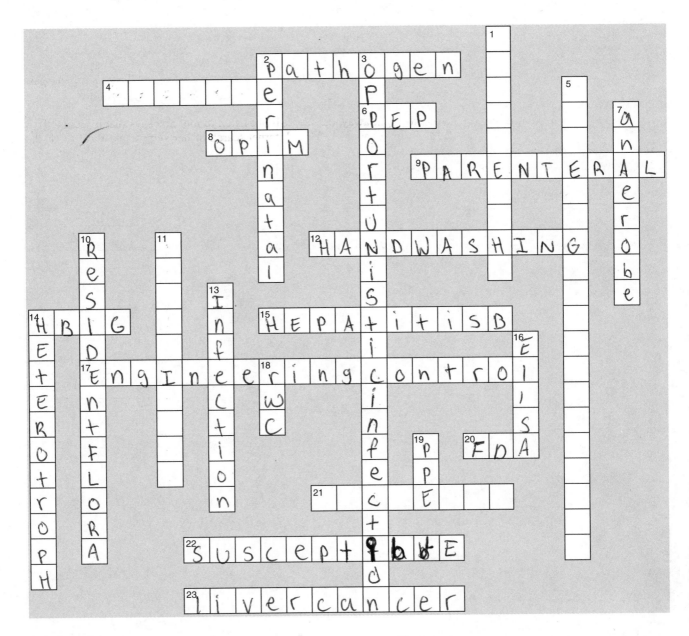

Across
- 2 MO that causes disease
- 4 Acute viral hepatitis B symptom
- 6 After exposure, may prevent disease
- 8 Vaginal secretions (ex)
- 9 Piercing of the skin barrier
- 12 No. 1 aseptic practice
- 14 Hepatitis B passive immunizing agent
- 15 No. 1 chronic viral disease in the United States
- 17 Health hazard eliminator
- 20 Protector of public health
- 21 Example of an MO
- 22 Lacking resistance
- 23 HBV serious complication

Down
- 1 Found in antimicrobial soap
- 2 Shortly before or after birth
- 3 AIDS-defining condition
- 5 Way to prevent an NSI
- 7 Grows best without oxygen
- 10 Normally live on the skin
- 11 Can live dry for 1 week
- 13 Body invasion by a pathogen
- 14 Eats "live stuff"
- 16 HIV screening test
- 18 Discard in a biohazard container
- 19 Scrubs are not this

Chapter **2** **Medical Asepsis and the OSHA Standard**

Name: _____

Directions:

a. Watch the indicated videos.
b. Mark each true statement with a T and each false statement with an F. For each false statement, change the wording of the question so that it becomes a true statement.

Video: Procedure 2-1: Handwashing

_____ 1. Resident florae are microorganisms that are picked up on the hands during your daily activities.

_____ 2. Transient florae are usually nonpathogenic and are attached loosely to your skin.

_____ 3. Transient flora can easily be removed by proper handwashing.

_____ 4. Handwashing is recommended when there is visible dirt on the hands.

_____ 5. Washing with a detergent soap breaks down and emulsifies dirt and oil on the skin.

_____ 6. You need to perform an antiseptic hand wash when you take a patient's pulse.

_____ 7. The faucets are usually the cleanest part of the sink.

_____ 8. Your hands will become dry and chapped if the water is hot or too cold.

_____ 9. Holding your arms in a downward position carries dirt away from your body and not up your arm.

_____ 10. Clean your fingernails with a manicure stick at least once each week.

_____ 11. Keep your fingernails short and avoid wearing artificial nails, which can trap dirt and microorganisms.

_____ 12. Dry your hands gently and thoroughly with a paper towel to prevent chapping of the hands.

Video: Procedure 2-2: Applying an Alcohol-Based Hand Rub

_____ 1. Alcohol-based hand rubs contain chlorine bleach, which is effective in removing transient flora from the hands.

_____ 2. Handwashing must be performed when you first arrive at the medical office to start your day, before eating, after using the restroom, and if your hands are visibly soiled.

_____ 3. Hand rubs can sting if you have a cut or abrasion.

_____ 4. After cleaning your hands 5 to 10 times with a hand rub, a buildup of emollients may occur, which can easily be removed by washing your hands with soap and water.

_____ 5. Microorganisms can lodge in the crevices and grooves of rings.

_____ 6. If you apply more than the recommended amount of hand rub, it will take a lot longer for your hands to dry.

_____ 7. If you do not completely cover all surfaces of your hands with the hand rub, the parts not covered will remain contaminated.

_____ 8. It should take about 2 minutes for your hands to dry if you have applied the correct amount of hand rub.

_____ 9. After applying a hand rub, your hands should be allowed to dry completely before you touch anything.

69

Video: Procedure 2-3: Application and Removal of Clean Disposable Gloves

_____ 1. OSHA requires that you wear gloves when it is anticipated that your hands will have contact with intact skin.

_____ 2. OSHA requires that you wear gloves when it is anticipated that your hands will have contact with mucous membranes.

_____ 3. Clean gloves reduce contamination from your hands by 20%.

_____ 4. Wearing gloves helps to protect you and your patients from infection.

_____ 5. It is important to change your gloves before and after each patient to prevent the spread of infection from one patient to next.

_____ 6. Rings can cause tears in your gloves.

_____ 7. The warm, dark, moist environment inside of a glove works to destroy microorganisms.

_____ 8. If your gloves are too small, they may rip as you are applying them.

_____ 9. If your gloves are too large, you may find it difficult to perform your tasks.

_____ 10. If you see a tear in one glove, remove both gloves, throw them away, and apply a new pair of gloves.

_____ 11. Used gloves are considered clean.

_____ 12. It is important to remove gloves in a way that does not contaminate your clean hands. This protects you from being infected with a pathogen.

_____ 13. If one of your gloves has blood or infectious materials on it, you should remove that glove last.

_____ 14. If your gloves are visibly contaminated with blood or other potentially infectious materials, they must be discarded in a biohazard sharps container.

_____ 15. If your gloves are not visibly contaminated, they can be discarded in a regular waste container.

Video: The OSHA Bloodborne Pathogens Standard

_____ 1. OSHA stands for the Occupational Safety and Health Administration.

_____ 2. The OSHA Standard consists of regulations designed to prevent the risk of exposure to infections diseases.

_____ 3. Other potentially infectious materials include tears and sweat.

_____ 4. The Exposure Control Plan spells out the protective control measures that must be followed to eliminate or minimize employee exposure to bloodborne pathogens and other potentially infectious materials.

_____ 5. OSHA training must be provided to employees when they initially begin working and at least annually thereafter.

_____ 6. The Exposure Control Plan must be updated every 2 years.

_____ 7. Engineering controls include safer medical devices and biohazard sharps containers.

_____ 8. Biohazard containers must be properly labeled with the biohazard symbol and must be available and accessible.

_____ 9. Work practice controls reduce the likelihood of exposure by altering the manner in which the technique is performed.

_____ 10. If your hands or other skin surfaces come in contact with blood or other potentially infectious material, immediately wash the area thoroughly with soap and water.

_____ 11. Food or drink can be stored in refrigerators, freezers, or cabinets, or on countertops where blood or other potentially infectious materials are present.

_____ 12. The first step to take if you are exposed to blood or other potentially infectious materials is to report the incident to your physician-employer.

_____ 13. Personal protective equipment is clothing or equipment that protects an individual from contact with blood or other potentially infectious materials.

_____ 14. Wear gloves when it is reasonably anticipated that your hands will have contact with blood and other potentially infectious materials.

_____ 15. Standard prescription eyeglasses are an example of personal protective equipment.

_____ 16. All personal protective equipment must be removed before leaving the office.

_____ 17. For the decontamination of blood spills, OSHA recommends the use of a 10% solution of household bleach in water.

_____ 18. Biohazard sharps containers must be located as close and possible to the area of use.

_____ 19. It is recommended that sharps containers be replaced when they are half full.

_____ 20. Employees who decline the hepatitis B vaccination must sign a hepatitis B waiver form documenting their refusal.

Notes

Medical Asepsis

Procedure 2-1: Handwashing. Perform the handwashing procedure. List five medically aseptic steps that must be followed during this procedure.

1. _____
   _____

2. _____
   _____

3. _____
   _____

4. _____
   _____

5. _____
   _____

Procedure 2-2: Alcohol-Based Hand Rub. Apply an alcohol-based hand rub. Practice applying a gel and a foam hand rub. List the brand names of the hand rubs you applied, and list the ingredients contained in them.

_____

_____

Procedure 2-3: Clean Disposable Gloves. Apply and remove clean disposable gloves. What size gloves fit you best?

_____

_____

EVALUATION OF COMPETENCY

Procedure 2-1: Handwashing

Name: _____   Date: _____

Evaluated by: _____   Score: _____

Performance Objective

Outcome:	Perform handwashing.
Conditions:	Using a sink.
Standards:	Given liquid soap and paper towels.
	Time: 5 minutes. Student completed procedure in _____ minutes.
	Accuracy: Satisfactory score on the Performance Evaluation Checklist.

Performance Evaluation Checklist

Trial 1	Trial 2	Point Value	Performance Standards
		•	Removed watch or pushed it up on the forearm.
		•	Removed rings.
		▷	Stated the reason for removing rings.
		•	Stood at sink with clothing away from edge of sink.
		•	Turned on faucets with paper towel.
		▷	Explained the reason for turning on faucets with paper towel.
		•	Adjusted the water to a warm temperature.
		•	Discarded towel into trash can.
		•	Wet hands and forearms with water.
		•	Held hands lower than elbows at all times.
		▷	Explained why the hands should be held lower than elbows.
		•	Did not touch the inside of sink with hands.
		•	Applied soap to hands.
		•	Washed palms and backs of hands with 10 circular motions and friction.
		▷	Explained why circular motions and friction are needed to wash hands.
		•	Washed fingers with 10 circular motions.
		•	Washed fingers while interlaced using friction and circular motions.
		•	Rinsed well (keeping hands lower than elbows).
		•	Washed wrists and forearms using friction and circular motions.
		•	Cleaned fingernails using manicure stick.

Trial 1	Trial 2	Point Value	Performance Standards
		•	Rinsed arms and hands.
		•	Repeated handwashing procedure (if necessary).
		•	Dried hands gently and thoroughly.
		▷	Stated the reason for drying hands gently and completely.
		•	Turned off faucets using paper towel.
		•	Did not touch sink area with bare hands.
		▷	Explained the reason for not touching sink area with bare hands.
		✶	Completed the procedure within 5 minutes.
			Totals

Evaluation of Student Performance

EVALUATION CRITERIA			COMMENTS
Symbol	**Category**	**Point Value**	
✶	Critical Step	16 points	
•	Essential Step	6 points	
▷	Theory Question	2 points	

Score calculation: 100 points

− _____ points missed

_____ Score

Satisfactory score: 85 or above

CAAHEP Competencies Achieved

Psychomotor (Skills)

☑ III. 2. Practice Standard Precautions.

☑ III. 4. Perform handwashing.

☑ IX. 8. Apply local, state, and federal health care legislation and regulation appropriate to the medical assisting practice setting.

Affective (Behavior)

☑ IX. 3. Recognize the importance of local, state, and federal legislation and regulations in the practice setting.

ABHES Competencies Achieved

☑ 4. f. Comply with federal, state, and local health laws and regulations.

☑ 9. b. Apply principles of aseptic techniques and infection control.

☑ 9. i. Use standard precautions.

Procedure 2-2: Applying an Alcohol-Based Hand Rub

Name: _____   Date: _____

Evaluated by: _____   Score: _____

Performance Objective

Outcome:	Apply an alcohol-based hand rub.
Conditions:	Given an alcohol-based hand rub.
Standards:	Time: 2 minutes. Student completed procedure in _____ minutes.
	Accuracy: Satisfactory score on the Performance Evaluation Checklist.

Performance Evaluation Checklist

Trial 1	Trial 2	Point Value	Performance Standards
		•	Inspected the hands to make sure they are not visibly soiled.
		▷	Stated the procedure to follow if the hands are visibly soiled.
		•	Removed watch or pushed it up on the forearm.
		•	Removed rings.
			Applied the alcohol-based hand rub to the palm of one hand as follows:
		•	*Gel or lotion:* Applied an amount of gel or lotion approximately equal to the size of a dime.
		•	*Foam:* Applied an amount of foam approximately equal to the size of a walnut.
		▷	Explained why it is important not to use more than the recommended amount of hand rub.
		•	Thoroughly spread the hand rub over the surface of both hands up to one-half inch above the wrist.
		•	Spread the hand rub around and under the fingernails.
		▷	Explained why it is important to cover the entire surface of the hands.
		•	Rubbed the hands together until they were dry.
		•	Did not touch anything until the hands were dry.
		✶	Completed the procedure within 2 minutes.
			Totals

EVALUATION CRITERIA			COMMENTS
Symbol	**Category**	**Point Value**	
∗	Critical Step	16 points	
•	Essential Step	6 points	
▷	Theory Question	2 points	

Score calculation: 100 points

$$- \underline{\qquad} \text{ points missed}$$

$$\underline{\qquad} \text{ Score}$$

Satisfactory score: 85 or above

CAAHEP Competencies Achieved

Psychomotor (Skills)

☑ III. 2. Practice Standard Precautions.

☑ IX. 8. Apply local, state, and federal health care legislation and regulation appropriate to the medical assisting practice setting.

Affective (Behavior)

☑ IV. IX. 3. Recognize the importance of local, state, and federal legislation and regulations in the practice setting.

ABHES Competencies Achieved

☑ 4. f. Comply with federal, state, and local health laws and regulations.

☑ 8. 9. b. Apply principles of aseptic techniques and infection control.

☑ 8. 9. i. Use standard precautions.

Procedure 2-3: Application and Removal of Clean Disposable Gloves

Name: _____ Date: _____

Evaluated by: _____ Score: _____

Performance Objective

Outcome:	Apply and remove clean disposable gloves.
Conditions:	Given the appropriate sized clean disposable gloves.
Standards:	Time: 5 minutes. Student completed procedure in _____ minutes.
	Accuracy: Satisfactory score on the Performance Evaluation Checklist.

Performance Evaluation Checklist

Trial 1	Trial 2	Point Value	Performance Standards
			Application of clean gloves
		•	Removed all rings.
		▷	Stated why rings should be removed.
		•	Sanitized the hands.
		•	Chose the appropriate sized gloves.
		▷	Explained what can happen if the gloves are too small or too large.
		•	Applied the gloves.
		•	Adjusted the gloves so that they fit comfortably.
		•	Inspected the gloves for tears.
		▷	Stated the procedure to follow if a glove is torn.
			Removal of clean gloves
		•	Grasped the outside of the left glove 1 to 2 inches from the top with the gloved right hand.
		•	Slowly pulled left glove off the hand.
		•	Pulled the left glove free, and scrunched it into a ball with the gloved right hand.
		•	Placed the index and middle fingers of the left hand on the inside of the right glove.
		•	Did not allow the clean hand to touch outside of the glove.

Trial 1	Trial 2	Point Value	Performance Standards
		•	Pulled the glove off the right hand enclosing the balled-up left glove.
		•	Discarded both gloves in an appropriate waste container.
		▷	Stated when gloves should be discarded in a biohazardous waste container.
		•	Sanitized the hands.
		▷	Stated why the hands should be sanitized after removing gloves.
		✱	Completed the procedure in 5 minutes.
			Totals

Evaluation of Student Performance

EVALUATION CRITERIA			COMMENTS
Symbol	**Category**	**Point Value**	
✱	Critical Step	16 points	
•	Essential Step	6 points	
▷	Theory Question	2 points	

Score calculation: 100 points

−_____ points missed

_____ Score

Satisfactory score: 85 or above

CAAHEP Competencies Achieved

Psychomotor (Skills)

☑ III. 2. Practice Standard Precautions.

☑ IX. 8. Apply local, state, and federal health care legislation and regulation appropriate to the medical assisting practice setting.

Affective (Behavior)

☑ IX. 3. Recognize the importance of local, state, and federal legislation and regulations in the practice setting.

ABHES Competencies Achieved

☑ 4. f. Comply with federal, state, and local health laws and regulations.

☑ 9. b. Apply principles of aseptic techniques and infection control.

☑ 9. i. Use standard precautions.

3 | Sterilization and Disinfection

√ After Completing	Date Due	Textbook Pages	TEXTBOOK ASSIGNMENTS	Possible Points	Points You Earned
		84–115	Read Chapter 3 Sterilization and Disinfection		
		87 113	Read Case Study 1 Case Study 1 questions	5	
		97 113	Read Case Study 2 Case Study 2 questions	5	
		101 113	Read Case Study 3 Case Study 3 questions	5	
			Total points		

√ After Completing	Date Due	Study Guide Pages	STUDY GUIDE ASSIGNMENTS (CTA = Critical Thinking Activity)	Possible Points	Points You Earned
		85	Pretest	10	
		86	Term Key Term Assessment	17	
		86–89	Evaluation of Learning questions	31	
		90–91	CTA A: Material Safety Data Sheet	17	
		91–93	CTA B: Obtaining a Material Data Safety Sheet	10	
		93	CTA C: Sanitization	8	
		94	CTA D: Storage of a Chemical Disinfectant	4	
		94–95	CTA E: Sterilization	10	
		96–98	CTA F: What Comes Next? Game (Record points earned)		
			Evolve Site: Chapter 3 What Happens Now? (Record points earned)		
			Evolve Site: Chapter 3 Quiz Show (Record points earned)		

√ After Completing	Date Due	Study Guide Pages	STUDY GUIDE ASSIGNMENTS (CTA = Critical Thinking Activity)	Possible Points	Points You Earned
			Evolve Site: Chapter 3 Nutrition Nugget: Food Labels	10	
			Evolve Site: Apply Your Knowledge questions	10	
		99–100	Video Evaluation	36	
		85	Posttest	10	
			ADDITIONAL ASSIGNMENTS		
			Total points		

√ When Assigned by Your Instructor	Study Guide Pages	Practices Required	LABORATORY ASSIGNMENTS (Procedure Number and Name)	Score*
	101	3	Practice for Competency *e* 3-1: Sanitization of Instruments Textbook reference: pp. 92–95	
	103–105		Evaluation of Competency 3-1: Sanitization of Instruments	*
	101	3	Practice for Competency 3-2: Chemical Disinfection of Articles Textbook reference: pp. 98–99	
	107–108		Evaluation of Competency 3-2: Chemical Disinfection of Articles	*
	101	Paper: 3 Muslin: 3	Practice for Competency *e* 3-3: Wrapping Instruments Using Paper or Muslin Textbook reference: pp. 104–105	
	109–110		Evaluation of Competency 3-3: Wrapping Instruments Using Paper or Muslin	*
	101	3	Practice for Competency *e* 3-4: Wrapping Instruments Using a Pouch Textbook reference: pp. 105–106	
	111–112		Evaluation of Competency 3-4: Wrapping Instruments Using a Pouch	*
	101	3	Practice for Competency *e* 3-5: Sterilizing Articles in the Autoclave Textbook reference: pp. 110–112	
	113–114		Evaluation of Competency 3-5: Sterilizing Articles in the Autoclave	*
			ADDITIONAL ASSIGNMENTS	

Notes

Name: _____   Date: _____

True or False

_____ 1. A bacterial spore consists of a hard, thick-walled capsule that can resist adverse conditions.

_____ 2. The purpose of sanitization is to remove all microorganisms and spores from a contaminated article.

_____ 3. According to OSHA, gloves do not need to be worn during the sanitization process.

_____ 4. Glutaraldehyde (Cidex) is a high-level disinfectant.

_____ 5. OSHA recommends a 10% bleach solution for decontaminating blood spills.

_____ 6. Sterilization is the process of destroying all forms of microbial life except for bacterial spores.

_____ 7. Autoclave tape indicates whether an autoclaved item is sterile.

_____ 8. The wrapper used to autoclave articles should prevent contaminants from getting in during handling and storage.

_____ 9. Tap water should be used in the autoclave.

_____ 10. The inside of the autoclave should be wiped every day with a damp cloth.

? POSTTEST

True or False

_____ 1. The agent used to destroy microorganisms on an article depends on the size of the article.

_____ 2. The purpose of the Hazard Communications Standard is to make sure that employees do not use hazardous chemicals in the workplace.

_____ 3. The Hazard Communications Standard requires that the label of a hazardous chemical include information on how to store and handle the chemical.

_____ 4. Stethoscopes must be decontaminated using a high-level disinfectant.

_____ 5. Protective eyewear must be worn when working with isopropyl alcohol.

_____ 6. The shelf life of a disinfectant indicates how long a disinfectant retains its effectiveness.

_____ 7. The best means of determining the effectives of the sterilization process are biologic indicators.

_____ 8. The proper time for sterilizing an article in the autoclave depends on what is being autoclaved.

_____ 9. A pack that has been in the storage cupboard for 4 weeks should be resterilized.

_____ 10. Ethylene oxide gas is used by medical manufacturers to sterilize disposable items.

Directions: Match each medical term (numbers) with its definition (letters).

_____ 1. Antiseptic

_____ 2. Autoclave

_____ 3. Contaminate

_____ 4. Critical item

_____ 5. Decontamination

_____ 6. Detergent

_____ 7. Disinfectant

_____ 8. Hazardous chemical

_____ 9. Incubate

_____ 10. Load

_____ 11. Material Safety Data Sheet

_____ 12. Noncritical item

_____ 13. Sanitization

_____ 14. Semicritical item

_____ 15. Spore

_____ 16. Sterilization

_____ 17. Thermolabile

A. To provide proper conditions for growth and development
B. To soil, stain, or pollute; to make impure
C. Easily affected or changed by heat
D. A substance that kills disease-producing microorganisms but not their spores (usually applied to living tissues)
E. An item that comes in contact with intact skin but not mucous membranes
F. A hard, thick-walled capsule formed by some bacteria that contains only the essential parts of the protoplasm of the bacterial cell
G. An item that comes in contact with sterile tissue or the vascular system
H. An apparatus for the sterilization of materials, using steam under pressure
I. An agent that cleanses by emulsifying dirt and oil
J. An item that comes in contact with nonintact skin or intact mucous membranes
K. The articles that are being sterilized
L. An agent used to destroy pathogenic microorganisms but not their spores (usually applied to inanimate objects)
M. A sheet that provides information regarding a chemical and its hazards, and measures to take to avoid injury and illness when handling the chemical
N. A process to remove organic matter from an article and to lower the number of microorganisms to a safe level as determined by public health requirements
O. The process of destroying all forms of microbial life, including bacterial spores
P. The use of physical or chemical means to remove or destroy pathogens on an item so that it is no longer capable of transmitting disease, making it safe to handle
Q. Any chemical that presents a threat to the health and safety of an individual coming into contact with it

EVALUATION OF LEARNING

Directions: Fill in each blank with the correct answer.

1. How does one determine what type of physical or chemical agent to use to destroy microorganisms on an article?

_____

_____

2. List two diseases that are caused by bacteria that produce spores.

_____

_____

3. What is the purpose of the Hazard Communication Standard?

_____

_____

4. List four examples of hazardous chemicals that may be used in the medical office.

_____

_____

5. What information must be included on a hazardous chemical label as required by the Hazard Communication Standard?

_____

_____

6. List and describe the information that must be included in a Material Safety Data Sheet.

_____

_____

_____

_____

_____

_____

_____

_____

7. What is the purpose of sanitizing an article?

_____

_____

8. What is the advantage of using the ultrasound method to clean instruments?

_____

_____

9. Why should gloves be worn during the sanitization procedure?

_____

_____

10. What is the definition of high-level disinfection?

_____

_____

11. List one example of an item that requires high-level disinfection. List one example of a high-level disinfectant.

_____

_____

12. List two examples of items that can be disinfected through intermediate-level disinfection. List one example of an intermediate-level disinfectant.

_____

_____

_____

13. List two examples of items that are disinfected by low-level disinfection.

_____

14. What disinfectant does OSHA recommend for the decontamination of blood spills?

_____

15. Why is it important to remove all organic matter from an article before it is disinfected?

_____

_____

16. Explain the difference between the shelf life and use life of a chemical disinfectant.

_____

_____

_____

17. What is the purpose of the pressure used in the autoclaving process?

_____

_____

18. Why is it important that all air be removed from the autoclave during the sterilization process?

_____

_____

19. What are the most common temperature and pressure used to sterilize materials with the autoclave?

_____

_____

20. What information does the CDC recommend be recorded in an autoclave log regarding each cycle?

_____

_____

_____

21. What is the function of a sterilization indicator?

_____

_____

22. What is the purpose of wrapping articles to be autoclaved?

_____

_____

23. List two properties of a good wrapper for use in autoclaving.

_____

_____

24. List three examples of wrapping material used for the autoclave, and identify an advantage of each type.

_____

_____

_____

25. Why is more time needed to autoclave a large minor office surgery pack?

_____

_____

26. What is *event-related sterility*?

_____

_____

27. Describe the care an autoclave should receive on a daily basis.

_____

_____

_____

28. Why is a longer exposure period needed to ensure sterilization when using the dry-heat oven?

_____

_____

29. What effect does moist heat have on instruments with sharp cutting edges?

_____

30. How does the medical manufacturing industry use ethylene oxide gas sterilization?

_____

_____

_____

31. What guidelines must be followed when using cold sterilization?

_____

_____

_____

_____

A. Material Safety Data Sheet

Refer to the Material Safety Data Sheet (MSDS) in the textbook (see Fig. 3-2), and answer the following questions.

1. When was this MSDS last revised?

_____

2. Is glutaraldehyde soluble in water?

_____

3. Describe the appearance and odor of glutaraldehyde.

_____

4. What is the pH of glutaraldehyde?

_____

5. Is glutaraldehyde flammable?

_____

6. Is glutaraldehyde stable?

_____

7. What conditions should be avoided with glutaraldehyde?

_____

8. How can glutaraldehyde enter the body?

_____

_____

9. What symptoms occur if glutaraldehyde does the following?

   a. Comes in contact with the skin

   _____

   b. Is splashed into the eyes

   _____

   c. Is inhaled

   _____

   d. Is ingested

   _____

10. What preexisting conditions can an individual possess that can be aggravated by glutaraldehyde?

_____

11. Does glutaraldehyde cause cancer?

_____

12. What are the emergency and first aid procedures for glutaraldehyde for the following?

a. Skin

_____

_____

b. Eyes

_____

_____

c. Inhalation

_____

_____

d. Ingestion

_____

_____

13. What should be done if glutaraldehyde is spilled?

_____

_____

_____

14. What is the disposal method for glutaraldehyde?

_____

_____

_____

15. How should glutaraldehyde be stored?

_____

_____

_____

16. What type of ventilation is needed when working with glutaraldehyde?

_____

17. What skin and eye protection should be taken with glutaraldehyde?

_____

_____

B. Obtaining a Material Safety Data Sheet

Obtain an MSDS for one of the following hazardous chemicals, and answer the questions.
To locate an MSDS on the Internet, enter the name of the chemical into a search engine along with the abbreviation "MSDS." (Example: Cidex MSDS)

- Cidex
- MetriCide

- Cidex OPA
- CaviCide
- MadaCide
- Wavicide
- Sporox II
- Vesphene
- Envirocide
- Clorox bleach

1. What is the chemical name of this hazardous chemical?

   _____

2. What is the trade or brand name of this chemical?

   _____

3. Who manufactures this chemical?

   _____

4. What number would you call if an emergency occurred with this chemical?

   _____

5. What type of symptoms occur if this chemical does the following?

   a. Comes in contact with the skin

      _____

   b. Is splashed into the eyes

      _____

   c. Is inhaled

      _____

   d. Is ingested

      _____

6. What are the emergency and first aid procedures for this chemical?

   _____

   _____

7. What should be done if this chemical is spilled?

   _____

   _____

8. What is the disposal method for this chemical?

   _____

   _____

9. How should this chemical be stored?

_____

_____

10. What type of protection should be taken when working with this chemical?

_____

_____

C. Sanitization

For each of the following situations involving sanitization, write **C** if the technique is correct and **I** if the technique is incorrect. If the situation is correct, state the principle underlying the technique. If the situation is incorrect, explain what could happen if the technique were performed in the incorrect manner.

_____ 1. A contaminated surgical instrument is left in the examination room.

_____

_____

_____ 2. The medical assistant does not wear gloves when sanitizing surgical instruments.

_____

_____

_____ 3. The medical assistant piles instruments while preparing them for sanitization.

_____

_____

_____ 4. The medical assistant forgets to read the MSDS before decontaminating some surgical instruments in Cidex.

_____

_____

_____ 5. The medical assistant uses laundry detergent to sanitize surgical instruments.

_____

_____

_____ 6. Dried blood is not completely cleansed from hemostatic forceps before they are sterilized in the autoclave.

_____

_____

_____ 7. The medical assistant checks all instruments for proper working condition before sterilizing them.

_____

_____

_____ 8. The medical assistant lubricates hemostatic forceps with a steam-penetrable lubricant before sterilizing them.

_____

_____

D. Storage of a Chemical Disinfectant

You have just received a 0.5-gallon container of Cidex Plus. You look at the label on the container and notice the following:

- Expiration date: 8/7/16
- Use life: 28 days
- Reuse life: 28 days

Based on this information, answer the following questions.

1. If the Cidex Plus is left unopened on the shelf, when would it expire and need to be discarded?

   _____

2. You open and activate the Cidex Plus on 9/1/14. What date should you write on the container?

   _____

3. You next fill a disinfectant container with the Cidex Plus and disinfect some articles in it. On what date would the Cidex Plus be unusable and need to be disposed?

   _____

4. On what date would you need to discard the rest of the container of Cidex Plus if it is not used?

   _____

E. Sterilization

For each of the following situations involving sterilization of articles in the autoclave, write **C** if the technique is correct and **I** if the technique is incorrect. If the situation is correct, state the principle underlying the technique. If the situation is incorrect, explain what might happen if the technique were performed in the incorrect manner.

_____ 1. The medical assistant opens a hemostat before placing it in a sterilization pouch.

                _____

                _____

_____ 2. Tap water is used to fill the water reservoir of the autoclave.

                _____

                _____

_____ 3. When loading the autoclave, the medical assistant places glass jars in an upright position.

                _____

                _____

_____ 4. The medical assistant places four sterilization pouches on top of each other in the autoclave.

                _____

                _____

_____ 5. The medical assistant places small packs to be sterilized approximately 1 to 3 inches apart in the autoclave.

                _____

                _____

_____ 6. Spore strips are placed in the autoclave where steam will penetrate them most easily.

_____

_____

_____ 7. The medical assistant begins timing the load in the autoclave after the proper temperature of 250° F has been reached.

_____

_____

_____ 8. The medical assistant removes the load from the autoclave while it is still wet.

_____

_____

_____ 9. The medical assistant notices a tear in one of the wrappers while removing articles from the autoclave. He or she rewraps and resterilizes the article.

_____

_____

_____ 10. The medical assistant notices that a sterilized wrapped article stored on the storage shelf has opened up. He or she retapes the pack and places it back on the storage shelf.

_____

_____

F. What Comes Next? Game

Object: The object of the game is to achieve sterilization of an article by determining the correct sequence of events in the sanitization and sterilization procedure.

Directions:

1. Cut out the game cards on the following page.
2. Make your cards unique by coloring and decorating them.
3. Review the sequence of steps in the sanitization and sterilization procedures.
4. Get into a group of three students.
5. Hold your game cards with the steps facing you.
6. Each player places the first step in the sanitization or sterilization procedure face down on the table.
7. When all players have placed a card on the table, turn the cards over.
8. Award yourself 5 points if you have correctly determined the proper step in the sequence. If you have a question regarding the correct answer, consult your instructor.
9. In turn, each player can earn an additional 5 points by stating a fact about that step in the procedure. For example, if the step is "Apply Gloves," a corresponding fact is that clean gloves and utility gloves must be worn during the sanitization procedure.
10. Keep track of your points on the Score Card provided.
11. Keep the cards in their proper sequence on the table, and continue the game until all of the game cards have been used.

WHAT COMES NEXT?

SCORE CARD

Name: _____

Recording Points:

Cross off a number each time you properly sequence a game card (starting with 5 and continuing in sequence). Cross off another number if you are able to state a fact about the step in the procedure. Your total points will be equal to the last number you crossed off. Record this number in the space provided, and check the level that you achieved.

Game Card Points:

		Total points: _____
5	75	
10	80	**LEVEL:**
15	85	
20	90	≤100 to 120 points: **Sterile**—You got rid of all MOs and spores!
25	95	≤80 to 100 points: **Aseptic**—You got rid of the pathogenic MOs.
30	100	≤60 to 80 points: **Contaminated**—Your article is still contaminated.
35	105	
40	110	
45	115	
50	120	
55	125	
60	130	
65	135	
70	140	

	Decontaminate instruments	Check working order and lubricate instruments	Store instruments
	Rinse contaminated instruments	Dry instruments	Operate the autoclave
	Apply gloves	Thoroughly rinse instruments	Load the autoclave
	Read MSDS	Clean instruments manually	Wrap instruments

**What
comes
next?**

**What
comes
next?**

**What
comes
next?**

**What
comes
next?**

**What
comes
next?**

**What
comes
next?**

**What
comes
next?**

**What
comes
next?**

**What
comes
next?**

Name: _____

Directions:

a. Watch the indicated videos.
b. Mark each true statement with a T and each false statement with an F. For each false statement, change the wording of the question so that it becomes a true statement.

Video: Procedure 3-1: Sanitization of Instruments

_____ 1. Before surgical instruments can be sterilized in the autoclave, they must first be sanitized.

_____ 2. Sanitization involves a series of steps designed to remove all microorganisms and spores from an article.

_____ 3. An MSDS provides information regarding a chemical, its hazards, and measures to take to prevent injury and illness when handling the chemical.

_____ 4. After removing used instruments from an examining room, immediately rinse them thoroughly under hot running water to remove organic material.

_____ 5. Instruments undergoing sanitization should be decontaminated by disinfecting them in an EPA-approved chemical disinfectant.

_____ 6. The instrument disinfectant container should be labeled with the name of the disinfectant and today's date.

_____ 7. An instrument cleaning agent that has expired loses its potency and should not be used.

_____ 8. A wire brush should be used to clean the surface of each instrument.

_____ 9. After cleaning each instrument, rinse it thoroughly with warm water.

_____ 10. If the instrument is not completely dry following sanitization, stains may occur on the instrument.

_____ 11. An instrument should be rinsed after a lubricant has been applied to it.

_____ 12. The manufacturer's instructions specify how to dispose of the instrument cleaning solution.

Video: Procedure 3-3 and 3-4: Wrapping Instruments

_____ 1. The purpose of wrapping an instrument is to protect it from recontamination during handling and storage.

_____ 2. If a minor office surgery setup is being wrapped, a double layer of sterilization paper is often used.

_____ 3. The wrapping material consists of a substance that prevents steam from reaching the instrument during the sterilization process.

_____ 4. If the sterilization strips are outdated, they may provide inaccurate results.

_____ 5. An instrument should be placed in the center of the sterilization wrapping paper with the longest part of the instrument pointing toward the two side corners.

_____ 6. If an instrument has a movable joint, it should be placed in a slightly closed position when wrapping an instrument.

_____ 7. A sterilization indicator strip is placed in the center of the pack next to the instrument.

_____ 8. The pack should be marked with the date of the sterilization and your initials.

_____ 9. If a sterilization indicator does not change appropriately, the item is not sterile and must not be used.

_____ 10. Autoclave tape turns from white to black, which indicates that the autoclaved item is sterile.

Video: Procedure 3-5: Sterilizing Articles in the Autoclave

_____ 1. Sterilization of articles in the autoclave destroys all microorganisms and spores.

_____ 2. The autoclave is typically operated at 15 pounds of pressure at a temperature of 212° F.

_____ 3. A surgical instrument requires a longer sterilizing time than a minor office surgery pack.

_____ 4. Before an article can be sterilized in the autoclave, it must first be sanitized.

_____ 5. Water contained in the water reservoir of the autoclave is converted to steam during the sterilization process.

_____ 6. Warm tap water must be used in the autoclave because it prevents corrosion of the stainless steel chamber of the autoclave.

_____ 7. Small packs should be placed 1 to 3 inches apart, and large packs should be placed 2 to 4 inches apart in the autoclave to provide for adequate steam penetration.

_____ 8. Pouches should be placed on an autoclave tray with the plastic side up and the paper side facing down.

_____ 9. An autoclave load is dried by cracking open the door approximately 6 inches.

_____ 10. The autoclave packs must dry fully; otherwise, microorganisms can move through the moisture on a wet wrap and contaminate the sterile article inside.

_____ 11. If an autoclaved pack shows any damage, such as holes or tears, the article should be rewrapped and resterilized.

_____ 12. Store the packs in a clean, dustproof area with the most recently sterilized packs placed in front of previously sterilized packs.

_____ 13. Daily care of the autoclave includes scrubbing the interior of the autoclave and the trays with scouring powder.

_____ 14. The rubber door gasket should be inspected for damage that could prevent a good seal.

PRACTICE FOR COMPETENCY

Sterilization and Disinfection

1. **Procedure 3-1: Sanitizing Instruments.** Sanitize instruments. In the space provided, indicate the following:

   A. Name of the disinfectant

   _____

   B. Name of the instrument cleaner

   _____

   _____

   C. Names of instruments sanitized

   _____

   _____

2. **Procedure 3-2: Chemical Disinfection of Articles.** Chemically disinfect contaminated articles. In the space provided, indicate the following:

   A. Name of the disinfectant

   _____

   B. Names of articles disinfected

   _____

   _____

   _____

3. **Procedures 3-3 and 3-4: Wrapping Articles for the Autoclave.** Wrap articles for autoclaving. In the space provided, list the information you indicated on the label of each pack that includes the contents of the pack, the date, and your initials. Information indicated on the label of the wrapped article:

   _____

   _____

   _____

   _____

   _____

   _____

   _____

4. **Procedure 3-5: Sterilizing Articles in the Autoclave.** Sterilize articles in the autoclave. In the space provided, indicate the articles you sterilized.

   _____

   _____

   _____

   _____

Notes

EVALUATION OF COMPETENCY

Procedure 3-1: Sanitization of Instruments

Name: _____   Date: _____

Evaluated by: _____   Score: _____

Performance Objective

Outcome:	Sanitize instruments.
Conditions:	Given the following: disposable gloves, utility gloves, contaminated instruments, chemical disinfectant and MSDS, disinfectant container, cleaning solution and MSDS, basin, nylon brush, wire brush, paper towels, cloth towel, and instrument lubricant.
Standards:	Time: 10 minutes. Student completed procedure in _____ minutes.
	Accuracy: Satisfactory score on the Performance Evaluation Checklist.

Performance Evaluation Checklist

Trial 1	Trial 2	Point Value	Performance Standards
		•	Reviewed the MSDS for hazardous chemicals being used.
		•	Applied gloves.
		•	Transported the contaminated instruments to the cleaning area.
		•	Applied heavy-duty utility gloves over the disposable gloves.
		▷	Stated the purpose of the utility gloves.
		•	Separated sharp instruments and delicate instruments from other instruments.
		▷	Explained why instruments should be separated.
		•	Immediately rinsed the instruments thoroughly under warm running water.
		▷	Stated why the instruments should be rinsed immediately.
			Decontaminated the instruments.
		•	Checked the expiration date of the chemical disinfectant.
		▷	Explained why an expired disinfectant should not be used.
		•	Observed all personal safety precautions listed on the label.
		•	Followed label directions for proper mixing and use of the disinfectant.
		•	Labeled the disinfecting container with the name of the disinfectant and the reuse expiration date.
		•	Poured the disinfectant into the labeled container.
		•	Completely submerged the articles in the disinfectant.
		•	Covered the disinfectant container.

103

Trial 1	Trial 2	Point Value	Performance Standards
		▷	Stated the reason for covering the container.
		•	Disinfected the articles for 10 minutes.
		▷	Explained the reason for decontaminating the instruments.
			Cleaned the instruments: manual method.
		•	Checked the expiration date of the cleaning agent.
		•	Observed all personal safety precautions.
		•	Followed label directions for proper use and mixing of the cleaning agent.
		•	Removed articles from disinfectant and placed them in the cleaning solution.
		•	Cleaned the surface of the instruments with a nylon brush.
		•	Cleaned grooves, crevices, or serrations with a wire brush.
		•	Removed stains using commercial stain remover.
		•	Scrubbed the instruments until they were visibly clean.
		▷	Explained why all organic matter must be removed.
			Cleaned the instruments: ultrasound method.
		•	Prepared the cleaning solution in the ultrasonic cleaner.
		•	Observed all personal safety precautions listed on label.
		•	Removed the articles from the disinfectant.
		•	Separated instruments of dissimilar metals.
		•	Properly placed the instruments in the ultrasonic cleaner.
		•	Positioned hinged instruments in an open position.
		▷	Stated why hinged instruments must be in an open position.
		•	Ensured that sharp instruments did not touch other instruments.
		•	Checked to make sure all instruments were fully submerged.
		•	Placed the lid on the ultrasonic cleaner.
		•	Turned on the ultrasonic cleaner.
		•	Cleaned the instruments for the length of time recommended by the manufacturer.
		•	Removed the instruments from the machine.
		•	Rinsed each instrument thoroughly with warm water for 20 to 30 seconds.
		▷	Explained why instruments should be rinsed thoroughly.
		•	Dried each instrument with a paper towel.
			Completed the procedure.
		•	Placed instrument on a towel for additional drying.
		▷	Stated the reason for drying the instruments.
		•	Checked each instrument for defects and proper working condition.
		•	Lubricated hinged instruments in an open position.
		•	Opened and closed the instrument to distribute the lubricant.
		•	Placed the lubricated instrument on a towel to drain.

Trial 1	Trial 2	Point Value	Performance Standards
		▷	Stated the reason for lubricating instruments.
		•	Disposed of the cleaning solution according to the manufacturer's instructions.
		•	Removed both sets of gloves.
		•	Sanitized hands.
		•	Wrapped the instruments.
		•	Sterilized the instruments in the autoclave.
		✶	Completed the procedure within 10 minutes.
			Totals

Evaluation of Student Performance

EVALUATION CRITERIA			COMMENTS
Symbol	**Category**	**Point Value**	
✶	Critical Step	16 points	
•	Essential Step	6 points	
▷	Theory Question	2 points	

Score calculation: 100 points

   − _____ points missed

   _____ Score

Satisfactory score: 85 or above

CAAHEP Competencies Achieved

Psychomotor (Skills)

☑ III. 5. Prepare items for autoclaving.

ABHES Competencies Achieved

☑ 9. b. Apply principles of aseptic techniques and infection control.

Notes

EVALUATION OF COMPETENCY

Procedure 3-2: Chemical Disinfection of Articles

Name: _____ Date: _____

Evaluated by: _____ Score: _____

Performance Objective

Outcome:	Chemically disinfect articles.
Conditions:	Given the following: disposable gloves, utility gloves, contaminated articles, chemical disinfectant and MSDS, disinfectant container, and paper towels.
Standards:	Time: 10 minutes. Student completed procedure in _____ minutes.
	Accuracy: Satisfactory score on the Performance Evaluation Checklist.

Performance Evaluation Checklist

Trial 1	Trial 2	Point Value	Performance Standards
		•	Applied gloves and sanitized the articles.
		•	Reviewed the MSDS for the chemical disinfectant.
		▷	Described what information is included on an MSDS.
		•	Checked the expiration date of the disinfectant.
		▷	Explained why an expired disinfectant should not be used.
		•	Observed all personal safety precautions listed on the container label.
		•	Followed the directions on the label for proper use and reuse of the disinfectant.
		•	Completely immersed articles in the chemical disinfectant.
		•	Covered disinfectant container.
		▷	Stated the reason for covering the container.
		•	Disinfected articles for the proper length of time as indicated on the label of the container.
		•	Rinsed the articles thoroughly.
		▷	Stated the reason for rinsing the articles.
		•	Dried the articles.
		•	Properly disposed of the disinfectant.
		▷	Stated the purpose of proper disposal of the disinfectant.
		•	Removed gloves.
		•	Sanitized hands.
		•	Properly stored the articles.
		★	Completed the procedure within 10 minutes.
			Totals

EVALUATION CRITERIA			COMMENTS
Symbol	**Category**	**Point Value**	
✶	Critical Step	16 points	
•	Essential Step	6 points	
▷	Theory Question	2 points	

Score calculation: 100 points

− _____ points missed

_____ Score

Satisfactory score: 85 or above

CAAHEP Competencies Achieved

Psychomotor (Skills)

☑ XI. 1. Comply with safety signs, symbols, and labels.

ABHES Competencies Achieved

☑ b. Apply principles of aseptic techniques and infection control.

Procedure 3-3: Wrapping Instruments Using Paper or Muslin

Name: _____   Date: _____

Evaluated by: _____   Score: _____

Performance Objective

Outcome:	Wrap an instrument for autoclaving.
Conditions:	Given the following: sanitized instrument, wrapping material, sterilization indicator strip, autoclave tape, and a permanent marker.
Standards:	Time: 5 minutes. Student completed procedure in _____ minutes.
	Accuracy: Satisfactory score on the Performance Evaluation Checklist.

Performance Evaluation Checklist

Trial 1	Trial 2	Point Value	Performance Standards
		•	Sanitized hands.
		•	Assembled equipment.
		•	Selected the appropriate-sized wrapping material.
		•	Checked the expiration date on the sterilization indicator box.
		▷	Stated why outdated strips should not be used.
		•	Placed wrapping material on clean, flat surface.
		•	Turned the wrap in a diagonal position.
		•	Placed instrument in the center of wrapping material.
		•	Placed instruments with movable joints in an open position.
		▷	Stated why instruments with movable joints must be placed in an open position.
		•	Placed a sterilization indicator in the center of the pack.
		•	Folded wrapping material up from the bottom and doubled back a small corner.
		•	Folded over one edge of wrapping material and doubled back the corner.
		•	Folded over the other edge of wrapping material and doubled back the corner.
		•	Folded the pack up from the bottom and secured with autoclave tape.
		•	Ensured that the pack was firm enough for handling, but loose enough to permit proper circulation of steam.
		▷	Stated why instruments are wrapped for autoclaving.
		•	Labeled and dated the pack. Included your initials.
		▷	Stated the purpose of dating the pack.
		✶	Completed the procedure within 5 minutes.
			Totals

Evaluation of Student Performance

EVALUATION CRITERIA			COMMENTS
Symbol	**Category**	**Point Value**	
✱	Critical Step	16 points	
•	Essential Step	6 points	
▷	Theory Question	2 points	

Score calculation: 100 points

− _____ points missed

_____ Score

Satisfactory score: 85 or above

CAAHEP Competencies Achieved

Psychomotor (Skills)

☑ III. 5. Prepare items for autoclaving.

ABHES Competencies Achieved

☑ 9. h. Wrap items for autoclaving.

Procedure 3-4: Wrapping Instruments Using a Pouch

Name: _____   Date: _____

Evaluated by: _____   Score: _____

Performance Objective

Outcome:	Wrap an instrument for autoclaving.
Conditions:	Given the following: sanitized instrument, sterilization pouch, and a permanent marker.
Standards:	Time: 5 minutes. Student completed procedure in _____ minutes.
	Accuracy: Satisfactory score on the Performance Evaluation Checklist.

Performance Evaluation Checklist

Trial 1	Trial 2	Point Value	Performance Standards
		•	Sanitized hands.
		•	Assembled equipment.
		•	Selected the appropriate-sized pouch.
		•	Placed the pouch on a clean, flat surface.
		•	Labeled and dated the pack. Included your initials.
		•	Inserted the instrument into the open end of the pouch.
		•	Sealed the pouch.
		•	Sterilized the pack in the autoclave.
		▷	Stated how long the pack is sterile once it has been autoclaved.
		✶	Completed the procedure within 5 minutes.
			Totals

Evaluation of Student Performance

EVALUATION CRITERIA			COMMENTS
Symbol	**Category**	**Point Value**	
✶	Critical Step	16 points	
•	Essential Step	6 points	
▷	Theory Question	2 points	
Score calculation: 100 points			
− _____ points missed			
_____ Score			
Satisfactory score: 85 or above			

CAAHEP Competencies Achieved
Psychomotor (Skills)
☑ III. 5. Prepare items for autoclaving.

ABHES Competencies Achieved
☑ 9. h. Wrap items for autoclaving.

EVALUATION OF COMPETENCY

Procedure 3-5: Sterilizing Articles in the Autoclave

Name: _____   Date: _____

Evaluated by: _____   Score: _____

Performance Objective

Outcome:	Sterilize articles in the autoclave.
Conditions:	Using an autoclave.
Standards:	Time: 10 minutes. Student completed procedure in _____ minutes.
	Accuracy: Satisfactory score on the Performance Evaluation Checklist.

Performance Evaluation Checklist

Trial 1	Trial 2	Point Value	Performance Standards
		•	Assembled equipment.
		•	Checked the water level in the autoclave.
		•	Properly loaded the autoclave.
		▷	Stated how far apart to place small packs and large packs.
		▷	Explained how to position pouches in the autoclave.
			Manually operated the autoclave.
		•	Determined the sterilizing time for the type of articles being autoclaved.
		•	Turned on the autoclave.
		•	Filled the chamber with water.
		•	Closed and latched the door.
		•	Set the timing control.
			Stated when the timer should be set.
		•	Vented the chamber of steam.
		•	Dried the load.
		▷	Stated the reason for drying the load.
			Automatically operated the autoclave.
		•	Closed and latched the door.
		•	Turned on the autoclave.
		•	Determined the sterilization program.
		•	Pressed the appropriate program button.
		•	Pressed the start button.
		▷	Stated the purpose of each control or indicator on the autoclave.
			Completed the procedure.
		•	Turned off the autoclave.

Trial 1	Trial 2	Point Value	Performance Standards
		•	Removed the load with heat-resistant gloves.
		▷	Stated the reason for using heat-resistant gloves.
		•	Inspected the packs as they were removed for damage.
		▷	Explained what should be done if a pack is torn.
		•	Checked the sterilization indicators on the outside of the packs.
		•	Recorded information in the autoclave log.
		•	Stored the articles in a clean dust-proof area.
		•	Placed the most recently sterilized packs behind previously sterilized packs.
		•	Maintained appropriate daily care of the autoclave.
		▷	Described the care the autoclave should receive each day.
		✳	Completed the procedure within 10 minutes.
			Totals

Evaluation of Student Performance

EVALUATION CRITERIA			COMMENTS
Symbol	**Category**	**Point Value**	
✳	Critical Step	16 points	
•	Essential Step	6 points	
▷	Theory Question	2 points	

Score calculation: 100 points

−　　　　　points missed

　　　　Score

Satisfactory score: 85 or above

CAAHEP Competencies Achieved

Psychomotor (Skills)

☑ III. 6. Perform sterilization procedures.

Affective (Behavior)

☑ IX. 3. Recognize the importance of local, state, and federal legislation and regulations in the practice setting.

ABHES Competencies Achieved

☑ 9. o. (4) Perform sterilization techniques.

4 Vital Signs

√ After Completing	Date Due	Textbook Pages	TEXTBOOK ASSIGNMENTS	Possible Points	Points You Earned
		116–171	Read Chapter 4: Vital Signs		
		136 166	Read Case Study 1 Case Study 1 questions	5	
		140 166	Read Case Study 2 Case Study 2 questions	5	
		152 166	Read Case Study 3 Case Study 3 questions	5	
			Total points		

√ After Completing	Date Due	Study Guide Pages	STUDY GUIDE ASSIGNMENTS (CTA = Critical Thinking Activity)	Possible Points	Points You Earned
		119	Pretest	10	
		120–122 122–123	Term Key Term Assessment A. Definitions B. Word Parts (Add 1 point for each medical term)	55 30	
		123–132	Evaluation of Learning questions	90	
		132–134	CTA A: Measurement of Body Temperature	18	
		135	CTA B: Alterations in Body Temperature	5	
		135	CTA C: Pulse Sites	6	
		135–136	CTA D: Pulse and Respiratory Rates	3	
		136–137	CTA E: Pulse Oximetry	18	
		137–138	CTA F: Blood Pressure Measurement	6	
		138	CTA G: Proper BP Cuff Selection	12	
		139	CTA H: Reading Blood Pressure Values	24	
			Evolve Site: Chapter 4 Under Pressure: Blood Pressure Readings (Record points earned)		

√ After Completing	Date Due	Study Guide Pages	STUDY GUIDE ASSIGNMENTS (CTA = Critical Thinking Activity)	Possible Points	Points You Earned
		139–140	CTA I: Interpreting Blood Pressure Readings	10	
		140–141	CTA J: Hypertension	20	
		142	CTA K: Crossword Puzzle	30	
			Evolve Site: Chapter 4: Road to Recovery Game Vital Signs Terminology (Record points earned)		
			Evolve Site: Chapter 4 Animations (2 points each)	16	
			Evolve Site: Chapter 4 Nutrition Nugget: DASH	10	
			Evolve Site: Apply Your Knowledge questions	11	
		143–146	Video Evaluation	86	
		119	Posttest	10	
			ADDITIONAL ASSIGNMENTS		
			Total points		

√ When Assigned by Your Instructor	Study Guide Pages	Practices Required	LABORATORY ASSIGNMENTS	Score*
	147	5	Practice for Competency 4-1: Measuring Oral Body Temperature with an Electronic Thermometer Textbook reference: pp. 126–128	
	149–150		Evaluation of Competency 4-1: Measuring Oral Body Temperature with an Electronic Thermometer	*
	147	3	Practice for Competency 4-2: Measuring Axillary Body Temperature with an Electronic Thermometer Textbook reference: pp. 128–129	
	151–152		Evaluation of Competency 4-2: Measuring Axillary Body Temperature with an Electronic Thermometer	*
	147	3	Practice for Competency 4-3: Measuring Rectal Body Temperature with an Electronic Thermometer Textbook reference: pp. 130–131	
	153–154		Evaluation of Competency 4-3: Measuring Rectal Body Temperature with an Electronic Thermometer	*
	147	5	Practice for Competency 4-4: Measuring Aural Body Temperature with a Tympanic Membrane Thermometer Textbook reference: pp. 131–133	
	155–156		Evaluation of Competency 4-4: Measuring Aural Body Temperature with a Tympanic Membrane Thermometer	*
	147	5	Practice for Competency 4-5: Measuring Temporal Body Temperature Textbook reference: pp. 134–136	
	157–158		Evaluation of Competency 4-5: Measuring Temporal Body Temperature	*
	148	10	Practice for Competency 4-6: Measuring Pulse and Respiration Textbook reference: pp. 146–147	
	159–160		Evaluation of Competency 4-6: Measuring Pulse and Respiration	*

√ When Assigned by Your Instructor	Study Guide Pages	Practices Required	LABORATORY ASSIGNMENTS	Score*
	148	5	**e** Practice for Competency 4-7: Measuring Apical Pulse Textbook reference: p. 148	
	161–162		Evaluation of Competency 4-7: Measuring Apical Pulse	*
	148	5	**e** Practice for Competency 4-8: Performing Pulse Oximetry Textbook reference: pp. 149–150	
	163–165		Evaluation of Competency 4-8: Performing Pulse Oximetry	*
	148	10	**e** Practice for Competency 4-9: Measuring Blood Pressure Textbook reference: pp. 162–164	
	167–169		Evaluation of Competency 4-9: Measuring Blood Pressure	*
			ADDITIONAL ASSIGNMENTS	

Name: _____ Date _____

True or False

___T___ 1. The heat-regulating center of the body is the medulla.

___T___ 2. A vague sense of body discomfort, weakness, and fatigue that often marks the onset of a disease is known as the blahs.

___F___ 3. If an axillary temperature of 100° F was taken orally, it would register as 101° F.

_____ 4. If the lens of a tympanic membrane thermometer is dirty, the reading may be falsely low.

_____ 5. Chemical thermometers should be stored in the freezer.

___F___ 6. The femoral pulse site can be used to assess circulation to the foot.

___T___ 7. The term used to describe an irregularity in the heart's rhythm is *dysrhythmia*.

___T___ 8. Pulse oximetry provides the physician with information on the amount of oxygen being delivered to the tissues.

_____ 9. Blood pressure measures the contraction and relaxation of the heart.

___T___ 10. When taking blood pressure, the stethoscope is placed over the brachial artery.

POSTTEST

True or False

___F___ 1. A temperature of 100° F is classified as a low-grade fever.

___T___ 2. The rectal site should not be used to take the temperature of a newborn.

___F___ 3. A tympanic membrane thermometer should not be used to measure temperature on a patient who has a normal amount of cerumen in the ear.

___F___ 4. A temporal artery temperature reading is the same as an oral reading.

___T___ 5. Excessive pressure should not be applied when measuring a pulse because it could obstruct the pulse.

___T___ 6. A child has a faster pulse rate than an adult.

___F___ 7. The normal respiratory rate of an adult ranges between 10 and 18 respirations per minute.

___F___ 8. The term used to describe a bluish discoloration of the skin due to a lack of oxygen is *hypoxia*.

___F___ 9. The oxygen saturation level of a healthy individual falls between 85% and 90%.

_____ 10. When measuring blood pressure, the patient's arm should be positioned above the level of the heart.

A. Definitions
Temperature

Directions: Match each medical term (numbers) with its definition (letters).

O __ 1. Afebrile
G __ 2. Antipyretic
D __ 3. Axilla
J __ 4. Celsius scale
M __ 5. Conduction
E __ 6. Convection
N __ 7. Crisis
B __ 8. Disinfectant
H __ 9. Fahrenheit scale
L __ 10. Febrile
F __ 11. Fever
K __ 12. Frenulum linguae
A __ 13. Hyperpyrexia
C __ 14. Hypothermia
P __ 15. Malaise
I __ 16. Radiation

A. An extremely high fever
B. An agent used to destroy disease-producing microorganisms but not necessarily their spores (usually applied to inanimate objects)
C. A body temperature that is below normal
D. The armpit
E. The transfer of energy, such as heat, through air currents
F. A body temperature that is above normal (pyrexia)
G. An agent that reduces fever
H. A temperature scale on which the freezing point of water is 32° and the boiling point of water is 212°
I. The transfer of energy, such as heat, in the form of waves
J. A temperature scale on which the freezing point of water is 0° and the boiling point is 100°
K. The midline fold that connects the undersurface of the tongue with the floor of the mouth
L. Pertaining to fever
M. The transfer of energy from one object to another by direct contact
N. A sudden falling of an elevated body temperature to normal
O. Without fever; the body temperature is normal
P. A vague sense of body discomfort, weakness, and fatigue often marking the onset of a disease and continuing through the course of the illness

Pulse

Directions: Match each medical term (numbers) with its definition (letters).

D __ 1. Antecubital space
F __ 2. Aorta
B __ 3. Bounding pulse
J __ 4. Bradycardia
I __ 5. Dysrhythmia
A __ 6. Intercostal
G __ 7. Pulse rhythm
C __ 8. Pulse volume
E __ 9. Tachycardia
H __ 10. Thready pulse

A. Between the ribs
B. A pulse with an increased volume that feels very strong and full
C. The strength of the heartbeat
D. The space located at the front of the elbow
E. An abnormally fast heart rate (more than 100 beats per minute)
F. The major trunk of the arterial system of the body
G. The time interval between heartbeats
H. A pulse with a decreased volume that feels weak and thin
I. An irregular rhythm
J. An abnormally slow heart rate (less than 60 beats per minute)

Respiration and Pulse Oximetry

Directions: Match each medical term (numbers) with its definition (letters).

H___ 1. Alveolus

D___ 2. Apnea

R___ 3. Bradypnea

K___ 4. Cyanosis

N___ 5. Dyspnea

O___ 6. Eupnea

A___ 7. Exhalation

S___ 8. Hyperpnea

Q___ 9. Hyperventilation

G___ 10. Hypopnea

C___ 11. Hypoxemia

B___ 12. Hypoxia

J___ 13. Inhalation

M___ 14. Orthopnea

F___ 15. Pulse oximeter

I___ 16. Pulse oximetry

L___ 17. Sao$_2$

O___ 18. Spo$_2$

E___ 19. Tachypnea

A. The act of breathing out
B. A reduction in the oxygen supply to the tissues of the body
C. A decrease in the oxygen saturation of the blood; may lead to hypoxia
D. The temporary cessation of breathing
E. An abnormal increase in the respiratory rate of more than 20 respirations per minute
F. A computerized device consisting of a probe and monitor used to measure the oxygen saturation of arterial blood
G. An abnormal decrease in the rate and depth of respiration
H. A thin-walled air sac of the lungs in which the exchange of oxygen and carbon dioxide takes place
I. The use of a pulse oximeter to measure the oxygen saturation of arterial blood
J. The act of breathing in
K. A bluish discoloration of the skin and mucous membranes first observed in the nailbeds and lips
L. Abbreviation for the percentage of hemoglobin that is saturated with oxygen in arterial blood
M. The condition in which breathing is easier when an individual is in a standing or sitting position
N. Shortness of breath or difficulty in breathing
O. Abbreviation for the percentage of hemoglobin that is saturated with oxygen in arterial blood as measured by a pulse oximeter
P. Normal respiration
Q. An abnormally fast and deep type of breathing usually associated with acute anxiety conditions
R. An abnormal decrease in the respiratory rate of less than 10 respirations per minute
S. An abnormal increase in the rate and depth of respiration

Blood Pressure

Directions: Match each medical term (numbers) with its definition (letters).

_____ 1. Diastole

_____ 2. Diastolic pressure

_____ 3. Hypertension

_____ 4. Hypotension

_____ 5. Meniscus

_____ 6. Pulse pressure

_____ 7. Sphygmomanometer

_____ 8. Stethoscope

_____ 9. Systole

_____ 10. Systolic pressure

A. The curved surface on a column of liquid in a tube
B. High blood pressure
C. The point of maximum pressure on the arterial walls
D. The phase in the cardiac cycle in which the heart relaxes between contractions
E. An instrument for measuring arterial blood pressure
F. The point of lesser pressure on the arterial walls
G. Low blood pressure
H. The phase in the cardiac cycle in which the ventricles contract, sending blood out of the heart and into the aorta and pulmonary aorta
I. An instrument for amplifying and hearing sounds produced by the body
J. The difference between the systolic and diastolic pressures

B. Word Parts

Directions: Indicate the meaning of each word part in the space provided. List as many medical terms as possible that incorporate the word part in the space provided.

Word Part	Meaning of Word Part	Medical Terms That Incorporate Word Part
1. anti-		
2. pyr/o		
3. -ic		
4. -pnea		
5. brady-		
6. cardi/o		
7. -ia		
8. a-		
9. cyan/o		
10. -osis		
11. dys-		
12. eu-		
13. -ex		
14. hyper-		
15. hypo-		
16. tension		

17. therm/o		
18. ox/i		
19. in-		
20. inter-		
21. cost/o		
22. -al		
23. -mal		
24. -meter		
25. orth/o		
26. -metry		
27. sphygm/o		
28. steth/o		
29. -scope		
30. tachy-		

EVALUATION OF LEARNING

Temperature

Directions: Fill in each blank with the correct answer.

1. Define a vital sign.

_____

_____

_____

2. What are the four vital signs?

_____

_____

_____

_____

3. What general guidelines should be followed when measuring vital signs?

_____

_____

_____

_____

4. List four ways in which heat is produced in the body.

_____

_____

_____

_____

5. List four ways in which heat is lost from the body.

_____

_____

_____

_____

6. What is the normal body temperature range?

_____

7. What is a fever?

_____

_____

8. How do diurnal variations affect body temperature?

_____

_____

9. How do emotional states affect the body temperature?

_____

10. How does vigorous physical exercise affect body temperature?

_____

11. What symptoms occur with a fever?

_____

_____

12. Describe the following fever patterns:
   a. Continuous fever

_____

_____

   b. Intermittent fever

_____

_____

   c. Remittent fever

_____

_____

13. What is the subsiding stage of a fever?

_____

14. What four sites are used for taking body temperature?

_____

15. List three instances in which the axillary site for taking body temperature would be preferred over the oral site.

_____

_____

_____

16. Why does the rectal method for taking body temperature provide a very accurate temperature measurement?

_____

_____

_____

17. When can the rectal method be used to take body temperature?

_____

_____

18. When can the aural method be used to take body temperature?

_____

_____

19. How does a temperature taken through the rectal and axillary method compare (in terms of degrees) with a temperature taken through the oral method?

_____

_____

20. List and describe the four types of thermometers available for taking body temperature.

_____

_____

_____

21. Describe the advantages of a tympanic membrane thermometer.

_____

_____

22. Explain how a tympanic membrane thermometer measures body temperature.

_____

_____

_____

23. The tympanic membrane thermometer should not be used to measure temperature on patients with what types of conditions?

_____

_____

24. Explain how to clean the lens of a tympanic membrane thermometer.

_____

_____

25. List two reasons why the temporal artery is a good site to measure body temperature.

_____

_____

26. How does the temperature obtained through the temporal site compare with oral, rectal, and axillary body temperature?

_____

_____

_____

27. List four factors that can result in a falsely low temperature reading when using the temporal artery thermometer.

_____

_____

28. Where should a chemical thermometer be stored? Explain why.

_____

_____

Pulse

Directions: Fill in each blank with the correct answer.

1. What causes the pulse to occur?

_____

_____

_____

2. What is the unit of measurement for pulse rate?

_____

3. How does physical activity affect the pulse rate?

_____

4. What is the most common site for taking the pulse?

_____

5. List two reasons for taking the pulse at the apical pulse site.

_____

_____

6. Where is the apex of the heart located?

_____

_____

7. When is the brachial artery used as a pulse site?

_____

8. When is the carotid artery used as a pulse site?

_____

9. When is the femoral artery used as a pulse site?

_____

10. What two pulse sites can be used to assess circulation to the foot?

_____

11. List two reasons for measuring the pulse rate.

_____

_____

12. State the normal range for a pulse rate for an adult.

_____

13. What is the normal pulse range for the following age groups?
    a. Infant _____
    b. Toddler _____
    c. Preschooler _____
    d. School-aged child _____
    e. Adult after age 60 _____

14. What is the normal pulse range for a well-trained athlete?

_____

15. What may cause tachycardia?

_____

16. If the rhythm and volume of a patient's pulse are normal, the medical assistant records the information as

_____

Respiration

Directions: Fill in each blank with the correct answer.

1. What is the purpose of respiration?

   _____

   _____

2. What is the purpose of inhalation?

   _____

   _____

3. What is the purpose of exhalation?

   _____

   _____

4. What is included in one complete respiration?

   _____

   _____

5. The exchange of oxygen and carbon dioxide between the body cells and blood is known as

   _____

6. What is the name of the control center for involuntary respiration?

   _____

7. Why must respiration be taken without the patient's awareness?

   _____

8. What is the normal respiratory rate (range) for a normal adult?

   _____

9. List two factors that can increase the respiratory rate.

   _____

   _____

10. Describe a normal rhythm for respiration.

    _____

    _____

11. What can cause hyperventilation?

    _____

12. What type of patient may experience hypopnea?

    _____

128

13. Where is cyanosis first observed?

_____

_____

14. What can cause cyanosis?

_____

15. What are two conditions in which dyspnea may occur?

_____

_____

16. Describe the character of normal breath sounds.

_____

_____

17. Describe the character of the following abnormal breath sounds:

a. Crackles

_____

_____

b. Rhonchi

_____

_____

c. Wheezes

_____

_____

Pulse Oximetry

Directions: Fill in each blank with the correct answer.

1. What is the purpose of pulse oximetry?

_____

_____

2. What is the function of hemoglobin?

_____

3. What is the oxygen saturation level of a healthy individual?

_____

4. What can occur if the oxygen saturation level falls between 85% and 90%?

_____

_____

5. List three patient conditions that can cause a decreased SpO_2 value.

_____

_____

_____

6. When can pulse oximetry be used for the short-term continuous monitoring of a patient?

_____

_____

_____

7. What is the purpose of the pulse oximeter power-on self-test (POST)?

_____

_____

8. What type of site must be used for applying a pulse oximeter probe?

_____

_____

9. How can dark fingernail polish cause a falsely low SpO_2 reading?

_____

_____

10. How can patient movement cause an inaccurate SpO_2 reading?

_____

_____

11. What type of patient may make it difficult to properly align the oximeter probe?

_____

_____

12. List three conditions that can cause poor peripheral blood flow.

_____

_____

13. Why must a reusable oximeter probe be free of all dirt and grime before it is used?

_____

_____

Blood Pressure

Directions: Fill in each blank with the correct answer.

1. What does blood pressure measure?

_____

_____

2. Why is the diastolic pressure lower than the systolic pressure?

_____

_____

_____

3. What is considered normal blood pressure for an adult?

_____

4. State the blood pressure range for each of the following:

   a. Prehypertension: _____

   b. Hypertension, stage 1: _____

   c. Hypertension, stage 2: _____

5. Why should blood pressure readings always be interpreted using the patient's baseline blood pressure?

_____

_____

6. How does age affect blood pressure?

_____

7. How do diurnal variations affect the blood pressure?

_____

_____

8. What are the two types of stethoscope chest pieces and the use of each?

_____

_____

_____

_____

9. What are the parts of a sphygmomanometer?

_____

_____

10. List the two types of sphygmomanometers.

_____

11. When would each of the following cuffs be used to measure blood pressure?

   a. Child: _____

   b. Adult: _____

   c. Thigh: _____

12. Explain how to determine the proper cuff size for a patient.

_____

_____

13. What may occur if blood pressure is taken using a cuff that is too small or too large?

_____

_____

14. How should blood pressure be measured if the patient's arm circumference is greater than 50 cm (20 inches)?

_____

_____

_____

15. List the five phases included in the Korotkoff sounds, and describe what type of sound is heard during each phase.

_____

_____

_____

_____

_____

16. List five advantages of an automated blood pressure monitor.

_____

_____

_____

_____

_____

_____

CRITICAL THINKING ACTIVITIES

A. Measurement of Body Temperature

For each of the following situations involving the measurement of body temperature, write **C** if the technique is correct and **I** if the technique is incorrect. If the situation is correct, state the principle underlying the technique. If the situation is incorrect, explain what might happen if the technique were performed in the incorrect manner.

Electronic Thermometer

_____ 1. The medical assistant takes a patient's oral temperature immediately after the patient has consumed a cup of coffee.

_____

_____

_____ 2. The medical assistant instructs the patient not to talk while his or her oral temperature is being measured.

_____

_____

_____ 3. The medical assistant forgets to lubricate the rectal probe before taking a patient's rectal temperature.

_____

_____

_____ 4. An axillary temperature reading is recorded as follows: 102.2° F.

_____

_____

_____ 5. The medical assistant discards a used rectal probe in a regular waste container.

_____

_____

_____ 6. The medical assistant's bare fingers accidentally touch a used oral probe cover while discarding it.

_____

_____

Tympanic Membrane Thermometer

_____ 1. A tympanic membrane thermometer is used to take the temperature of a patient with impacted cerumen.

_____

_____

_____ 2. A thermometer with a dirty probe lens is used to take the patient's temperature.

_____

_____

_____ 3. The ear canal is straightened before taking a patient's aural temperature.

_____

_____

_____ 4. The medical assistant does not seal the opening of the ear canal with the probe when taking aural temperature.

_____

_____

_____ 5. The probe is positioned toward the opposite temple when taking aural temperature.

_____

_____

_____ 6. The medical assistant waits 30 seconds before taking the patient's temperature in the same ear.

_____

_____

Temporal Artery Thermometer

_____ 1. The medical assistant checks to make sure the probe lens is clean and intact before using a temporal artery thermometer.

_____

_____

_____ 2. The medical assistant brushes hair away from the patient's forehead before measuring the patient's temperature.

_____

_____

_____ 3. The medical assistant slides the temporal artery probe across the patient's forehead while continually depressing the scan button.

_____

_____

_____ 4. The medical assistant quickly scans the patient's forehead during temporal artery temperature measurement.

_____

_____

_____ 5. After scanning the forehead, the medical assistant records the patient's temporal artery temperature reading.

_____

_____

_____ 6. The medical assistant cleans the temporal artery thermometer by immersing it in warm, sudsy water.

_____

_____

B. Alterations in Body Temperature

Label the diagram below with the terms that describe the body temperature alteration.

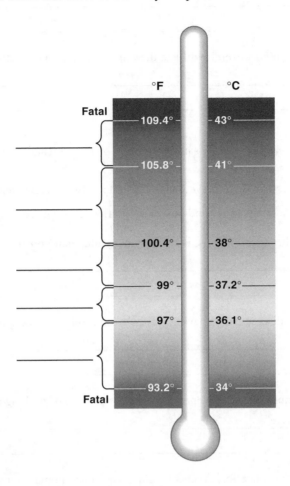

C. Pulse Sites

Locate the pulse at the following sites, and record the pulse rates below:

1. Brachial pulse _____

2. Temporal pulse _____

3. Carotid pulse _____

4. Femoral pulse _____

5. Popliteal pulse _____

6. Dorsalis pedis pulse _____

D. Pulse and Respiratory Rates

Take the pulse and respiration of a person before and after vigorous exercise, and record the results.

1. Before vigorous exercise

_____

_____

2. After vigorous exercise

_____

_____

3. Compare the results, and explain how exercise affects the pulse and respiratory rates.

_____

_____

E. Pulse Oximetry

Your physician asks you to measure the oxygen saturation level of the patients listed. For each situation, answer the following questions:

    a. What would you do in each situation to prevent an inaccurate pulse oximetry reading?

    b. What occurs with each of these situations and how does it affect the SpO_2 reading?

1. Kelly Collins, a patient with chronic bronchitis, is wearing navy blue nail polish.

_____

_____

2. Melvin Hosey has Parkinson's disease and is having difficulty controlling tremors in his hands.

_____

_____

3. Scott Kimes, a patient with emphysema, frequently experiences periods of prolonged coughing.

_____

_____

4. Nicole Lowe has returned to the office for a recheck of her viral pneumonia. You are getting ready to measure her oxygen saturation and notice that bright sunlight is coming through the window where she is seated and shining on her hand.

_____

_____

5. Rebecca Bensie, a patient on oxygen therapy, is morbidly obese, and you are having trouble properly aligning the oximeter probe on her finger.

_____

_____

6. Doug Habbershaw, a patient with peripheral vascular disease, has come to the office for a health checkup.

_____

_____

7. Emily Lacey has come to the office because she has been experiencing dyspnea. Her hands are very cold, and it is interfering with the pulse oximetry procedure.

_____

_____

8. Susan Boone, a patient with asthma, is wearing artificial fingernails.

_____

_____

9. Frank Stewart, a patient with congestive heart failure, is at the office to have a mole removed from his back. There are bright overhead lights in the room, and they cannot be turned off because the physician needs to have good lighting to perform the surgery.

_____

_____

10. Wanda Weaver is having a sebaceous cyst removed from her chest and has been sedated for the procedure. You have applied an automatic blood pressure cuff to her right arm. The physician asks you to apply an oximeter probe to continuously monitor her oxygen saturation level during the procedure.

_____

_____

11. Which control, indicator, or display is involved when the following occurs?

a. The oximeter is searching for a pulse. _____

b. The oximeter cannot find a pulse. _____

c. The oximeter is portraying the strength of the pulse. _____

d. The pulse is audibly broadcasted by a beeping sound. _____

e. The oximeter displays the oxygen saturation level. _____

f. The oximeter displays the pulse rate. _____

g. The battery is low. _____

h. You turn the oximeter off. _____

F. Blood Pressure Measurement

Using the principles outlined in the Procedure for Measuring Blood Pressure, explain what happens under the following circumstances:

1. The blood pressure is taken on a patient who has just undergone vigorous physical exercise.

_____

2. The blood pressure is taken on a patient with tight sleeves.

_____

_____

3. An adult cuff is used to measure blood pressure on a young child.

_____

_____

4. The rubber bladder is not centered over the brachial artery.

_____

_____

5. The cuff is placed ½ inch above the bend in the elbows.

_____

_____

6. The manometer is viewed from a distance of 4 feet.

_____

_____

G. Proper BP Cuff Selection

Measurements of the arm circumference (in cm) are given for various patients. Using Table 4-9 on page 156 of your textbook, indicate what size of blood pressure cuff (child, small adult, adult, large adult, or adult thigh) should be used with each of these patients.

1. 47 cm _____

2. 20 cm _____

3. 32 cm _____

4. 16 cm _____

5. 38 cm _____

6. 27 cm _____

7. 52 cm _____

8. 24 cm _____

Measure the arm circumference of four classmates with a cm tape measure, and record the values below. Next to each value, indicate what size blood pressure cuff should be used with each of these individuals.

1. _____

2. _____

3. _____

4. _____

H. Reading Blood Pressure Values

Read and record the following blood pressure measurements in the space provided.

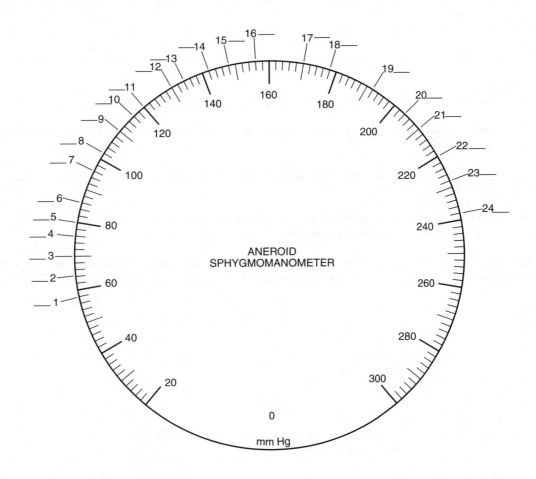

ANEROID SPHYGMOMANOMETER

I. Interpreting Blood Pressure Readings

Classify each of the following blood pressure readings into its appropriate category. The readings are based on the average of two or more properly measured, seated blood pressure readings taken at each of two or more visits.

Normal

Prehypertension

Hypertension: Stage 1

Hypertension: Stage 2

1. 90/66 _____

2. 126/76 _____

3. 146/88 _____

4. 120/88 _____

5. 120/80 _____

6. 158/102 _____

7. 134/82 _____

8. 180/106 _____

9. 104/60 _____

10. 148/94 _____

J. Hypertension

Create a profile of an individual who is at risk for hypertension following these guidelines:

1. Using colored pencils, crayons, or markers, draw a figure of an individual exhibiting risk factors for hypertension. Be as creative as possible.

2. Do not use any text in your drawing other than to label items you have drawn in your picture (e.g., cigarettes). A picture is worth a thousand words!

3. Include at least six risk factors for hypertension in your drawing. The Hypertension Patient Teaching Box in your textbook (page 153) can be used as a reference source.

4. In the classroom, choose a partner and trade drawings. Identify the risk factors for hypertension in your partner's drawing. Discuss with your partner what this person could do to lower his or her chances of developing hypertension.

K. Crossword Puzzle: Vital Signs

Directions: Complete the crossword puzzle using the clues presented below. All of your answers can be found in a box or a table in your textbook.

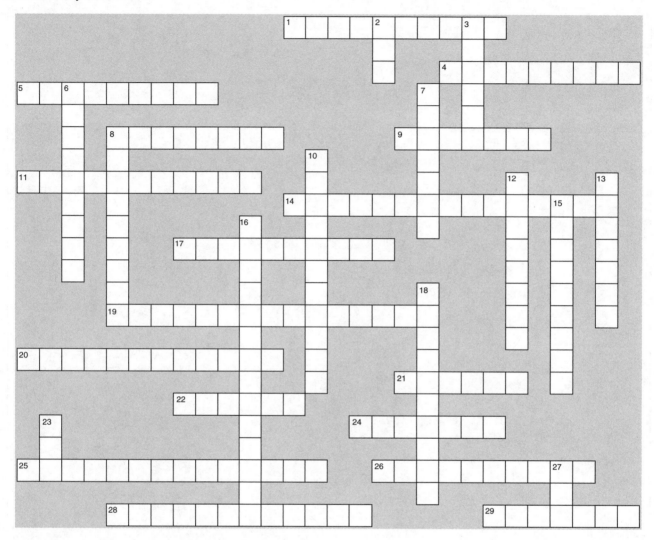

Across

1 Diaphragm or bell
4 Angled stethoscope earpieces
5 BP sounds
8 Has an S-shape
9 European temp measurement
11 Fever reducer
14 Fever increases this by 7%
17 U.S. temp measurement
19 Lowers pulse rate over time
20 Above 140/90
21 High BP might cause this
22 2400 mg or less per day
24 Asthma breath sounds
25 Center BP cuff over this
26 Risk factor for high BP
28 Cools body
29 Cracked earpieces can cause this

Down

2 Pulse range for exercising
3 Body temperature increaser
6 Fever that occurs with the flu
7 Invented the stethoscope
8 COPD example
10 Profuse perspiration
12 Do this after aerobic exercise
13 Leading cause of COPD
15 Fever causer
16 Drug to help COPD
18 BP position for patient's arm
23 220 minus your age
27 Good cholesterol

Name: _____

Directions:

a. Watch the indicated videos.

b. Mark each true statement with a T and each false statement with an F. For each false statement, change the wording of the question so that it becomes a true statement.

Video: Procedure 4-1: Measuring Oral Body Temperature with an Electronic Thermometer

_____ 1. The mouth has a rich blood supply under the tongue.

_____ 2. The temperature of the body varies depending on where the temperature is taken.

_____ 3. The oral probe of an electronic thermometer is red.

_____ 4. Hot and cold liquids change the temperature of the mouth resulting in an inaccurate temperature reading.

_____ 5. The probe cover prevents the transmission of microorganisms from one patient to another.

_____ 6. The patient should be instructed to keep the mouth closed during the procedure to keep out cooler air that may influence the reading.

_____ 7. The used probe cover must be discarded in a biohazard waste container.

Video: Procedure 4-2: Measuring Axillary Body Temperature with an Electronic Thermometer

_____ 1. The axillary site is used for mouth-breathing patients and those who have oral inflammation or have had oral surgery.

_____ 2. The axillary site is a good site to use to take the temperature of a toddler or preschooler.

_____ 3. The axillary temperature is approximately 1 degree higher than the same patient's oral temperature.

_____ 4. The probe of the thermometer should be placed in the center of the patient's axilla.

_____ 5. The arm should be held close to the body to prevent air currents from interfering with the reading.

_____ 6. The symbol ® should be charted next to the reading to tell the physician that this was an axillary temperature.

Video: Procedure 4-3: Measuring Rectal Body Temperature with an Electronic Thermometer

_____ 1. Rectal temperature can be taken on newborns.

_____ 2. The rectal area is a good site for measuring temperature because the rectum has a rich blood supply and it is a closed cavity.

_____ 3. Sterile gloves must be worn when measuring rectal temperature.

_____ 4. Older children and adults should be placed in the supine position for rectal temperature measurement.

_____ 5. Lubricant applied to the probe cover makes it easier to insert the probe into the rectum.

_____ 6. Never force insertion of the rectal thermometer probe to prevent damage to the rectal mucosa.

_____ 7. It is important to remove the probe from the rectum in the same direction in which it was inserted.

_____ 8. The used probe cover should be discarded in a regular waste container.

Video: Procedure 4-4: Measuring Aural Body Temperature

_____ 1. Aural temperature can be taken on a patient with an inflamed ear canal.

_____ 2. A normal amount of cerumen does not affect an aural temperature reading.

_____ 3. A tympanic membrane thermometer has a sensor that takes a picture of the infrared waves given off by the tympanic membrane.

_____ 4. An inaccurate aural temperature reading may occur if the patient has been lying on his or her ear.

_____ 5. Recent swimming or bathing does not affect an aural temperature reading.

_____ 6. A dirty or damaged tympanic thermometer lens can cause a falsely high reading.

_____ 7. If the lens is dirty, it should be gently cleaned with a water-based lubricant and wiped dry with a cotton swab.

_____ 8. The ear canal is straightened in adults and children older than 3 years by gently pulling the ear auricle upward and backward.

_____ 9. The tip of the probe should be pointed toward the opposite temple to allow the sensor to obtain a clear view of the tympanic membrane.

_____ 10. If the temperature appears to be too low, take the reading again, making sure to use proper technique.

_____ 11. Store the thermometer in its storage base to protect the lens from damage and dirt.

Video: Procedure 4-5: Measuring Temporal Body Temperature

_____ 1. The temporal artery runs across the forehead and down the side of the neck.

_____ 2. The temporal artery reading is about the same as the oral site.

_____ 3. The forehead needs to be fully exposed to the environment to obtain an accurate reading.

_____ 4. A dirty, damaged lens can lead to a falsely high temperature reading.

_____ 5. Hair covering the forehead traps body heat resulting in a falsely high temperature reading.

_____ 6. The probe should be positioned on the center of the patient's forehead, midway between the eyebrow and the hairline.

_____ 7. The scan button should be depressed the entire time you are scanning.

_____ 8. Quickly slide the probe in a straight line across the forehead until you reach the hairline.

_____ 9. The probe should be kept flat against the skin of the forehead while scanning.

_____ 10. Rapid beeping and blinking of the thermometer indicate that the temperature is rising.

_____ 11. Once you reach the hairline, lift the probe and gently place it behind the earlobe, keeping the scan button depressed.

_____ 12. If the temperature needs to be taken again, you must wait 10 seconds.

Video: Procedure 4-6: Measuring Radial Pulse and Respiration

_____ 1. The radial pulse is located on the inner aspect of the wrist, just below the thumb.

_____ 2. When measuring the pulse rate, you should also assess the rhythm and volume of the pulse.

_____ 3. The forearm should be positioned at heart level when measuring the pulse and respiration.

_____ 4. The index finger should not be used to measure pulse because it has a pulse of its own.

_____ 5. If you apply too much pressure when taking pulse, you may close off the artery and be unable to feel the pulse.

_____ 6. If the rhythm is irregular, you should measure the pulse for 5 minutes.

_____ 7. Inform the patient when you begin measuring the patient's respirations.

_____ 8. One complete respiration includes one inhalation and one exhalation.

_____ 9. The normal resting pulse rate for an adult ranges from 60 to 100 beats per minute.

_____ 10. The respiratory rate of a normal healthy adult ranges from 8 to 16 respirations per minute.

Video: Procedure 4-7: Measuring Apical Pulse

_____ 1. The apical pulse has a stronger beat and is easier to measure than the other pulse sites.

_____ 2. An apical pulse is usually measured on infants and children up to 3 years of age.

_____ 3. The apical pulse site is located in the fourth intercostal space at the junction of the left midclavicular line.

_____ 4. A diaphragm chest piece allows you to hear the sounds better when taking apical pulse.

_____ 5. Apical pulse can be measured with the patient in a sitting or lying down position.

_____ 6. To make it easier to hear the heartbeat, insert the earpieces in your ears with the earpieces directed slightly forward.

_____ 7. Each lubb-dupp sound represents one heartbeat.

Video: Procedure 4-8: Performing Pulse Oximetry

_____ 1. Pulse oximetry is used to measure the oxygen saturation level of the blood.

_____ 2. Pulse oximetry provides information on the amount of carbon dioxide that is being expelled from the body.

_____ 3. The oxygen saturation level of most healthy individuals falls between 85% and 99%.

_____ 4. An oxygen saturation level below 70% is life-threatening.

_____ 5. The patient should be seated comfortably with the lower arm firmly supported.

_____ 6. Dark fingernail polish will not interfere with the pulse oximetry reading.

_____ 7. The fleshy tip of the finger should cover the LED window, and the tip of the finger should touch the end of the probe stop.

_____ 8. The cable should be positioned so that it lies across the back of the hand and parallel to the arm.

_____ 9. To ensure an accurate reading, instruct the patient to remain still and breathe normally.

_____ 10. The pulse oximeter also measures the patient's blood pressure.

Video: Procedure 4-9: Measuring Blood Pressure

_____ 1. Several readings, taken on different occasions, provide a good index of an individual's baseline blood pressure.

_____ 2. Blood pressure is a measurement of the number of times the heart beats each minute.

_____ 3. The phase in the cardiac cycle that represents the highest point of blood pressure in the body is known as the diastolic pressure.

_____ 4. The standard unit for measuring blood pressure is millimeters of mercury.

_____ 5. The first sound that is heard is phase I of the Korotkoff sounds and is recorded as the systolic pressure.

_____ 6. The last sound you hear is known as phase V of the Korotkoff sounds and is recorded as the diastolic pressure.

_____ 7. Signs that may influence the blood pressure reading include fear, pain, and recent physical activity.

_____ 8. A sleeve that is too tight has no effect on the blood pressure reading.

_____ 9. A cuff that is too small may cause the blood pressure reading to be falsely low.

_____ 10. The brachial artery is located near the center of the antecubital space, but slightly to the little-finger side of the arm.

_____ 11. The bladder of the cuff should be centered over the brachial pulse site.

_____ 12. The cuff should be positioned so that the lower edge is about 4 inches above the bend in the elbow.

_____ 13. Good contact of the diaphragm with the skin makes it easier to hear the Korotkoff sounds.

_____ 14. The pressure in the cuff should be released at a steady rate of 2 to 3 mm per second.

_____ 15. If you do not obtain an accurate measurement, wait 30 seconds before making another attempt on the same arm.

Measuring Body Temperature

Measure body temperature with each of the following types of thermometers, and record results in the chart provided.

Procedures 4-1, 4-2, and 4-3: Electronic Thermometer (Oral, Axillary, and Rectal)

Procedure 4-4: Tympanic Membrane Thermometer (Aural)

Procedure 4-5: Temporal Artery Thermometer

CHART	
Date	

Measuring Pulse, Respiration, and Oxygen Saturation

Procedure 4-6: Pulse and Respiration. Measure the radial pulse and respiration. Describe the rhythm and volume of the pulse. Describe the rhythm and depth of the respirations. Record the results in the chart provided.

Procedure 4-7: Apical Pulse. Measure the apical pulse. Describe the rhythm and volume of the pulse. Record the results in the chart provided.

Procedure 4-8: Pulse Oximetry. Measure the oxygen saturation level and record the results in the chart provided.

Measuring Blood Pressure

Procedure 4-9: Blood Pressure. Measure blood pressure. Record the results in the chart provided.

CHART	
Date	

Procedure 4-1: Measuring Oral Body Temperature with an Electronic Thermometer

Name: _____   Date: _____

Evaluated by: _____   Score: _____

Performance Objective

Outcome:	Measure oral body temperature.
Conditions:	Given the following: electronic thermometer and oral probe, probe cover, and a waste container.
Standards:	Time: 5 minutes. Student completed procedure in _____ minutes.
	Accuracy: Satisfactory score on the Performance Evaluation Checklist.

Performance Evaluation Checklist

Trial 1	Trial 2	Point Value	Performance Standards
		•	Sanitized hands.
		•	Assembled equipment.
		•	Removed thermometer from its storage base.
		•	Attached oral probe to thermometer unit.
		•	Inserted probe into the thermometer.
		•	Greeted the patient and introduced yourself.
		•	Identified the patient and explained the procedure.
		•	Asked the patient whether he or she has ingested hot or cold beverages.
		▷	Explained what to do if the patient has recently ingested a hot or cold beverage.
		•	Removed probe from the thermometer.
		▷	Explained what occurs when probe is removed from the thermometer.
		•	Attached probe cover to probe.
		▷	Stated the purpose of the probe cover.
		•	Correctly inserted the probe in patient's mouth.
		•	Instructed the patient to keep the mouth closed.
		▷	Explained why the mouth should be kept closed.
		•	Held probe in place until an audible tone was heard.
		•	Noted patient's temperature reading on display screen.
		•	Removed probe from patient's mouth.
		•	Discarded probe cover in a regular waste container.
		•	Did not allow fingers to come in contact with cover.
		•	Returned probe to the thermometer unit.
		▷	Stated what occurs when probe is returned to the thermometer.

149

Trial 1	Trial 2	Point Value	Performance Standards
		•	Returned the thermometer unit to its storage base.
		•	Sanitized hands.
		•	Charted the results correctly.
		✷	The temperature recording was identical to the reading on the display screen.
		▷	Stated the normal body temperature range for an adult (97° F to 99° F).
		✷	Completed the procedure within 5 minutes.
			Totals

CHART	
Date	

Evaluation of Student Performance

EVALUATION CRITERIA			COMMENTS
Symbol	**Category**	**Point Value**	
✷	Critical Step	16 points	
•	Essential Step	6 points	
▷	Theory Question	2 points	

Score calculation: 100 points

−   _____ points missed

_____ Score

Satisfactory score: 85 or above

CAAHEP Competencies Achieved

Psychomotor (Skills)

☑ I. 1. Obtain vital signs.

Affective (Behavior)

☑ I. 1. Apply critical thinking skills in performing patient assessment and care.

ABHES Competencies Achieved

☑ 9. c. Take vital signs.

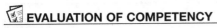

EVALUATION OF COMPETENCY

Procedure 4-2: Measuring Axillary Body Temperature with an Electronic Thermometer

Name: _____   Date: _____

Evaluated by: _____   Score: _____

Performance Objective

Outcome:	Measure axillary body temperature.
Conditions:	Given the following: electronic thermometer and oral probe, probe cover, and a waste container
Standards:	Time: 5 minutes. Student completed procedure in _____ minutes.
	Accuracy: Satisfactory score on the Performance Evaluation Checklist.

Performance Evaluation Checklist

Trial 1	Trial 2	Point Value	Performance Standards
		•	Sanitized hands.
		•	Assembled equipment.
		•	Removed thermometer from its storage base.
		•	Attached oral probe to thermometer unit.
		•	Inserted probe into the thermometer.
		•	Greeted the patient and introduced yourself.
		•	Identified the patient and explained the procedure.
		•	Removed clothing from patient's shoulder and arm.
		•	Made sure that the axilla was dry.
		•	Removed probe from the thermometer.
		•	Attached probe cover to probe.
		•	Placed probe in the center of the patient's axilla.
		•	Ensured that the arm was held close to the body.
		▷	Explained why the arm must be held close to the body.
		•	Held probe in place until an audible tone was heard.
		•	Removed probe from patient's axilla.
		•	Noted patient's temperature reading on display screen.
		•	Discarded probe cover in a regular waste container.
		•	Did not allow fingers to come in contact with cover.
		•	Returned probe to the thermometer unit.
		•	Returned the thermometer unit to its storage base.
		•	Sanitized hands.
		•	Charted the results correctly.

151

Trial 1	Trial 2	Point Value	Performance Standards
		*	Temperature recording was identical to the reading on the display screen.
		*	Completed the procedure within 5 minutes.
			Totals

CHART	
Date	

Evaluation of Student Performance

EVALUATION CRITERIA			COMMENTS
Symbol	**Category**	**Point Value**	
*	Critical Step	16 points	
•	Essential Step	6 points	
▷	Theory Question	2 points	

Score calculation:　　100 points

　　　　　−＿＿＿＿ points missed
　　　　　＿＿＿＿ Score

Satisfactory score: 85 or above

CAAHEP Competencies Achieved

Psychomotor (Skills)

☑ I. 1. Obtain vital signs.

Affective (Behavior)

☑ I. 1. Apply critical thinking skills in performing patient assessment and care.

ABHES Competencies Achieved

☑ 9. c. Take vital signs.

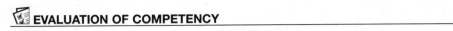

Procedure 4-3: Measuring Rectal Body Temperature with an Electronic Thermometer

Name: _____   Date: _____

Evaluated by: _____   Score: _____

Performance Objective

Outcome:	Measure rectal body temperature.
Conditions:	Given the following: electronic thermometer, rectal probe, probe cover, lubricant, disposable gloves, tissues, and a waste container.
Standards:	Time: 5 minutes. Student completed procedure in _____ minutes.
	Accuracy: Satisfactory score on the Performance Evaluation Checklist.

Performance Evaluation Checklist

Trial 1	Trial 2	Point Value	Performance Standards
		•	Sanitized hands.
		•	Assembled equipment.
		•	Removed thermometer from its storage base.
		•	Attached rectal probe to thermometer unit.
		•	Inserted probe into the thermometer.
		•	Greeted the patient and introduced yourself.
		•	Identified the patient and explained the procedure.
		•	Applied gloves.
		▷	Stated the reason for applying gloves.
		•	Positioned and draped the patient.
		▷	Explained how to position an adult and an infant.
		•	Removed probe from the thermometer.
		•	Attached probe cover to probe.
		•	Applied lubricant up to a level of 1 inch.
		▷	Stated the purpose of the lubricant.
		•	Instructed patient to lie still.
		•	Separated the buttocks and properly inserted the thermometer.
		▷	Stated how far the thermometer should be inserted for adults, children, and infants.
		•	Held probe in place until an audible tone was heard.
		•	Removed the probe in the same direction as it was inserted.
		•	Noted patient's temperature reading on display screen.
		•	Discarded probe cover in a regular waste container.
		▷	Explained why the cover can be discarded in a regular waste container.
		•	Returned probe to the thermometer unit.

Trial 1	Trial 2	Point Value	Performance Standards
		•	Returned the thermometer unit to its storage base.
		•	Wiped the anal area with tissues.
		•	Removed gloves and sanitized hands.
		•	Charted the results correctly.
		✳	The temperature recording was identical to the reading on the display screen.
		✳	Completed the procedure within 5 minutes.
			Totals

CHART	
Date	

Evaluation of Student Performance

EVALUATION CRITERIA			COMMENTS
Symbol	**Category**	**Point Value**	
✳	Critical Step	16 points	
•	Essential Step	6 points	
▷	Theory Question	2 points	

Score calculation: 100 points

− _____ points missed

_____ Score

Satisfactory score: 85 or above

CAAHEP Competencies Achieved

Psychomotor (Skills)

☑ I. 1. Obtain vital signs.

Affective (Behavior)

☑ I. 1. Apply critical thinking skills in performing patient assessment and care.

ABHES Competencies Achieved

☑ 9. c. Take vital signs.

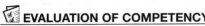

EVALUATION OF COMPETENCY

Procedure 4-4: Measuring Aural Body Temperature with a Tympanic Membrane Thermometer

Name: _____ Date: _____

Evaluated by: _____ Score: _____

Performance Objective

Outcome:	Measure aural body temperature.
Conditions:	Given the following: tympanic membrane thermometer, probe cover, and a waste container.
Standards:	Time: 5 minutes. Student completed procedure in _____ minutes.
	Accuracy: Satisfactory score on the Performance Evaluation Checklist.

Performance Evaluation Checklist

Trial 1	Trial 2	Point Value	Performance Standards
		•	Sanitized hands.
		•	Assembled equipment.
		•	Greeted the patient and introduced yourself.
		•	Identified the patient and explained the procedure.
		•	Removed thermometer from its storage base.
		•	Checked to make sure the probe lens was clean and intact.
		▷	Stated what might occur if the lens was dirty.
		•	Attached a cover on the probe.
		▷	Explained the purpose of the probe cover.
		•	Observed the screen to determine whether the thermometer is ready to use.
		•	Held the thermometer in the dominant hand.
		•	Straightened the patient's ear canal with the nondominant hand.
		▷	Explained the purpose of straightening the ear canal.
		•	Inserted the probe into the patient's ear canal and sealed the opening without causing the patient discomfort.
		•	Pointed the tip of the probe toward the opposite temple.
		▷	Stated the reason for pointing the probe toward the opposite temple.
		•	Asked the patient to remain still.
		•	Depressed the activation button for 1 full second or until an audible tone is heard.
		•	Removed the thermometer from the ear canal and noted the patient's temperature on the display screen.
		▷	Stated what should be done if the temperature seems too low.
		•	Disposed of the probe cover in a waste container.
		•	Replaced the thermometer in its storage base.
		▷	Explained the reason for storing the thermometer in its base.

Trial 1	Trial 2	Point Value	Performance Standards
		•	Sanitized hands.
		•	Charted the results correctly.
		✳	The temperature recording was identical to the reading on the display screen.
		✳	Completed the procedure within 5 minutes.
			Totals
CHART			
Date			

Evaluation of Student Performance

EVALUATION CRITERIA			COMMENTS
Symbol	**Category**	**Point Value**	
✳	Critical Step	16 points	
•	Essential Step	6 points	
▷	Theory Question	2 points	

Score calculation: 100 points

      −_____ points missed

      _____ Score

Satisfactory score: 85 or above

CAAHEP Competencies Achieved

Psychomotor (Skills)

☑ I. 1. Obtain vital signs.

Affective (Behavior)

☑ I. 1. Apply critical thinking skills in performing patient assessment and care.

ABHES Competencies Achieved

☑ 9. c. Take vital signs.

EVALUATION OF COMPETENCY

Procedure 4-5: Measuring Temporal Body Temperature

Name: _____   Date: _____

Evaluated by: _____   Score: _____

Performance Objective

Outcome:	Measure temporal body temperature.
Conditions:	Given the following: temporal artery thermometer, disposable probe cover, antiseptic wipe, waste container.
Standards:	Time: 5 minutes. Student completed procedure in _____ minutes.
	Accuracy: Satisfactory score on the Performance Evaluation Checklist.

Performance Evaluation Checklist

Trial 1	Trial 2	Point Value	Performance Standards
		•	Sanitized the hands and assembled equipment.
		•	Greeted the patient and introduced yourself.
		•	Identified the patient and explained the procedure.
		•	Checked to make sure the probe lens is clean and intact.
		▷	Stated why the lens should be clean.
		•	Placed a disposable cover onto the probe or cleaned the probe with an antiseptic wipe and allowed it to dry.
		•	Selected an appropriate site (right or left side of the forehead).
		•	Brushed away any hair that was covering the scanning sites.
		▷	Explained why hair must be brushed away.
		•	Held the thermometer in the dominant hand with the thumb on the scan button.
		•	Gently positioned the probe of the thermometer on the center of the patient's forehead midway between the eyebrow and hairline.
		•	Depressed the scan button and kept it depressed for the entire measurement.
		▷	Stated why the scan button must be continually depressed.
		•	Slowly and gently slid the probe straight across the forehead midway between the eyebrow and the upper hairline.
		•	Continued until the hairline was reached, making sure to keep the probe flush against the forehead.
		•	Keeping the button depressed, lifted the probe from the forehead and placed it behind the earlobe for 1 to 2 seconds.
		▷	Stated why the probe is placed behind the earlobe.
		•	Released the scan button and noted the temperature on the display screen.
		•	Disposed of the probe cover in a regular waste container.
		•	Wiped the probe with an antiseptic wipe and allowed it to dry.

Trial 1	Trial 2	Point Value	Performance Standards
		•	Sanitized hands.
		•	Charted the results correctly.
		✱	The temperature recording was identical to the reading on the display screen.
		•	Stored the thermometer in a clean, dry area.
		✱	Completed the procedure within 5 minutes.
			Totals

CHART

Date	

Evaluation of Student Performance

EVALUATION CRITERIA			COMMENTS
Symbol	**Category**	**Point Value**	
✱	Critical Step	16 points	
•	Essential Step	6 points	
▷	Theory Question	2 points	

Score calculation: 100 points

− _____ points missed

_____ Score

Satisfactory score: 85 or above

CAAHEP Competencies Achieved

Psychomotor (Skills)

☑ I. 1. Obtain vital signs.

Affective (Behavior)

☑ I. 1. Apply critical thinking skills in performing patient assessment and care.

ABHES Competencies Achieved

☑ 9. c. Take vital signs.

Procedure 4-6: Measuring Pulse and Respiration

Name: _____   Date: _____

Evaluated by: _____   Score: _____

Performance Objective

Outcome:	Measure radial pulse and respiration.
Conditions:	Using a watch with a second hand.
Standards:	Time: 5 minutes. Student completed procedure in _____ minutes.
	Accuracy: Satisfactory score on the Performance Evaluation Checklist.

Performance Evaluation Checklist

Trial 1	Trial 2	Point Value	Performance Standards
		•	Sanitized hands.
		•	Greeted the patient and introduced yourself.
		•	Identified the patient and explained the procedure.
		•	Observed patient for any signs that might affect the pulse rate or respiratory rate.
		▷	Stated two factors that would increase the pulse rate.
		•	Positioned the patient in a comfortable seated position.
		•	Placed three middle fingertips over the radial pulse site.
		▷	Explained why the pulse should not be taken with the thumb.
		•	Applied moderate, gentle pressure until the pulse was felt.
		▷	Stated what will occur if too much pressure is applied over the radial artery.
		•	Counted the pulse for 30 seconds and made a mental note of the number.
		•	Determined the rhythm and volume of the pulse.
		▷	Stated when the pulse should be measured for a full minute.
		•	Continued to hold the fingers on the patient's wrist.
		▷	Explained why respirations should be taken without the patient's awareness.
		•	Observed the rise and fall of patient's chest.
		•	Counted the number of respirations for 30 seconds and made a mental note of the number.
		▷	Stated what makes up one respiration.
		•	Determined the rhythm and depth of the respirations.
		•	Observed the patient's color.
		•	Sanitized hands.
		•	Multiplied the pulse and respiration values by 2.
		•	Charted the results correctly.
		✶	The pulse rate was within ±2 beats of the evaluator's reading.

Trial 1	Trial 2	Point Value	Performance Standards
		∗	The respiratory rate was within 1 respiration of the evaluator's measurement.
		▷	Stated the normal adult range for the pulse rate (60 to 100 beats/min).
		▷	Stated the normal adult range for the respiratory rate (12 to 20 respirations/min).
		∗	Completed the procedure within 5 minutes.
			Totals

CHART	
Date	

Evaluation of Student Performance

EVALUATION CRITERIA			COMMENTS
Symbol	**Category**	**Point Value**	
∗	Critical Step	16 points	
•	Essential Step	6 points	
▷	Theory Question	2 points	

Score calculation: 100 points

− _____ points missed

_____ Score

Satisfactory score: 85 or above

CAAHEP Competencies Achieved

Psychomotor (Skills)

☑ I. 1. Obtain vital signs.

Affective (Behavior)

☑ I. 1. Apply critical thinking skills in performing patient assessment and care.

ABHES Competencies Achieved

☑ 9. c. Take vital signs.

160

Chapter **4** Vital Signs

Procedure 4-7: Measuring Apical Pulse

Name: _____   Date: _____

Evaluated by: _____   Score: _____

Performance Objective

Outcome:	Measure apical pulse.
Conditions:	Given the following: stethoscope and antiseptic wipe.
Standards:	Using a watch with a second hand.
	Time: 5 minutes. Student completed procedure in _____ minutes.
	Accuracy: Satisfactory score on the Performance Evaluation Checklist.

Performance Evaluation Checklist

Trial 1	Trial 2	Point Value	Performance Standards
		•	Sanitized hands.
		•	Greeted the patient and introduced yourself.
		•	Identified the patient and explained the procedure.
		•	Observed the patient for any signs that might affect the pulse rate.
		•	Assembled equipment.
		•	Rotated the chest piece to the bell position.
		•	Cleaned earpieces and chest piece with antiseptic wipe.
		▷	Stated the reason for cleaning stethoscope with an antiseptic.
		•	Asked the patient to unbutton or remove his or her shirt.
		•	Positioned patient in a sitting or lying position.
		•	Warmed chest piece of the stethoscope.
		▷	Explained the reason for warming chest piece.
		•	Inserted earpieces of stethoscope in a forward position in the ears.
		▷	Explained why the earpieces must be directed forward.
		•	Placed the chest piece over the apex of the heart.
		▷	Described the location of the apex of the heart.
		•	Counted the number of heartbeats for 30 seconds and multiplied by 2.
		✱	The reading was within ±2 beats of the evaluator's reading.
		•	Sanitized hands.
		•	Charted the results correctly.
		•	Cleaned earpieces and chest piece with an antiseptic wipe.
		✱	Completed the procedure within 5 minutes.
			Totals

CHART	
Date	

Evaluation of Student Performance

EVALUATION CRITERIA			COMMENTS
Symbol	**Category**	**Point Value**	
✳	Critical Step	16 points	
•	Essential Step	6 points	
▷	Theory Question	2 points	

Score calculation: 100 points

$$-\ \underline{\qquad}\ \text{points missed}$$

$\underline{\qquad}$ Score

Satisfactory score: 85 or above

CAAHEP Competencies Achieved

Psychomotor (Skills)

☑ I. 1. Obtain vital signs.

Affective (Behavior)

☑ I. 1. Apply critical thinking skills in performing patient assessment and care.

ABHES Competencies Achieved

☑ 9. c. Take vital signs.

Procedure 4-8: Performing Pulse Oximetry

Name: _____   Date: _____

Evaluated by: _____   Score: _____

Performance Objective

Outcome:	Perform pulse oximetry.
Conditions:	Given the following: handheld pulse oximeter, reusable finger probe, and an antiseptic wipe.
Standards:	Time: 5 minutes. Student completed procedure in _____ minutes.
	Accuracy: Satisfactory score on the Performance Evaluation Checklist.

Performance Evaluation Checklist

Trial 1	Trial 2	Point Value	Performance Standards
		•	Sanitized hands and assembled equipment.
		•	Ensured the probe opened and closed smoothly and that the windows were clean.
		•	Disinfected the probe windows and platforms and allowed them to dry.
		▷	Stated the purpose of disinfecting the probe windows.
		•	If necessary, connected the probe to the cable.
		•	Connected the cable to the monitor.
		•	Did not lift or carry the monitor by the cable.
		•	Greeted the patient and introduced yourself.
		•	Identified the patient and explained the procedure.
		•	Seated the patient in a chair with the lower arm supported and the palm facing down.
		▷	Explained why the arm should be supported.
		•	Selected an appropriate finger to apply the probe.
		•	Observed the patient's finger to make sure it is free of dark fingernail polish or an artificial nail.
		•	Checked to make sure the patient's fingertip is clean.
		•	Checked to make sure the patient's finger is not cold.
		▷	Explained what to do if the patient's finger is cold
		•	Made sure that ambient light will not interfere with the measurement.
		▷	Explained why ambient light should be avoided.
		•	Positioned the probe securely on the fingertip with the fleshy tip of the finger covering the window.
		•	Allowed the cable to lie across the back of the hand and parallel to the arm of the patient.
		•	Instructed the patient to remain still and to breathe normally.
		▷	Stated why the patient must remain still.

Trial 1	Trial 2	Point Value	Performance Standards
		•	Turned on the pulse oximeter.
		•	Waited while the oximeter went through its power-on self-test (POST).
		▷	Explained the purpose of the POST.
		•	Allowed several seconds for the oximeter to detect the pulse and calculate the oxygen saturation.
		•	Ensured that the pulse strength indicator fluctuates with each pulsation and that the pulse signal is strong.
		▷	Stated what should be done if the oximeter is unable to locate a pulse.
		•	Left the probe in place until the oximeter displayed a reading.
		•	Noted the oxygen saturation value and pulse rate.
		✳	The reading was identical to the evaluator's reading.
		▷	Stated the normal oxygen saturation level of a healthy adult (95% to 99%).
		▷	Stated what should be done if the oxygen saturation level is less than 95%.
		•	Removed the probe from the patient's finger and turned off the oximeter.
		•	Sanitized hands.
		•	Charted the results correctly.
		•	Disconnected the cable from the monitor.
		•	Disinfected the probe with an antiseptic wipe.
		•	Properly stored the monitor in a clean dry area.
		✳	Completed the procedure within 5 minutes.
			Totals
CHART			
Date			

Evaluation of Student Performance

EVALUATION CRITERIA			COMMENTS
Symbol	Category	Point Value	
✳	Critical Step	16 points	
•	Essential Step	6 points	
▷	Theory Question	2 points	

Score calculation: 100 points

− _____ points missed

_____ Score

Satisfactory score: 85 or above

CAAHEP Competencies Achieved
Psychomotor (Skills)
☑ I. 1. Obtain vital signs.
Affective (Behavior)
☑ I. 1. Apply critical thinking skills in performing patient assessment and care.

ABHES Competencies Achieved
☑ 9. c. Take vital signs.

Notes

Procedure 4-9: Measuring Blood Pressure

Name: _____   Date: _____

Evaluated by: _____   Score: _____

Performance Objective

Outcome:	Measure blood pressure.
Conditions:	Given the following: stethoscope, sphygmomanometer, and an antiseptic wipe.
Standards:	Time: 5 minutes.　　Student completed procedure in _____ minutes.
	Accuracy: Satisfactory score on the Performance Evaluation Checklist.

Performance Evaluation Checklist

Trial 1	Trial 2	Point Value	Performance Standards
		•	Sanitized hands.
		•	Assembled equipment.
		•	Rotated the chest piece to the diaphragm position.
		•	Cleaned earpieces and chest piece of stethoscope with an antiseptic wipe.
		•	Greeted the patient and introduced yourself.
		•	Identified the patient and explained the procedure.
		•	Observed patient for any signs that might influence the blood pressure reading.
		▷	Stated signs that would influence the blood pressure reading.
		•	Determined how high to pump the cuff (palpated systolic pressure or checking the patient's chart).
		•	Positioned patient in a sitting position with the legs uncrossed.
		•	Made sure that the patient's arm was uncovered.
		▷	Explained why blood pressure should not be taken over clothing.
		•	Positioned patient's arm at heart level with the palm facing up.
		•	Selected the proper cuff size.
		▷	Explained how to determine the proper cuff size.
		•	Located the brachial pulse with the fingertips.
		▷	Stated the location of the brachial pulse.
		•	Centered bladder over the brachial pulse site.
		▷	Explained why the bladder should be centered over the brachial pulse site.
		•	Placed cuff on patient's arm 1 to 2 inches above bend in elbow.
		•	Wrapped cuff smoothly and snugly around patient's arm and secured it.
		•	Positioned self and/or manometer for direct viewing and at a distance of no more than 3 feet.
		•	Instructed the patient not to talk.

Trial 1	Trial 2	Point Value	Performance Standards
		•	Inserted earpieces of stethoscope in a forward position in the ears.
		•	Located the brachial pulse again.
		•	Placed diaphragm of the stethoscope over the brachial pulse site to make a tight seal.
		▷	Explained why there should be good contact of the chest piece with the skin.
		•	Made sure chest piece was not touching cuff.
		▷	Explained why the chest piece should not touch the cuff.
		•	Closed valve on bulb by turning thumbscrew to the right.
		•	Rapidly pumped air into cuff up to a level of approximately 30 mm Hg above the palpated or previously measured systolic pressure.
		•	Released pressure at a moderate, steady rate by turning thumbscrew to the left.
		•	Heard and noted the first clear tapping sound (systolic pressure).
		•	Continued to deflate the cuff for another 10 mm Hg.
		•	Heard and noted the point on the scale at which the sounds ceased (diastolic pressure).
		•	Quickly and completely deflated cuff to zero and removed earpieces from ears.
		▷	Stated how long to wait before taking the blood pressure again on the same arm.
		•	Carefully removed cuff from patient's arm.
		•	Sanitized hands.
		•	Charted the results correctly.
		✶	The reading was within ±2 mm Hg of the evaluator's reading.
		▷	Stated the normal blood pressure for an adult (less than 120/80 mm Hg).
		•	Cleaned earpieces and chest piece with an antiseptic wipe.
		✶	Completed the procedure within 5 minutes.
			Totals
CHART			
Date			

Evaluation of Student Performance

EVALUATION CRITERIA			COMMENTS
Symbol	**Category**	**Point Value**	
✷	Critical Step	16 points	
•	Essential Step	6 points	
▷	Theory Question	2 points	

Score calculation: 100 points

− _____ points missed

_____ Score

Satisfactory score: 85 or above

CAAHEP Competencies Achieved

Psychomotor (Skills)

☑ I. 1. Obtain vital signs.

Affective (Behavior)

☑ I. 1. Apply critical thinking skills in performing patient assessment and care.

ABHES Competencies Achieved

☑ 9. c. Take vital signs.

Notes

5 The Physical Examination

CHAPTER ASSIGNMENTS

√ After Completing	Date Due	Textbook Pages	TEXTBOOK ASSIGNMENTS	Possible Points	Points You Earned
		172–212	Read Chapter 5: The Physical Examination		
		177 209	Read Case Study 1 Case Study 1 questions	5	
		178 209	Read Case Study 2 Case Study 2 questions	5	
		206 178–179	Read Case Study 3 Case Study 3 questions	5	
			Total points		

√ After Completing	Date Due	Study Guide Pages	STUDY GUIDE ASSIGNMENTS (CTA = Critical Thinking Activity)	Possible Points	Points You Earned
		175	Pretest	10	
		176 176	Term Key Term Assessment A. Definitions B. Word Parts (Add 1 point for each medical term)	17 9	
		177–180	Evaluation of Learning questions	31	
		180	CTA A: Preparation of the Examining Room	10	
		181	CTA B: Reading Weight Measurements	15	
			Evolve Site: Chapter 5 By the Pound: Measuring Weight (Record points earned)		
		182	CTA C: Reading Height Measurements	11	
			Evolve Site: Chapter 5 Feet and Inches: Measuring Height (Record points earned)		
		183	CTA D: Calculating BMI	12	
		183–184	CTA E: Patient Positions	10	
			Evolve Site: Chapter 5 Let's Get Physical (Record points earned)		
		184	CTA F: Examination Techniques	10	

171

√ After Completing	Date Due	Study Guide Pages	STUDY GUIDE ASSIGNMENTS (CTA = Critical Thinking Activity)	Possible Points	Points You Earned
		185	CTA G: Crossword Puzzle	25	
			e Evolve Site: Chapter 5 Nutrition Nugget: Cultural Foods	10	
			e Evolve Site: Apply Your Knowledge questions	10	
		187–189	*e* Video Evaluation	54	
		175	Posttest	10	
			ADDITIONAL ASSIGNMENTS		
			Total points		

√ When Assigned by Your Instructor	Study Guide Pages	Practices Required	LABORATORY ASSIGNMENTS (Procedure Number and Name)	Score*
	191–192	5	Practice for Competency 5-1: Measuring Weight and Height Textbook reference: pp. 182–184	
	193–195		Evaluation of Competency 5-1: Measuring Weight and Height	*
	191–192	3	Practice for Competency 5-A: Body Mechanics Textbook reference: pp. 185–187	
	197–199		Evaluation of Competency 5-A: Body Mechanics	*
	191–192	3	Practice for Competency 5-2: Sitting Position Textbook reference: p. 188	
	201–202		Evaluation of Competency 5-2: Sitting Position	*
	191–192	3	Practice for Competency 5-3: Supine Position Textbook reference: p. 189	
	203–204		Evaluation of Competency 5-3: Supine Position	*
	191–192	3	Practice for Competency 5-4: Prone Position Textbook reference: p. 190	
	205–206		Evaluation of Competency 5-4: Prone Position	*
	191–192	3	Practice for Competency 5-5: Dorsal Recumbent Position Textbook reference: p. 191	
	207–208		Evaluation of Competency 5-5: Dorsal Recumbent Position	*
	191–192	3	Practice for Competency 5-6: Lithotomy Position Textbook reference: pp. 192–193	
	209–211		Evaluation of Competency 5-6: Lithotomy Position	*

√ When Assigned by Your Instructor	Study Guide Pages	Practices Required	LABORATORY ASSIGNMENTS (Procedure Number and Name)	Score*
	191–192	3	Practice for Competency 5-7: Sims Position Textbook reference: pp. 193–194	
	213–214		Evaluation of Competency 5-7: Sims' Position	*
	191–192	3	Practice for Competency 5-8: Knee-Chest Position Textbook reference: pp. 194–195	
	215–216		Evaluation of Competency 5-8: Knee-Chest Position	*
	191–192	3	Practice for Competency 5-9: Fowler's Position Textbook reference: pp. 195–196	
	217–218		Evaluation of Competency 5-9: Fowler's Position	*
	191–192	3	Practice for Competency 5-10: Wheelchair Transfer Textbook reference: pp. 197–200	
	219–221		Evaluation of Competency 5-10: Wheelchair Transfer	*
	191–192	3	Practice for Competency 5-11: Assisting with the Physical Examination Textbook reference: pp. 206–208	
	223–226		Evaluation of Competency 5-11: Assisting with the Physical Examination	*
			ADDITIONAL ASSIGNMENTS	

⁇ PRETEST

True or False

_____ 1. A complete patient examination consists of a physical examination and laboratory tests.

_____ 2. Arthritis is an example of a chronic illness.

_____ 3. An otoscope is used to examine the eyes.

_____ 4. A patient should be identified by name and date of birth.

_____ 5. The reason for weighing a prenatal patient is to determine the baby's due date.

_____ 6. The height of an adult is measured during every office visit.

_____ 7. The lithotomy position is used to examine the vagina.

_____ 8. Inspection involves the observation of the patient for any signs of disease.

_____ 9. Measuring blood pressure is an example of auscultation.

_____ 10. The supine position is used to examine the back.

⁇ POSTTEST

True or False

_____ 1. The prognosis is what is wrong with the patient.

_____ 2. A risk factor means that a patient will develop a certain disease.

_____ 3. Electrocardiography is an example of a therapeutic procedure.

_____ 4. The function of a speculum is to open a body orifice for viewing.

_____ 5. The process of measuring the patient is called mensuration.

_____ 6. A reason for weighing a child is to determine drug dosage.

_____ 7. The purpose of draping a patient is to make it easier for the physician to examine the patient.

_____ 8. Sims' position is used for flexible sigmoidoscopy.

_____ 9. Measuring pulse is an example of percussion.

_____ 10. BMI is the acronym for *body mass index*.

A. Definitions

Directions: Match each medical term (numbers) with its definition (letters).

_____ 1. Audiometer

_____ 2. Auscultation

_____ 3. Bariatrics

_____ 4. Body mechanics

_____ 5. Clinical diagnosis

_____ 6. Diagnosis

_____ 7. Differential diagnosis

_____ 8. Inspection

_____ 9. Mensuration

_____ 10. Ophthalmoscope

_____ 11. Otoscope

_____ 12. Palpation

_____ 13. Percussion

_____ 14. Percussion hammer

_____ 15. Prognosis

_____ 16. Speculum

_____ 17. Symptom

A. An instrument for examining the interior of the eye

B. A tentative diagnosis obtained through the evaluation of the health history and the physical examination, without the benefit of laboratory or diagnostic tests

C. An instrument for opening a body orifice or cavity for viewing

D. An instrument used to measure hearing

E. The process of measuring a patient

F. The scientific method for determining and identifying a patient's condition

G. The process of tapping the body to detect signs of disease

H. The process of observing a patient to detect any signs of disease

I. Any change in the body or its functioning that indicates that a disease might be present

J. The process of listening to the sounds produced within the body to detect signs of disease

K. A determination of which of two or more diseases with similar symptoms is producing the patient's symptoms

L. An instrument for examining the external ear canal and tympanic membrane

M. The process of feeling with the hands to detect signs of disease

N. An instrument with a rubber head, used for testing reflexes

O. The probable course and outcome of a patient's condition and the patient's prospects for recovery

P. The branch of medicine that deals with the treatment and control of obesity and diseases associated with obesity

Q. Utilization of the correct muscles to maintain proper balance, posture, and body alignment to accomplish a task safely and efficiently

B. Word Parts

Directions: Indicate the meaning of each word part in the space provided. List as many medical terms as possible that incorporate the word part in the space provided.

Word Part	Meaning of Word Part	Medical Terms That Incorporate Word Part
1. audi/o		
2. -meter		
3. bar/o		
4. -iatrics		
5. dia-		
6. -gnosis		
7. ophthalm/o		
8. -scope		
9. ot/o		

EVALUATION OF LEARNING

Directions: Fill in each blank with the correct answer.

1. What are the three parts of a complete patient examination?

_____

_____

2. List two functions of the patient examination.

_____

_____

3. What is the purpose of establishing a final diagnosis?

_____

_____

4. Why is there a space for indicating the clinical diagnosis on the laboratory request form?

_____

_____

5. What is a *risk factor*?

_____

_____

6. What is an acute illness? List two examples of acute illnesses.

_____

_____

7. What is a chronic illness? List two examples of chronic illnesses.

_____

_____

8. What is the difference between a therapeutic procedure and a diagnostic procedure?

_____

_____

_____

9. How should a patient be identified?

_____

_____

10. Why is it important to properly identify the patient?

_____

_____

11. How can patient apprehension be reduced during a physical examination?

_____

_____

12. Why should patients be asked whether they need to void before the physical examination?

_____

_____

13. What are two examples of locations for placing a paper-based patient record (PPR) for review by the physician?

_____

_____

14. What is the purpose for measuring weight?

_____

_____

15. Why is it important to use proper body mechanics?

_____

_____

16. What are the four curvatures of the vertebral column, and what is their purpose?

_____

_____

17. What body mechanics principles should be followed for each of the following?

   a. Physical condition of the body

   _____

   _____

   b. Reaching for something

   _____

   _____

   c. Working height

   _____

   _____

   d. Storing heavy and lighter items on shelves

   _____

   _____

   e. Retrieving an item from an overhead shelf

   _____

   _____

f. Lifting an object

_____

_____

g. Transferring a patient

_____

_____

h. Patient who starts to fall

_____

_____

i. Uncertainty about your ability to lift a heavy object

_____

_____

18. What is the purpose of positioning and draping?

_____

_____

_____

19. Indicate three types of examinations for which the supine position is used.

_____

_____

20. Indicate two types of examinations for which the lithotomy position is used.

_____

_____

21. Indicate one type of examination for which the knee-chest position is used.

_____

_____

22. What is the purpose of a wheelchair?

_____

_____

23. What is the purpose of a transfer belt for both the patient and the medical assistant?

_____

_____

24. What should the medical assistant do if he or she does not think it is possible to transfer a patient from a wheelchair to the examining table?

_____

_____

25. What is performed during a complete physical examination?

_____

_____

26. What is the advantage of using EMR software to record the results of a physical examination?

_____

_____

27. What are four types of assessments that can be made through inspection?

_____

_____

28. What are four types of assessments that can be made through palpation?

_____

_____

29. What can be assessed through the use of percussion?

_____

_____

30. What type of assessments can be made using auscultation?

_____

_____

31. What type of stethoscope chest piece should be used to assess the heart?

_____

CRITICAL THINKING ACTIVITIES

A. Preparation of the Examining Room

For each of the following examining room preparation guidelines, indicate the problems that may result if the guideline is not followed.

	Preparation	Problems if not Performed
1.	Ensure the examining room is well lit.	
2.	Restock supplies that are getting low.	
3.	Empty waste containers frequently.	
4.	Replace biohazard containers as necessary.	
5.	Make sure room is well ventilated.	
6.	Maintain room temperature that is comfortable for the patient.	
7.	Clean and disinfect examining table daily.	
8.	Change the examining table paper after each patient.	
9.	Check equipment and instruments to make sure they are in proper working condition.	
10.	Know how to operate and care for each piece of equipment and instrument.	

B. Reading Weight Measurements

The diagram is an illustration of a portion of the calibration bar of an upright balance beam scale. In the spaces provided, record the weight measurements indicated on the calibration bar. In all cases, assume that the lower weight is resting in the 100-lb notched groove.

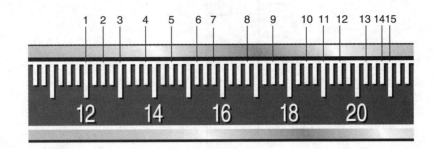

1. _____

2. _____

3. _____

4. _____

5. _____

6. _____

7. _____

8. _____

9. _____

10. _____

11. _____

12. _____

13. _____

14. _____

15. _____

C. Reading Height Measurements

The diagram is an illustration of a portion of the calibration rod of an upright balance beam scale. In the spaces provided, indicate the height measurement in feet and inches indicated on the calibration rod.

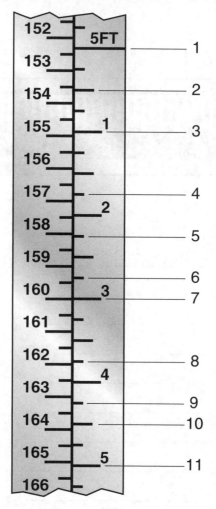

1. _____

2. _____

3. _____

4. _____

5. _____

6. _____

7. _____

8. _____

9. _____

10. _____

11. _____

D. Calculating Body Mass Index

1. Using the *Highlight on Body Mass Index* box on page 182 of your textbook, calculate and interpret your BMI and record the results below.

_____

2. Calculate the BMI of the following individuals, and record the value in the space provided. Interpret each BMI value according to the information indicated in *Highlight on Interpreting Body Weight* as follows: underweight, healthy weight, overweight, obesity (I), obesity (II), extreme obesity (III).

	Weight	Height	BMI	Interpretation of BMI
1.	146	5'5"		
2.	175	5'6"		
3.	110	5'9"		
4.	122	5'1"		
5.	260	6'		
6.	180	6'8"		
7.	330	5'11"		
8.	150	5'4"		
9.	170	5'2"		
10.	151	6'4"		

3. List the diseases that an individual with an above-normal BMI has an increased chance of developing.

_____

_____

_____

_____

E. Patient Positions

In which position would you place the patient for the following examinations or procedures?

1. Measurement of rectal temperature of an adult _____

2. Examination of the back _____

3. Measurement of vital signs _____

4. Pelvic examination _____

5. Examination of the upper extremities _____

6. Examination of the eyes, ears, nose, and throat _____

7. Examination of the breasts _____

8. Flexible sigmoidoscopy _____

9. Administration of an enema _____

10. Examination of the upper body of a patient with emphysema _____

F. Examination Techniques

List the examination technique (e.g., inspection, palpation, percussion, auscultation) that is used in each of the following situations.

1. A patient with a stutter _____

2. Taking the radial pulse _____

3. Finding the location of the apical pulse _____

4. Taking the apical pulse _____

5. Taking respiration (may be two answers, depending on method) _____

6. A patient with cracked lips _____

7. Checking for lumps in the breast _____

8. Checking reflexes _____

9. Obtaining the fetal heart rate _____

10. A patient with a fever (may be several methods) _____

G. Crossword Puzzle: The Physical Examination

Directions: Complete the crossword puzzle using the clues presented below.

Across
1 Eye examiner
5 Ear examiner
7 BMI: below 18.5
9 BMI: 25 to 29.9
10 "Listen to heart" position
14 Measuring the patient
16 I am listening
20 Metric unit of height
22 Metric unit of weight
23 Curative procedure
24 Reflex tester
25 Can cause premature death

Down
2 Hearing tester
3 Flex sigmoid position
4 Face-down
6 Orifice opener
8 What is the probable outcome?
11 What is wrong with you?
12 Before you measure weight
13 GYN position
15 Five feet in inches
17 Severe and intense condition
18 Provides warmth and modesty
19 Long-time illness
21 Face-up

Notes

Name: _____

Directions:
a. Watch the indicated videos.
b. Mark each true statement with a T and each false statement with an F. For each false statement, change the wording of the question so that it becomes a true statement.

Video: Procedure 5-1: Measuring Weight and Height

_____ 1. The process of measuring a patient is known as mensuration.

_____ 2. Changes in weight and height often help the physician diagnose a patient's condition and prescribe treatment.

_____ 3. The height and weight of prenatal patients is measured during each prenatal visit.

_____ 4. If the scale is not balanced, the weight measurement will be inaccurate.

_____ 5. The patient's weight should be taken with the shoes on.

_____ 6. If the lower weight is not seated firmly in its groove when measuring weight, the reading will be inaccurate.

_____ 7. Read the weight results to the nearest quarter pound.

_____ 8. When measuring height, instruct the patient to stand erect and to look up.

_____ 9. When measuring height, the measuring bar should form a 90-degree angle with the calibration rod.

_____ 10. The height should be charted in feet and inches to the nearest inch.

Video: Procedures 5-2 through 5-9: Positioning and Draping

_____ 1. Correct positioning allows for better access to the part that is undergoing examination or treatment.

_____ 2. The patient position selected depends on the type of examination or procedure being performed.

_____ 3. The patient is draped to provide comfort and warmth and to maintain modesty.

_____ 4. The sitting position is used to examine the back and buttocks.

_____ 5. The supine position is used to examine the head, chest, abdomen, and extremities.

_____ 6. The prone position is used to examine the back and to assess extension of the hip joint.

_____ 7. When placing the patient in the prone position, the patient should turn onto the stomach by rolling away from you.

_____ 8. The dorsal recumbent position is used for vaginal and rectal examinations and for the insertion of a urinary catheter.

_____ 9. The lithotomy position is used for vaginal, pelvic, and rectal examinations.

_____ 10. Stirrup covers provide a soft, warm, nonslip surface for the patient's feet.

_____ 11. The drape for the lithotomy position should be positioned lengthwise over the patient.

_____ 12. The stirrups for the lithotomy position should be level with the examining table and pulled out approximately 3 feet from the edge of the table.

_____ 13. For the lithotomy position, the patient should be instructed to slide her buttocks all the way down to the edge of the examining table.

_____ 14. To take the patient out of the lithotomy position, lift the patient's legs out of the stirrups one at a time, and place them on the table extension.

_____ 15. Sims' position is used to measure rectal temperature, to perform a flexible sigmoidoscopy, and to administer an enema.

_____ 16. The knee-chest position is used to examine the knees and chest.

_____ 17. The drape should be positioned diagonally with the knee-chest position.

_____ 18. Fowler's position is used to examine the upper body of patients with cardiovascular and respiratory problems.

_____ 19. For semi-Fowler's position, the table should be positioned at a 90-degree angle.

_____ 20. When sliding the table extension back into place, the patient's lower legs should be supported by the medical assistant.

Video: Procedure 5-10: Wheelchair Transfer

_____ 1. A wheelchair helps individuals remain mobile when they cannot walk or have difficulty walking.

_____ 2. A transfer belt provides a secure grip by the medical assistant and helps to control the patient's movements.

_____ 3. The medical assistant should not perform the transfer if he or she thinks that a musculoskeletal injury may result.

_____ 4. The transfer belt should be wrapped snugly around the patient's waist under his or her clothing.

_____ 5. The patient's weaker side should be positioned next to the examining table.

_____ 6. The wheelchair should be positioned at a 90-degree angle to the end of the examining table.

_____ 7. The brakes of the wheelchair should be locked to prevent it from moving during the transfer.

_____ 8. The transfer belt should be grasped on either side of the patient's waist by using an overhand grasp.

_____ 9. The patient should be lifted from the wheelchair by bending from the waist and using the back muscles.

_____ 10. To transfer the patient back to the wheelchair, ask the patient to place his or her arms around your neck.

Video: Procedure 5-11: The Physical Examination

_____ 1. Arrange the instruments and supplies for a physical examination in a neat and orderly manner so that one item does not lie on top of another.

_____ 2. Each patient should be identified by his or her last name.

_____ 3. When obtaining information from a patient, seat yourself so that you are facing your patient at a distance of about 6 feet.

_____ 4. Information relayed to you by the patient is strictly confidential.

_____ 5. Normal body temperature falls between 96° F and 98° F.

_____ 6. An empty bladder makes the examination easier and is more comfortable for the patient.

_____ 7. To make the medical record available for review by the physician, it can be placed on a shelf near the outside of the examining room or in a holder mounted on the outside of the door.

_____ 8. To protect the patient's privacy, it is important to position the record so that the patient's identifiable information is hidden from view.

_____ 9. After handing the physician the ophthalmoscope, the lights must be turned up when the physician is ready to examine the eyes.

_____ 10. The otoscope is used to examine the nasal cavity.

_____ 11. A tongue depressor should be discarded in a regular waste container.

_____ 12. Hearing acuity is tested using a percussion hammer.

_____ 13. Instructions should be provided to a patient using medical terms.

_____ 14. Clean gloves should be applied to disinfect an examining table.

Notes

PRACTICE FOR COMPETENCY

Procedure 5-1: Weight and Height. Take weight and height measurements. Record results in the chart provided.

Procedure 5-A: Body Mechanics. Demonstrate proper body mechanics while standing, sitting, and lifting an object.

Procedures 5-2 to 5-9: Positioning and Draping. Position and drape an individual in each of the following positions: sitting, supine, prone, dorsal recumbent, lithotomy, Sims, knee-chest, and Fowler's.

Procedure 5-10: Wheelchair Transfer. Transfer a patient from a wheelchair to the examining table and from the examining table to a wheelchair.

Procedure 5-11: Assisting with the Physical Examination. Prepare the patient and assist with a physical examination. In the chart provided, record the results of the procedures you performed while assisting with the examination (e.g., vital signs, height, and weight).

CHART	
Date	

191

Chapter **5** **The Physical Examination**

CHART	
Date	

EVALUATION OF COMPETENCY

Procedure 5-1: Measuring Weight and Height

Name: _____   Date: _____

Evaluated by: _____   Score: _____

Performance Objective

Outcome:	Measure weight and height.
Conditions:	Given a paper towel.
	Using an upright balance scale.
Standards:	Time: 5 minutes. Student completed procedure in _____ minutes.
	Accuracy: Satisfactory score on the Performance Evaluation Checklist.

Performance Evaluation Checklist

Trial 1	Trial 2	Point Value	Performance Standards
			Weight
		•	Sanitized hands.
			Checked the balance scale for accuracy.
		•	Verified that the upper and lower weights were on zero.
		•	Looked at the indicator point to make sure the scale is balanced.
		▷	Stated what will be observed if the scale is balanced.
		▷	Explained what to do if the indicator point rests below the center.
		▷	Explained what to do if the indicator point rests above the center.
		▷	Stated what occurs if the scale is not balanced.
		•	Greeted the patient and introduced yourself.
		•	Identified the patient and explained the procedure.
		•	Instructed the patient to remove shoes and heavy outer clothing.
		•	Placed paper towel on the scale.
		•	Assisted the patient onto the scale.
		•	Instructed the patient not to move.
			Balanced the scale.
		•	Moved the lower weight to the groove that did not cause the indicator point to drop to the bottom of the balance area.

Trial 1	Trial 2	Point Value	Performance Standards
		▷	Stated why the lower weight should be seated firmly in its groove.
		•	Slid the upper weight slowly until the indicator point came to a rest at the center of the balance area.
		•	Read the results to the nearest quarter pound. Jotted down this value or made a mental note of it.
		✱	The reading was identical to the evaluator's reading.
		•	Asked the patient to step off the scale.
			Height
		•	Slid the calibration rod until it was above the patient's height.
		•	Opened the measuring bar to its horizontal position.
		•	Instructed the patient to step onto the scale platform with his or her back to the scale.
		•	Instructed the patient to stand erect and to look straight ahead.
		•	Carefully lowered the measuring bar until it rested gently on top of the patient's head.
		•	Verified that the bar was in a horizontal position.
		•	Instructed the patient to step down and put on his or her shoes.
		•	Read the marking to the nearest quarter inch. Jotted down this value or made a mental note of it.
		✱	The reading was identical to the evaluator's reading.
		•	Returned the measuring bar to its vertical position.
		•	Slid the calibration rod to its lowest position.
		•	Returned the weights to zero.
		•	Sanitized hands.
		•	Charted the results correctly.
		✱	Completed the procedure within 5 minutes.
			Totals
			CHART
Date			

Evaluation of Student Performance

EVALUATION CRITERIA			COMMENTS
Symbol	**Category**	**Point Value**	
✳	Critical Step	16 points	
•	Essential Step	6 points	
▷	Theory Question	2 points	

Score calculation: 100 points

$$- \underline{\qquad} \text{ points missed}$$

$$\underline{\qquad} \text{ Score}$$

Satisfactory score: 85 or above

CAAHEP Competencies Achieved

Psychomotor (Skills)

☑ IV. 6. Prepare a patient for procedures and/or treatments.

Affective (Behavior)

☑ IV. 1. Demonstrate empathy in communicating with patients, family, and staff.

☑ IV. 9. Recognize and protect personal boundaries in communicating with others.

ABHES Competencies Achieved

☑ 8. bb. Are impartial and show empathy when dealing with patients.

☑ 9. l. Prepare patient for examinations and treatments.

Notes

Chapter **5** **The Physical Examination**

EVALUATION OF COMPETENCY

Procedure 5-A: Body Mechanics

Name: _____   Date: _____

Evaluated by: _____   Score: _____

Performance Objective

Outcome:	Demonstrate proper body mechanics while standing, sitting, and lifting an object.
Conditions:	Using a chair.
	Given the following: object for lifting.
Standards:	Time: 10 minutes. Student completed procedure in _____ minutes.
	Accuracy: Satisfactory score on the Performance Evaluation Checklist.

Performance Evaluation Checklist

Trial 1	Trial 2	Point Value	Performance Standards
			Standing
		•	Wore comfortable, low-heeled shoes that provide good support.
		•	Held the head erect at the midline of the body.
		•	Maintained the back as straight as possible with the pelvis tucked inward.
		•	The chest is forward with the shoulders back and the abdomen drawn in and kept flat.
		▷	Stated the purpose of standing correctly.
		•	Knees are slightly flexed.
		•	Feet are pointing forward and parallel to each other about 3 inches apart.
		▷	Explained the reason for proper positioning of the feet.
		•	Arms are positioned comfortably at the side.
		•	Weight of the body is evenly distributed over both feet.
			Sitting
		•	Sat in a chair with a firm back.
		•	Back and buttocks are supported against the back of the chair.
		•	Body weight is evenly distributed over the buttocks and thighs.
		•	A small pillow or rolled towel is used.
		▷	Stated the use of the pillow or rolled towel.
		•	Feet are flat on the floor.
		•	Knees are level with the hips.
		▷	Explained what to do if prolonged sitting is required.

197

Trial 1	Trial 2	Point Value	Performance Standards
			Lifting
		•	Determined the weight of the object.
		▷	Stated the purpose of determining the weight of an object before lifting it.
		•	Stood in front of the object with the feet 6 to 8 inches apart.
		•	The toes are pointed outward and one foot is slightly forward.
		•	Tightened the stomach and gluteal muscles in preparation for the lift.
		•	Bent the body at the knees and hips.
		▷	Stated the purpose of bending the body at the knees and hips.
		•	Grasped the object firmly with both hands.
		•	Lifted the object smoothly with the leg muscles while keeping the back straight.
		▷	Stated why the leg muscles and not the back muscles should be used to lift the object.
		•	Held the object as close to the body as possible at waist level.
		▷	Stated why the object should not be lifted higher than the chest.
		•	Turned by pivoting the whole body.
		•	Made sure the area of transport of the object is dry and free of clutter.
		•	Lowered the object slowly while bending from the knees.
		✶	Completed the procedures within 10 minutes.
			Totals

Evaluation of Student Performance

EVALUATION CRITERIA			COMMENTS
Symbol	**Category**	**Point Value**	
✶	Critical Step	16 points	
•	Essential Step	6 points	
▷	Theory Question	2 points	
Score calculation: 100 points – ______ points missed ____ Score Satisfactory score: 85 or above			

CAAHEP Competencies Achieved

Psychomotor (Skills)

☑ XI.   3. Develop a personal (patient and employee) safety plan.

☑ XI. 11. Use proper body mechanics.

ABHES Competencies Achieved

☑ 4. e. Perform risk management procedures.

Notes

Procedure 5-2: Sitting Position

Name: _____   Date: _____

Evaluated by: _____   Score: _____

Performance Objective

Outcome:	Position and drape an individual in the sitting position.
Conditions:	Using an examining table.
	Given the following: a patient gown and a drape.
Standards:	Time: 5 minutes. Student completed procedure in _____ minutes.
	Accuracy: Satisfactory score on the Performance Evaluation Checklist.

Performance Evaluation Checklist

Trial	Trial 2	Point Value	Performance Standards
		•	Sanitized hands.
		•	Greeted the patient and introduced yourself.
		•	Identified the patient.
		•	Explained what type of examination or procedure will be performed.
		•	Provided the patient with a patient gown.
		•	Instructed the patient to remove clothing and to put on a patient gown with the opening in front.
		▷	Stated what qualities the disrobing facility should have.
		•	Pulled out the footrest and assisted the patient into a sitting position.
		•	The patient's buttocks and thighs were firmly supported on the edge of the table.
		•	Placed a drape over the patient's thighs and legs.
		•	Assisted the patient off the table after the examination.
		•	Returned the footrest to its normal position.
		•	Instructed the patient to get dressed.
		•	Discarded the gown and drape in a waste container.
		▷	Stated one use of the sitting position.
		✳	Completed the procedure within 5 minutes.
			Totals

Evaluation of Student Performance

EVALUATION CRITERIA			COMMENTS
Symbol	**Category**	**Point Value**	
✳	Critical Step	16 points	
•	Essential Step	6 points	
▷	Theory Question	2 points	

Score calculation: 100 points

    − _____ points missed
      _____ Score

Satisfactory score: 85 or above

CAAHEP Competencies Achieved

Psychomotor (Skills)

☑ IV. 6. Prepare a patient for procedures and/or treatments.

☑ XI. 11. Use proper body mechanics.

Affective (Behavior)

☑ IV. 4. Demonstrate awareness of the territorial boundaries of the person with whom communicating.

ABHES Competencies Achieved

☑ 9. l. Prepare patient for examinations and treatments.

Procedure 5-3: Supine Position

Name: _____   Date: _____

Evaluated by: _____   Score: _____

Performance Objective

Outcome:	Position and drape an individual in the supine position.
Conditions:	Using an examining table.
	Given the following: a patient gown and a drape.
Standards:	Time: 5 minutes. Student completed procedure in _____ minutes.
	Accuracy: Satisfactory score on the Performance Evaluation Checklist.

Performance Evaluation Checklist

Trial 1	Trial 2	Point Value	Performance Standards
		•	Sanitized hands.
		•	Greeted the patient and introduced yourself.
		•	Identified the patient.
		•	Explained what type of examination or procedure will be performed.
		•	Provided the patient with a patient gown.
		•	Instructed the patient to remove clothing and to put on a patient gown with the opening in front.
		•	Pulled out the footrest and assisted the patient into a sitting position.
		•	Placed a drape over the patient's thighs and legs.
		•	Asked the patient to move back on the table.
		•	Pulled out the table extension while supporting the patient's lower legs.
		•	Asked the patient to lie down on his or her back with the legs together.
		•	Placed the patient's arms above the head or alongside the body.
		•	Positioned the drape lengthwise over the patient.
		▷	Stated the purpose of the drape.
		•	Moved the drape according to the body parts being examined.
		•	Assisted the patient back into a sitting position after the examination.
		•	Slid the table extension back into place while supporting the patient's lower legs.
		•	Assisted the patient from the examining table.
		•	Returned the footrest to its normal position.
		•	Instructed the patient to get dressed.

Trial 1	Trial 2	Point Value	Performance Standards
		•	Discarded the gown and drape in a waste container.
		▷	Stated one use of the supine position.
		✳	Completed the procedure within 5 minutes.
			Totals

Evaluation of Student Performance

EVALUATION CRITERIA			COMMENTS
Symbol	**Category**	**Point Value**	
✳	Critical Step	16 points	
•	Essential Step	6 points	
▷	Theory Question	2 points	

Score calculation: 100 points

− _____ points missed

_____ Score

Satisfactory score: 85 or above

CAAHEP Competencies Achieved

Psychomotor (Skills)

☑ IV. 6. Prepare a patient for procedures and/or treatments.

☑ XI. 11. Use proper body mechanics.

Affective (Behavior)

☑ IV. 4. Demonstrate awareness of the territorial boundaries of the person with whom communicating.

ABHES Competencies Achieved

☑ 9. 1. Prepare patient for examinations and treatments.

e Procedure 5-4: Prone Position

Name: _____ Date: _____

Evaluated by: _____ Score: _____

Performance Objective

Outcome:	Position and drape an individual in the prone position.
Conditions:	Using an examining table.
	Given the following: a patient gown and a drape.
Standards:	Time: 5 minutes. Student completed procedure in _____ minutes.
	Accuracy: Satisfactory score on the Performance Evaluation Checklist.

Performance Evaluation Checklist

Trial 1	Trial 2	Point Value	Performance Standards
		•	Sanitized hands.
		•	Greeted the patient and introduced yourself.
		•	Identified the patient.
		•	Explained what type of examination or procedure will be performed.
		•	Provided the patient with a patient gown.
		•	Instructed the patient to remove clothing and to put on a patient gown with the opening in back.
		•	Pulled out the footrest and assisted the patient into a sitting position.
		•	Placed a drape over the patient's thighs and legs.
		•	Asked the patient to move back on the table.
		•	Pulled out the table extension while supporting the patient's lower legs.
		•	Asked the patient to lie down on his or her back.
		•	Positioned the drape lengthwise over the patient.
		•	Asked the patient to turn onto his or her stomach by rolling toward you.
		•	Provided assistance.
		▷	Stated the reason for providing assistance.
		•	Positioned the patient with his or her legs together and the head turned to one side.
		•	Placed the patient's arms above the head or alongside the body.
		•	Adjusted the drape as needed.
		•	Moved the drape according to the body parts being examined.
		•	Assisted the patient into the supine position after the examination.
		•	Assisted the patient into a sitting position.

Trial 1	Trial 2	Point Value	Performance Standards
		•	Slid the table extension back into place while supporting the patient's lower legs.
		•	Assisted the patient from the examining table.
		•	Returned the footrest to its normal position.
		•	Instructed the patient to get dressed.
		•	Discarded the gown and drape in a waste container.
		▷	Stated one use of the prone position.
		∗	Completed the procedure within 5 minutes.
			Totals

Evaluation of Student Performance

EVALUATION CRITERIA			COMMENTS
Symbol	**Category**	**Point Value**	
∗	Critical Step	16 points	
•	Essential Step	6 points	
▷	Theory Question	2 points	

Score calculation: 100 points

− _____ points missed

_____ Score

Satisfactory score: 85 or above

CAAHEP Competencies Achieved

Psychomotor (Skills)

☑ IV. 6. Prepare a patient for procedures and/or treatments.

☑ XI. 11. Use proper body mechanics.

Affective (Behavior)

☑ IV. 4. Demonstrate awareness of the territorial boundaries of the person with whom communicating.

ABHES Competencies Achieved

☑ 9. 1. Prepare patient for examinations and treatments.

e Procedure 5-5: Dorsal Recumbent Position

Name: _____   Date: _____

Evaluated by: _____   Score: _____

Performance Objective

Outcome:	Position and drape an individual in the dorsal recumbent position.
Conditions:	Using an examining table.
	Given the following: a patient gown and a drape.
Standards:	Time: 5 minutes. Student completed procedure in _____ minutes.
	Accuracy: Satisfactory score on the Performance Evaluation Checklist.

Performance Evaluation Checklist

Trial 1	Trial 2	Point Value	Performance Standards
		•	Sanitized hands.
		•	Greeted the patient and introduced yourself.
		•	Identified the patient.
		• ▷	Explained what type of examination or procedure will be performed.
		•	Provided the patient with a patient gown.
		•	Instructed the patient to remove clothing and to put on a patient gown with the opening in front.
		•	Pulled out the footrest and assisted the patient into a sitting position.
		•	Placed a drape over the patient's thighs and legs.
		•	Asked the patient to move back on the table.
		•	Pulled out the table extension while supporting the patient's lower legs.
		•	Asked the patient to lie down on his or her back.
		•	Placed the patient's arms above the head or alongside the body.
		•	Positioned the drape diagonally over the patient.
		•	Asked the patient to bend the knees and place each foot at the edge of the table with the soles of the feet flat on the table.
		•	Provided assistance.
		•	Pushed in the table extension and the footrest.
		•	Adjusted the drape as needed.
		•	Folded back the center corner of the drape when the physician was ready to examine the patient.

Trial 1	Trial 2	Point Value	Performance Standards
		•	Pulled out the footrest and the table extension after the examination.
		•	Assisted the patient back into a supine position and then into a sitting position.
		•	Slid the table extension back into place while supporting the patient's lower legs.
		•	Assisted the patient from the examining table.
		•	Returned the footrest to its normal position.
		•	Instructed the patient to get dressed.
		•	Discarded the gown and drape in a waste container.
		▷	Stated one use of the dorsal recumbent position.
		✳	Completed the procedure within 5 minutes.
			Totals

Evaluation of Student Performance

EVALUATION CRITERIA			COMMENTS
Symbol	**Category**	**Point Value**	
✳	Critical Step	16 points	
•	Essential Step	6 points	
▷	Theory Question	2 points	

Score calculation: 100 points

− _____ points missed

_____ Score

Satisfactory score: 85 or above

CAAHEP Competencies Achieved

Psychomotor (Skills)

☑ IV. 6. Prepare a patient for procedures and/or treatments.

☑ XI. 11. Use proper body mechanics.

Affective (Behavior)

☑ IV. 4. Demonstrate awareness of the territorial boundaries of the person with whom communicating.

ABHES Competencies Achieved

☑ 9. 1. Prepare patient for examinations and treatments.

EVALUATION OF COMPETENCY

Procedure 5-6: Lithotomy Position

Name: _____ Date: _____

Evaluated by: _____ Score: _____

Performance Objective

Outcome:	Position and drape an individual in the lithotomy position.
Conditions:	Using an examining table.
	Given the following: a patient gown and a drape.
Standards:	Time: 5 minutes. Student completed procedure in _____ minutes.
	Accuracy: Satisfactory score on the Performance Evaluation Checklist.

Performance Evaluation Checklist

Trial 1	Trial 2	Point Value	Performance Standards
		•	Sanitized hands.
		•	Greeted the patient and introduced yourself.
		•	Identified the patient.
		•	Explained what type of examination or procedure will be performed.
		•	Provided the patient with a patient gown.
		•	Instructed the patient to remove clothing and to put on a patient gown with the opening in front.
		•	Pulled out the footrest and assisted the patient into a sitting position.
		•	Placed a drape over the patient's thighs and legs.
		•	Asked the patient to move back on the table.
		•	Pulled out the table extension while supporting the patient's lower legs.
		•	Asked the patient to lie down on his or her back.
		•	Placed the patient's arms above the head or alongside the body.
		•	Positioned the drape diagonally over the patient.
		•	Pulled out the stirrups and positioned them at an angle.
		•	Positioned the stirrups so that they were level with the examining table and pulled out approximately 1 foot from the edge of the table.
		•	Asked the patient to bend the knees and place each foot into a stirrup.
		•	Provided assistance.
		•	Pushed in the table extension and the footrest.
		•	Instructed the patient to slide buttocks to the edge of the table and to rotate thighs outward as far as is comfortable.

Trial 1	Trial 2	Point Value	Performance Standards
		•	Repositioned the drape as needed.
		•	Folded back the center corner of the drape when the physician was ready to examine the genital area.
		•	After completion of the examination, pulled out the footrest and the table extension.
		•	Asked the patient to slide the buttocks back from the end of the table.
		•	Lifted the patient's legs out of the stirrups at the same time and placed them on the table extension.
		▷	Stated why both legs should be lifted at the same time.
		•	Returned stirrups to the normal position.
		•	Assisted the patient back into a sitting position.
		•	Slid the table extension back into place while supporting the patient's lower legs.
		•	Assisted the patient from the examining table.
		•	Returned the footrest to its normal position.
		•	Instructed the patient to get dressed.
		•	Discarded the gown and drape in a waste container.
		▷	Stated one use of the lithotomy position.
		✷	Completed the procedure within 5 minutes.
			Totals

Evaluation of Student Performance

EVALUATION CRITERIA			COMMENTS
Symbol	**Category**	**Point Value**	
✷	Critical Step	16 points	
•	Essential Step	6 points	
▷	Theory Question	2 points	

Score calculation: 100 points

− _____ points missed

_____ Score

Satisfactory score: 85 or above

CAAHEP Competencies Achieved

Psychomotor (Skills)

☑ IV. 6. Prepare a patient for procedures and/or treatments.

☑ XI. 11. Use proper body mechanics.

Affective (Behavior)

☑ IV. 4. Demonstrate awareness of the territorial boundaries of the person with whom communicating.

ABHES Competencies Achieved

☑ 9. l. Prepare patient for examinations and treatments.

Notes

Chapter **5** **The Physical Examination**

Procedure 5-7: Sims Position

Name: _____   Date: _____

Evaluated by: _____   Score: _____

Performance Objective

Outcome:	Position and drape an individual in Sims position.
Conditions:	Using an examining table.
	Given the following: a patient gown and a drape.
Standards:	Time: 5 minutes. Student completed procedure in _____ minutes.
	Accuracy: Satisfactory score on the Performance Evaluation Checklist.

Performance Evaluation Checklist

Trial 1	Trial 2	Point Value	Performance Standards
		•	Sanitized hands.
		•	Greeted the patient and introduced yourself.
		•	Identified the patient.
		•	Explained what type of examination or procedure will be performed.
		•	Provided the patient with a patient gown.
		•	Instructed the patient to remove clothing and to put on a patient gown with the opening in back.
		•	Pulled out the footrest and assisted the patient into a sitting position.
		•	Placed a drape over the patient's thighs and legs.
		•	Asked the patient to move back on the table.
		•	Pulled out the table extension while supporting the patient's lower legs.
		•	Asked the patient to lie down on his or her back.
		•	Positioned the drape lengthwise over the patient.
		•	Asked the patient to turn onto the left side.
		•	Provided assistance.
		•	Positioned the left arm behind the body and the right arm forward with the elbow bent.
		•	Assisted the patient in flexing the legs with the right leg flexed sharply and the left leg flexed slightly.
		•	Adjusted the drape by folding back the drape to expose the anal area when the physician was ready to examine the patient.
		•	Assisted the patient into a supine position and then into a sitting position following the examination.

Trial 1	Trial 2	Point Value	Performance Standards
		•	Slid the table extension back into place while supporting the patient's lower legs.
		•	Assisted the patient from the examining table.
		•	Returned the footrest to its normal position.
		•	Instructed the patient to get dressed.
		•	Discarded the gown and drape in a waste container.
		▷	Stated one use of Sims position.
		✳	Completed the procedure within 5 minutes.
			Totals

Evaluation of Student Performance

EVALUATION CRITERIA			COMMENTS
Symbol	**Category**	**Point Value**	
✳	Critical Step	16 points	
•	Essential Step	6 points	
▷	Theory Question	2 points	

Score calculation: 100 points

− _____ points missed

_____ Score

Satisfactory score: 85 or above

CAAHEP Competencies Achieved

Psychomotor (Skills)

☑ IV. 6. Prepare a patient for procedures and/or treatments.

☑ XI. 11. Use proper body mechanics.

Affective (Behavior)

☑ IV. 4. Demonstrate awareness of the territorial boundaries of the person with whom communicating.

ABHES Competencies Achieved

☑ 9. 1. Prepare patient for examinations and treatments.

Procedure 5-8: Knee-Chest Position

Name: _____   Date: _____

Evaluated by: _____   Score: _____

Performance Objective

Outcome:	Position and drape an individual in the knee-chest position.
Conditions:	Using an examining table.
	Given the following: a patient gown and a drape.
Standards:	Time: 5 minutes. Student completed procedure in _____ minutes.
	Accuracy: Satisfactory score on the Performance Evaluation Checklist.

Performance Evaluation Checklist

Trial 1	Trial 2	Point Value	Performance Standards
		•	Sanitized hands.
		•	Greeted the patient and introduced yourself.
		•	Identified the patient.
		•	Explained what type of examination or procedure will be performed.
		•	Provided the patient with a patient gown.
		•	Instructed the patient to remove clothing and to put on a patient gown with the opening in back.
		•	Pulled out the footrest and assisted the patient into a sitting position.
		•	Placed a drape over the patient's thighs and legs.
		•	Asked the patient to move back on the table.
		•	Pulled out the table extension while supporting the patient's lower legs.
		•	Assisted the patient into the supine position and then into the prone position.
		•	Positioned the drape diagonally over the patient.
		•	Asked the patient to bend the arms at the elbows and rest them alongside the head.
		•	Asked the patient to elevate the buttocks while keeping the back straight.
		•	Turned the patient's head to one side, with the weight of the body supported by the chest.
		•	Used a pillow for additional support, if needed.
		•	Separated the knees and lower legs approximately 12 inches.
		•	Adjusted the drape diagonally as needed.
		•	Folded back a small portion of the drape to expose the anal area when the physician was ready to examine the patient.

Trial 1	Trial 2	Point Value	Performance Standards
		•	Assisted the patient into a prone position and then into a supine position after the examination.
		•	Allowed the patient to rest in a supine position before sitting up.
		▷	Stated why the patient should be allowed to rest.
		•	Assisted the patient into a sitting position.
		•	Slid the table extension back into place while supporting the patient's lower legs.
		•	Assisted the patient from the examining table.
		•	Returned the footrest to its normal position.
		•	Instructed the patient to get dressed.
		•	Discarded the gown and drape in a waste container.
		▷	Stated one use of the knee-chest position.
		✱	Completed the procedure within 5 minutes.
			Totals

Evaluation of Student Performance

EVALUATION CRITERIA			COMMENTS
Symbol	**Category**	**Point Value**	
✱	Critical Step	16 points	
•	Essential Step	6 points	
▷	Theory Question	2 points	

Score calculation: 100 points

− _____ points missed

_____ Score

Satisfactory score: 85 or above

CAAHEP Competencies Achieved

Psychomotor (Skills)

☑ IV. 6. Prepare a patient for procedures and/or treatments.

☑ XI. 11. Use proper body mechanics.

Affective (Behavior)

☑ IV. 4. Demonstrate awareness of the territorial boundaries of the person with whom communicating.

ABHES Competencies Achieved

☑ 9. 1. Prepare patient for examinations and treatments.

Procedure 5-9: Fowler's Position

Name: _____ Date: _____

Evaluated by: _____ Score: _____

Performance Objective

Outcome:	Position and drape an individual in Fowler's position.
Conditions:	Using an examining table.
	Given the following: a patient gown and a drape.
Standards:	Time: 5 minutes. Student completed procedure in _____ minutes.
	Accuracy: Satisfactory score on the Performance Evaluation Checklist.

Performance Evaluation Checklist

Trial 1	Trial 2	Point Value	Performance Standards
		•	Sanitized hands.
		•	Greeted the patient and introduced yourself.
		•	Identified the patient.
		•	Explained what type of examination or procedure will be performed.
		•	Provided the patient with a patient gown.
		•	Instructed the patient to remove clothing and to put on a patient gown with the opening in front.
		•	Positioned the head of the table at a 45-degree angle for semi-Fowler's position or at a 90-degree angle for full Fowler's position.
		•	Pulled out the footrest and assisted the patient into a sitting position.
		•	Placed a drape over the patient's thighs and legs.
		•	Pulled out the table extension while supporting the patient's lower legs.
		•	Asked the patient to lean back against the table head.
		•	Provided assistance.
		•	Positioned the drape lengthwise over the patient.
		•	Moved the drape according to the body parts being examined.
		•	Assisted the patient into a sitting position after the examination.
		•	Slid the table extension back into place while supporting the patient's lower legs.
		•	Assisted the patient from the examining table.
		•	Instructed the patient to get dressed.
		•	Returned the head of the table and the footrest to their normal positions.
		•	Discarded the gown and drape in a waste container.

Trial 1	Trial 2	Point Value	Performance Standards
		▷	Stated one use of Fowler's position.
		✳	Completed the procedure within 5 minutes.
			Totals

Evaluation of Student Performance

EVALUATION CRITERIA			COMMENTS
Symbol	**Category**	**Point Value**	
✳	Critical Step	16 points	
•	Essential Step	6 points	
▷	Theory Question	2 points	

Score calculation: 100 points

− _____ points missed

_____ Score

Satisfactory score: 85 or above

CAAHEP Competencies Achieved

Psychomotor (Skills)

☑ IV. 6. Prepare a patient for procedures and/or treatments.

☑ XI. 11. Use proper body mechanics.

Affective (Behavior)

☑ IV. 4. Demonstrate awareness of the territorial boundaries of the person with whom communicating.

ABHES Competencies Achieved

☑ 9. 1. Prepare patient for examinations and treatments.

Procedure 5-10: Wheelchair Transfer

Name: _____ Date: _____

Evaluated by: _____ Score: _____

Performance Objective

Outcome:	Transfer a patient from a wheelchair to the examining table and from the examining table to a wheelchair.
Conditions:	Using an examining table and a wheelchair.
	Given the following: transfer belt.
Standards:	Time: 10 minutes. Student completed procedure in _____ minutes.
	Accuracy: Satisfactory score on the Performance Evaluation Checklist.

Performance Evaluation Checklist

Trial 1	Trial 2	Point Value	Performance Standards
			Transferring to the examining table:
		•	Sanitized hands.
		•	Greeted the patient and introduced yourself.
		•	Identified the patient and explained the procedure.
		•	Determined whether the patient has the mental and physical capability to perform the transfer.
		•	Estimated the weight of the patient and whether he or she can assist in the transfer.
		•	Assessed your ability to make the transfer safely.
		▷	Stated factors that would prevent you from making the transfer.
		•	Wrapped the transfer belt around the patient's waist and fastened it.
		•	The belt was snug with just enough space to allow the fingers to be inserted comfortably.
		▷	Stated why the belt should be snug.
		•	With the patient's stronger side next to the table, positioned the wheelchair at a 45-degree angle to the end of the examining table.
		•	If the table is height adjustable, adjusted it to the same height as the wheelchair or slightly lower.
		•	If the table is not height adjustable, pulled out the footrest.
		•	Locked the brakes of the wheelchair.
		▷	Stated why the brakes should be locked.
		•	Folded back the wheelchair footrests.
		•	Informed the patient what to do during the transfer.
		•	Made sure the patient's feet were flat on the floor.

Trial 1	Trial 2	Point Value	Performance Standards
		•	Stood in front of the patient with the feet 6 to 8 inches apart, with one foot slightly forward and the knees bent.
		•	Asked the patient to place his or her arms on the armrests of the wheelchair and to lean forward.
		•	Grasped the transfer belt on either side of the patient's waist using an underhand grasp.
		▷	Stated the purpose of the transfer belt.
		•	Instructed the patient to push off the armrests and into a standing position on the count of 3.
		•	Straightened the knees and assisted the patient to a standing position by pulling upward on the transfer belt.
		•	Kept the back straight and lifted with the knees, arms, and legs, and not the back.
		•	Pivoted and positioned the patient's buttocks and back of the legs toward the examining table.
		•	Instructed the patient to step backward onto the footrest, one foot at a time.
		•	Gradually lowered the patient into a sitting position on the examining table.
		•	Removed the transfer belt.
		•	Unlocked the wheelchair and moved it out of the way.
		•	Pushed in the footrest of the examining table.
		•	Stayed with the patient to prevent falls.
			Transferring to the wheelchair:
		•	Wrapped the transfer belt snugly around the patient's waist and fastened it.
		•	Positioned the wheelchair at a 45-degree angle to the end of the examining table.
		•	If the table is height adjustable, adjusted it to the same height as the wheelchair or slightly lower.
		•	If the table is not height adjustable, pulled out the footrest.
		•	Locked the wheelchair in place and folded back the footrests, if needed.
		•	Informed the patient what to do during the transfer.
		•	Stood in front of the patient with the feet 6 to 8 inches apart, with one foot slightly forward and the knees bent.
		•	Asked the patient to place his or her arms on your shoulders.
		•	Did not allow the patient to place his or her arms around your neck.
		•	Grasped the transfer belt on either side of the patient's waist using an underhand grasp.
		•	Instructed the patient to stand on the count of 3.
		•	Straightened your knees and assisted the patient to a standing position by pulling upward on the transfer belt.
		•	Instructed the patient to step down from the footrest, one foot at a time.
		•	Pivoted the patient until the back of the legs are against the seat of the wheelchair.

Trial 1	Trial 2	Point Value	Performance Standards
		•	Asked the patient to grasp the armrests of the wheelchair.
		•	Gradually lowered the patient into the wheelchair by bending at the knees.
		•	Removed the transfer belt and made sure the patient was comfortable.
		•	Repositioned the wheelchair footrests and assisted the patient in placing his or her feet in them.
		•	Unlocked the wheelchair.
		•	Pushed in the footrest of the examining table.
		✷	Completed the procedure within 10 minutes.
			Totals

Evaluation of Student Performance

EVALUATION CRITERIA			COMMENTS
Symbol	**Category**	**Point Value**	
✷	Critical Step	16 points	
•	Essential Step	6 points	
▷	Theory Question	2 points	

Score calculation: 100 points

− _____ points missed

_____ Score

Satisfactory score: 85 or above

CAAHEP Competencies Achieved

Psychomotor (Skills)

☑ IV. 6. Prepare a patient for procedures and/or treatments.

☑ XI. 11. Use proper body mechanics.

Affective (Behavior)

☑ IV. 4. Demonstrate awareness of the territorial boundaries of the person with whom communicating.

ABHES Competencies Achieved

☑ 5. b. Identify and respond appropriately when working/caring for patients with special needs.

☑ 9. l. Prepare patient for examinations and treatments.

☑ 9. q. Instruct patients with special needs.

Notes

Procedure 5-11: Assisting with the Physical Examination

Name: _____ Date: _____

Evaluated by: _____ Score: _____

Performance Objective

Outcome:	Prepare the patient and assist with a physical examination.
Conditions:	Using an examining table.
	Given the following: equipment for the type of examination to be performed, patient examination gown, and drapes.
Standards:	Time: 20 minutes. Student completed procedure in _____ minutes.
	Accuracy: Satisfactory score on the Performance Evaluation Checklist.

Performance Evaluation Checklist

Trial 1	Trial 2	Point Value	Performance Standards
		•	Prepared examination room.
		•	Sanitized hands.
		•	Assembled all necessary equipment.
		•	Arranged instruments in a neat and orderly manner.
		•	Obtained the patient's medical record.
		•	Went to the waiting room, and asked the patient to come back.
		•	Escorted the patient to the examination room.
		•	Asked the patient to be seated.
		•	Greeted the patient and introduced yourself.
		•	Identified the patient by full name and date of birth.
		▷	Stated why a calm and friendly manner should be used.
		•	Seated yourself facing the patient at a distance of 3 to 4 feet.
		•	Obtained and recorded patient symptoms.
		•	Measured vital signs and charted results.
		▷	Stated the adult normal range for temperature (97° F to 99° F), pulse (60 to 100 beats/min), respiration (12 to 20 breaths/min), and blood pressure (<120/80 mm Hg).

Trial 1	Trial 2	Point Value	Performance Standards
		•	Measured weight and height, and charted results.
		•	Asked the patient whether he or she needs to void.
		▷	Stated why the patient should be asked to void.
		•	Instructed the patient to remove all clothing and put on an examining gown.
		•	Informed the patient that the physician will be in soon.
		•	Left the room to provide the patient with privacy.
		•	Made the patient's medical record available to the physician.
		•	Checked to make sure patient is ready to be seen.
		•	Informed the physician that the patient is ready.
		•	*Assisted the physician:*
		•	Ensured the patient was in a sitting position on examination table.
		•	Handed the ophthalmoscope to the physician when requested.
		•	Dimmed the lights when the physician was ready to use the ophthalmoscope.
		▷	Stated why the lights are dimmed.
		▷	Stated the proper use of the ophthalmoscope.
		•	Handed the otoscope to the examiner when requested.
		▷	Stated the proper use of the otoscope.
		•	Handed the tongue depressor to the examiner when requested.
		•	Offered reassurance to patient as needed.
		•	Positioned patient as required for examination of the remaining body systems.
			Assisted and instructed the patient:
		•	Allowed the patient to rest in a sitting position before getting off the examining table.
		▷	Stated why the patient should be allowed to rest before getting off the table.
		•	Assisted the patient off the examining table.
		•	Instructed the patient to get dressed.
		•	Provided the patient with any necessary instructions.
		▷	Stated what type of instructions may need to be relayed to the patient.
		•	Sanitized hands and charted any instructions given to the patient.
		•	Escorted the patient to the reception area.
			Cleaned the examination room:
		•	Discarded paper on the examining table and unrolled a fresh length.

Trial 1	Trial 2	Point Value	Performance Standards
		•	Discarded all disposable supplies into an appropriate waste container.
		•	Checked to make sure ample supplies are available.
		•	Removed reusable equipment for sanitization, sterilization, or disinfection.
		✶	Completed the procedure within 20 minutes.
			Totals

CHART	
Date	

Evaluation of Student Performance

EVALUATION CRITERIA			COMMENTS
Symbol	**Category**	**Point Value**	
✶	Critical Step	16 points	
•	Essential Step	6 points	
▷	Theory Question	2 points	

Score calculation: 100 points

− _____ points missed

_____ Score

Satisfactory score: 85 or above

CAAHEP Competencies Achieved

Psychomotor (Skills)

☑ I. 10. Assist physician with patient care.

☑ IV. 5. Instruct patients according to their needs to promote health maintenance and disease prevention.

☑ IV. 6. Prepare a patient for procedures and/or treatments.

☑ IV. 12. Develop and maintain a current list of community resources related to patients' health care needs.

☑ V. 9. Perform routine maintenance of office equipment with documentation.

☑ XI. 11. Use proper body mechanics.

Affective (Behavior)

☑ I. 3. Demonstrate respect for diversity in approaching patients and families.

☑ IV. 2. Apply active listening skills.

☑ IV. 3. Use appropriate body language and other nonverbal skills in communicating with patients, family, and staff.

☑ IV. 8. Analyze communications in providing appropriate responses or feedback.

☑ IV. 10. Demonstrate respect for individual diversity, incorporating awareness of one's own biases in areas including gender, race, religion, age, and economic status.

☑ X. 3. Demonstrate awareness of diversity in providing patient care.

ABHES Competencies Achieved

☑ 6. g. Analyze the effect of hereditary, cultural, and environmental influences.

☑ 8. x. Maintain medical facility.

☑ 8. y. Perform routine maintenance of administrative and clinical equipment.

☑ 8. z. Maintain inventory equipment and supplies.

☑ 8. aa. Are attentive, listen, and learn.

☑ 8. cc. Communicate on the recipient's level of comprehension.

☑ 8. ii. Recognize and respond to verbal and nonverbal communication.

☑ 8. kk. Adapt to individualized needs.

☑ 9. k. Prepare and maintain examination and treatment area.

☑ 9. l. Prepare patient for examinations and treatments.

☑ 9. m. Assist physician with routine and specialty examinations and treatments.

☑ 9. p. Advise patients of office policies and procedures.

☑ 9. r. Teach patients methods of health promotion and disease prevention.

6 Eye and Ear Assessment and Procedures

CHAPTER ASSIGNMENTS

√ After Completing	Date Due	Textbook Pages	TEXTBOOK ASSIGNMENTS	Possible Points	Points You Earned
		213–239	Read Chapter 6: Eye and Ear Assessment and Procedures		
		218 237	Read Case Study 1 Case Study 1 questions	5	
		223 237	Read Case Study 2 Case Study 2 questions	5	
		229 237–238	Read Case Study 3 Case Study 3 questions	5	
			Total points		

√ After Completing	Date Due	Study Guide Pages	STUDY GUIDE ASSIGNMENTS (CTA = Critical Thinking Activity)	Possible Points	Points You Earned
		231	Pretest	10	
		232 232	Key Term Assessment A. Definitions B. Word Parts (Add 1 point for each medical term)	13 11	
		233–236	Evaluation of Learning questions	34	
			Evolve Site: Chapter 6 Eye-Dentify: Diagram of Eye (Record points earned)		
		236	CTA A: Measuring Distance Visual Acuity	6	
		236–237	CTA B: Interpreting Visual Acuity Results	4	
		237	CTA C: Charting Visual Acuity Results	4	
			Evolve Site: Chapter 6 Can You Hear Me Now?: Diagram of Ear (Record points earned)		
		237–238	CTA D: Ear Procedures	8	

√ After Completing	Date Due	Study Guide Pages	STUDY GUIDE ASSIGNMENTS (CTA = Critical Thinking Activity)	Possible Points	Points You Earned
		238	CTA E: Dear Gabby	10	
		239	CTA F: Crossword Puzzle	23	
		240–242	CTA G: Eye and Ear Conditions	40	
			e Evolve Site: Chapter 6 Animations (2 points each)	8	
			e Evolve Site: Chapter 6 Nutrition Nugget: Nutrition and the Older Adult	10	
			e Evolve Site: Apply Your Knowledge questions	10	
		243–246	*e* Video Evaluation	70	
		231	[?] Posttest	10	
			ADDITIONAL ASSIGNMENTS		
			Total points		

√ When Assigned by Your Instructor	Study Guide Pages	Practices Required	LABORATORY ASSIGNMENTS (Procedure Number and Name)	Score*
	247	5	Practice for Competency 6-1: Assessing Distance Visual Acuity—Snellen Chart Textbook reference: pp. 220–222	
	249–250		Evaluation of Competency 6-1: Assessing Distance Visual Acuity—Snellen Chart	*
	247–248	3	Practice for Competency 6-2: Assessing Color Vision—Ishihara Test Textbook reference: pp. 222–223	
	251–253		Evaluation of Competency 6-2: Assessing Color Vision—Ishihara Test	*
	247	3	Practice for Competency 6-3: Performing an Eye Irrigation Textbook reference: pp. 224–226	
	255–257		Evaluation of Competency 6-3: Performing an Eye Irrigation	*
	247	3	Practice for Competency 6-4: Performing an Eye Instillation Textbook reference: pp. 226–227	
	259–260		Evaluation of Competency 6-4: Performing an Eye Instillation	*
	247	3	Practice for Competency 6-5: Performing an Ear Irrigation Textbook reference: pp. 233–235	
	261–263		Evaluation of Competency 6-5: Performing an Ear Irrigation	*
	247	3	Practice for Competency 6-6: Performing an Ear Instillation Textbook reference: pp. 235–236	
	265–266		Evaluation of Competency 6-6: Performing an Ear Instillation	*
			ADDITIONAL ASSIGNMENTS	

Notes

Name: _____ 85 010 (☺) _____ Date: _____

True or False

True 1. The outer layer of the eye composed of white connective tissue is known as the *sclera*.

False 2. A person who is farsighted has a condition known as *myopia*.

False 3. An optometrist can perform eye surgery.

True 4. The Snellen eye test is conducted at a distance of 20 feet.

false 5. The eustachian tube connects the nasopharynx to the inner ear.

True 6. An eye instillation may be performed to treat an eye infection.

False 7. The function of cerumen is to inhibit the growth of pathogens.

True 8. The most specific type of hearing test is the tuning fork test.

True 9. Serous otitis media can result in a conductive hearing loss.

True 10. An ear instillation may be performed to treat an ear infection.

❓ **POSTTEST**

True or False

✓ *True* 1. The function of the lens is to permit the entrance of light rays into the eye.

✓ *T* 2. Visual acuity refers to sharpness of vision. ✗

✓ *T* 3. Presbyopia is a decrease in the elasticity of the lens as a result of the aging process. ✗

✓ *True* 4. An optician fills prescriptions for eyeglasses.

✓ *True* 5. The Snellen Big E chart is used with school-aged children.

✓ *True* 6. The most common color vision defects are congenital.

✓ *False* 7. The cochlea functions in maintaining equilibrium.

✓ *True* 8. The range of frequencies for normal speech is 300 to 4000 Hz.

T 9. Intense noise can result in a sensorineural hearing loss. ✗

T 10. Tympanometry is used to diagnose patients with auditory nerve damage. ✗

KEY TERM ASSESSMENT

A. Definitions

Directions: Match each medical term (numbers) with its definition (letters).

- **L** 1. Astigmatism
- **J** 2. Audiometer
- **E** 3. Canthus
- **I** 4. Cerumen
- **C** 5. Hyperopia
- **M** 6. Impacted
- **G** 7. Instillation
- **A** 8. Irrigation
- **F** 9. Myopia
- **H** 10. Otoscope
- **B** 11. Presbyopia
- **D** 12. Refraction
- **K** 13. Tympanic membrane

A. The washing of a body canal with a flowing solution
B. A decrease in the elasticity of the lens that occurs with aging, resulting in a decreased ability to focus on close objects
C. Farsightedness
D. The deflection or bending of light rays by a lens
E. The junction of the eyelids at either corner of the eye
F. Nearsightedness
G. The dropping of a liquid into a body cavity
H. An instrument for examining the external ear canal and tympanic membrane
I. Earwax
J. An instrument used to quantitatively measure hearing acuity for the various frequencies of sound waves
K. A thin, semitransparent membrane located between the external ear canal and the middle ear that receives and transmits sound waves
L. A refractive error that causes distorted and blurred vision for both near and far objects due to a cornea that is oval-shaped
M. Wedged firmly together so as to be immovable

B. Word Parts

Directions: Indicate the meaning of each word part in the space provided. List as many medical terms as possible that incorporate the word part in the space provided.

Word Part	Meaning of Word Part	Medical Terms That Incorporate Word Part
1. a-	without	
2. stigma/a	point	
3. -ism	state of	
4. audi/o	hearing	
5. -meter	instrument used to measure	
6. hyper-	above	
7. -opia	vision	
8. ot/o	Ear	
9. -scope	to view	
10. tympan/o	eardrum	
11. -ic	pertaining to	

232

Chapter 6 Eye and Ear Assessment and Procedures

Copyright © 2015, 2012, 2008, 2004, 2000, 1995, 1990 by Saunders, an imprint of Elsevier Inc. All rights reserved.

Directions: Fill in each blank with the correct answer.

1. What is the name of the tough white outer layer of the eye?

   Sclera

2. What is the function of the lens?

   focusing light rays on retina

3. What is the function of the retina?

   transmission of light rays to brain, by optic nerve, to be interpreted

4. What parts of the eye are covered with conjunctiva?

   eyelids and front of eye except cornea.

5. What is visual acuity?

   accuteness or sharpness of vision

6. What types of symptoms may be experienced with myopia?

   difficulty seeing objects at a distance, squinting, headaches as a result of eyestrain.

7. What methods can be used to correct myopia?

   glasses, contacts, or laser surger

8. What causes an individual with astigmatism to have distorted and blurred vision?

   Refractive error

9. What are each of the following eye professionals qualified to perform?

   a. Ophthalmologist

   Can prescribe ophthalmic and systemic meds and can perform eye surgery

   b. Optometrist

   measures & prescribe corrective lenses for of refractive errors disorders & diseases of eyes & prescribed opthalmic meds.

   c. Optician

   interprets and fills prescription for glasses and contacts

10. What condition can be detected by measuring distance visual acuity?

myopia

11. What type of patient would warrant use of the Snellen Big E eye chart? (Give two examples.)

non readers, non-English speaking people

12. Explain the significance of the top number and bottom number next to each line of letters of the Snellen eye chart.

distance (20 ft) at which test is being conducted

13. List two conditions that can be detected by measuring near visual acuity.

Hyperopia & presbyopia

14. Explain the difference between congenital and acquired color vision defects.

congenital born w/ color deficiency that is inhererited
acquired acquired afther birth resulting from eye or brain injury
disease, or certain drugs

15. What is a polychromatic plate?

primary colored Dots arranged to form a numeral against a
backgrand of similar Dots of contrasting colors

16. List three reasons for performing eye irrigation.

washing away ~~foreing~~ foreign bodies, ocular dischargers or
harmful chemicals, releive inflamation through application or
heat

17. List three reasons for performing eye instillation.

eye infections, soothe irritated eye, dilate pupil

18. What is the function of the ear auricle?

recieve and collect sound waves & to direct them toward external
auditory canal

19. What is the function of cerumen?

lubricate & protect ear

20. Explain why the external auditory canal must be straightened when viewing it with an otoscope.

~~the~~ because its S-shaped

21. What is the normal appearance of the tympanic membrane?

pearly gray, semitransparent

22. What is the purpose of the eustachian tube?

Air pressure ~~between~~ the external atmosphere & middle ear is stabilized

23. What is the function of the semicircular canals?

maintain equilibrium

24. What is the range of frequencies for normal speech?

300 - 4000 hz

25. List five conditions that may cause conductive hearing loss.

obstruction in external auditory canal, swelling from external otitis foreign ~~body~~ bodies, Serous otitis meadia, acute otitis media

26. List four conditions that may result in sensorineural hearing loss.

hereditary, presbycusis, noise exposure over time tumors

27. How is hearing acuity tested with the gross screening test?

ask patient to repeat a simple word or series of numbers whispered from a distance of 1-2 feet from the ear.

28. What are the names of the hearing acuity tests that require the use of a tuning fork?

Weber test and Rinne test

29. What information is obtained through audiometry?

~~scribbled out~~ how extensive a hearing loss is and which frequencies are involve

235

Chapter **6** **Eye and Ear Assessment and Procedures**

30. What information is obtained through tympanometry?

cause of hearing loss

31. List three reasons for performing ear irrigation.

Cleanse external audiotory canal to remove cerumen discharge of foreign body, releive Inflamation, releive pain

32. List three reasons for performing ear instillation.

~~Aat~~ soften ear wax, releive pain, treat infections

33. Explain how impacted cerumen is removed from the ear.

Ear irrigation

34. Explain how to straighten the external auditory canal in an adult and in children 3 years old or younger.

gently pull baackward and ~~upward~~ downward ~~ear~~ from the earlobe

CRITICAL THINKING ACTIVITIES

A. Measuring Distance Visual Acuity

For each of the following situations, write **C** if the technique is correct and **I** if the technique is incorrect.

_____ 1. The patient is not given an opportunity to study the Snellen chart before beginning the test.

_____ 2. The Snellen chart is positioned at the medical assistant's eye level.

_____ 3. The patient is instructed to use his hand to cover the eye that is not being tested.

_____ 4. The medical assistant instructs the patient to close the eye that is not being tested.

_____ 5. The first line that the medical assistant asks the patient to identify is the 20/20 line.

_____ 6. The medical assistant observes the patient for signs of squinting or leaning forward during the test.

B. Interpreting Visual Acuity Results

1. A patient has a distance visual acuity reading of 20/30 in the right eye. Using this information, answer the following questions:

   a. How far was the patient from the eye chart?

   b. At what distance would a person with normal acuity be able to read this line?

2. A patient has a distance visual acuity reading of 20/10 in the left eye. Using this information, answer the following questions:

a. How far was the patient from the eye chart?

_____

b. At what distance would a person with normal acuity be able to read this line?

_____

C. Charting Visual Acuity Results

Properly chart the distance visual acuity results in the spaces provided. In all cases, the line indicated is the smallest line the patient could read at a distance of 20 feet.

1. The patient read the line marked 20/30 with the right eye with two errors, and with the left eye, he read the line marked 20/30 with one error. The patient was wearing corrective lenses.

_____

_____

2. The patient read the line marked 20/20 with the right eye with one error, and with the left eye, he read the line marked 20/20 with no errors. The patient was wearing corrective lenses.

_____

_____

3. The patient read the line marked 20/40 with the right eye with two errors, and with the left eye, she read the line marked 20/30 with one error. The patient exhibited squinting and frowning during the test. The patient was not wearing corrective lenses.

_____

_____

4. The patient read the line marked 20/15 with the right eye with no errors, and with the left eye, she read the line marked 20/20 with one error. The patient was not wearing corrective lenses.

_____

_____

D. Ear Procedures

Explain the principle for each of the following procedures.

Ear Irrigation

1. Positioning the patient's head so that it is tilted toward the affected ear

_____

_____

2. Cleansing the outer ear before irrigating

_____

_____

3. Straightening the external auditory canal

_____

_____

4. Injecting the irrigating solution toward the roof of the ear canal

_____

_____

5. Making sure not to obstruct the canal opening

_____

_____

Ear Instillation

6. Positioning the patient's head so that it is tilted toward the unaffected ear

_____

_____

7. Instructing the patient to lie on the unaffected side after the instillation

_____

_____

8. Placing a cotton wick in the patient's ear

_____

_____

E. Dear Gabby

Gabby has a middle ear infection and is not feeling well. She wants you to fill in for her. In the space provided, respond to the following letter.

Dear Gabby:

I am dating the sweetest and dearest man. "Mike" has only one flaw. He likes loud music. He had those big boom boxes installed in his car. When we drive somewhere in his car, he blasts the music. Sometimes, when we are driving down a street, people even turn around to see where the loud music is coming from. The music hurts my ears, and I cannot think straight. My ears even start ringing when we go on a trip. When I am talking to Mike, he says I mumble, and I have to speak extra loud around him. I keep telling Mike that the loud music is going to damage our hearing, but he says that we are way too young for that and that only old people have trouble hearing. Please help me Gabby, because I love going on trips with Mike, but not if my ears hurt afterward.

Signed, Ears Are Ringing

_____

_____

_____

_____

_____

_____

_____

_____

_____

_____

_____

F. Crossword Puzzle: Eye and Ear Assessment and Procedures

Directions: Complete the crossword puzzle by using the clues provided below.

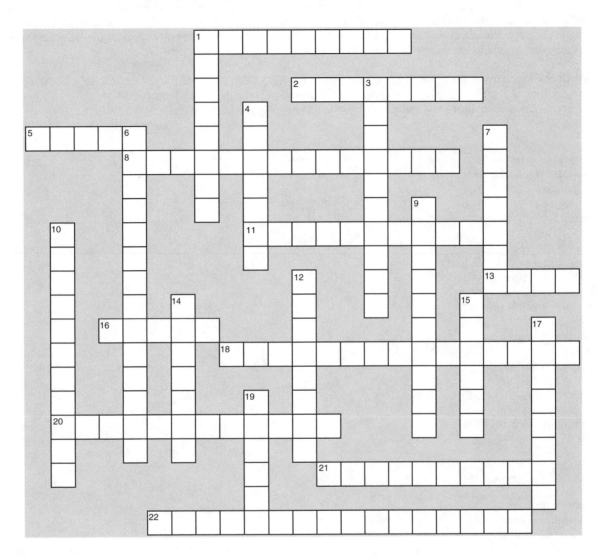

Across
1 Symptom of pink eye
2 Has an S-shape
5 Eye opening
8 Middle ear to the nasopharynx
11 Function of semicircular canals
13 Music that is too loud may cause this
16 An ossicle
18 Dr. that dx and tx eye disorders
20 Fixed stapes
21 Instrument that measures hearing
22 Drum in your ear

Down
1 Risk factor for eye disorders
3 Caught it!
4 Measurement unit for sound
6 20/200 OU c̄c
7 Earwax
9 Decreased lens elasticity
10 Controls shape of the lens
12 A cause of pink eye
14 Sound wave collector
15 Cannot see far away
17 Color-blind test
19 Transparent cover of the iris

G. Eye and Ear Conditions

1. You and your classmates work at a large clinic. It is National Eye and Ear Week. The physicians at your clinic ask you to develop for their patients informative, creative, and colorful brochures about eye and ear conditions. Choose a condition, and design a brochure using the blank Frequently Asked Questions (FAQ) brochure provided on the following page. Each student in the class should select a different topic. On a separate sheet of paper, write three true/false questions related to the information in your brochure.

2. Present your brochure to the class. After all the brochures have been presented, each student should ask his or her three questions to the entire class to see how well the class understands eye and ear conditions. (*Note:* You can take notes during the presentations and refer to them when answering the questions.)

Eye

1. Amblyopia (lazy eye)
2. Age-related macular degeneration
3. Astigmatism
4. Blepharitis
5. Cataracts
6. CMV retinitis
7. Corneal ulcer
8. Corneal abrasion
9. Strabismus (crossed-eyed)
10. Diabetic retinopathy
11. Drooping eyelids (ptosis)
12. Dry eyes
13. Floaters and spots
14. Glaucoma
15. Keratoconus
16. Ocular hypertension
17. Presbycusis
18. Retinal detachment
19. Retinitis pigmentosa
20. Stye

Ear

1. Acute mastoiditis
2. External otitis
3. Meniere's disease
4. Noise-induced hearing loss
5. Serous otitis media

FAQ ON:

Q: A:

Q: A:

Q: A:

Q: A:

Q:

A:

Q:

A:

Illustration

Q:

A:

Q:

A:

Name: _____

Directions:

a. Watch the indicated videos.
b. Mark each true statement with a T and each false statement with an F. For each false statement, change the wording of the question so that it becomes a true statement.

Video: Procedure 6-1: Assessing Distance Visual Acuity

_____ 1. The distance visual acuity test is performed to screen for the presence of hyperopia.

_____ 2. Preschool children, non–English-speaking people, and nonreaders are tested using a Snellen Big E chart.

_____ 3. The Snellen eye test is performed at a distance of 10 feet.

_____ 4. The patient should be instructed to wear his or her glasses or contact lenses for a distance visual acuity test unless they are for reading.

_____ 5. The occluder should be placed over the eye being tested.

_____ 6. Squinting in the eye being tested can temporarily improve vision and can lead to inaccurate test results.

_____ 7. During the test, you should check for squinting, head tilting, and eye watering.

_____ 8. If the patient misses more than three letters on a line, the previous line is recorded.

_____ 9. Chart whether or not the patient is wearing corrective lenses during the test.

_____ 10. The abbreviation for the right eye is OS.

Video: Procedure 6-2: Assessing Color Vision

_____ 1. The Ishihara test is a convenient and accurate method to detect congenital color blindness and red-green blindness.

_____ 2. Patients with color vision defects see no number at all or a different number on the plates.

_____ 3. Using natural lighting may change the shades of the colors on the plates, and this could cause an inaccurate reading.

_____ 4. The first plate is a practice plate that is designed to be read correctly by everyone.

_____ 5. Hold the first plate 60 inches away from the patient at a right angle to the patient's line of vision.

_____ 6. The patient should be given 15 seconds to identify each plate.

_____ 7. Do not allow the patient to touch the plate with his or her fingers because any dirt or grime on the fingers can alter the colors over time.

_____ 8. Chart an "X" if the patient reads a plate correctly.

_____ 9. Chart "Traceable" if the patient could correctly trace a winding line.

_____ 10. Store the book in a closed position to keep light from fading the colors on the plates.

Video: Procedure 6-3: Performing an Eye Irrigation

_____ 1. An eye irrigation involves washing the eye with a flowing solution.

_____ 2. An eye irrigation may be performed to wash away foreign particles, ocular discharges, or harmful chemicals.

_____ 3. If both eyes are to be irrigated, one set of equipment is used to prevent cross-infection from one eye to the other.

_____ 4. Normal saline, also known as sodium chloride, usually is used to irrigate the eye.

_____ 5. Check the solution label three times.

_____ 6. If the solution is outdated, it may produce undesirable effects.

_____ 7. Warm the solution to room temperature.

_____ 8. Palm the label of the container to prevent the solution from dripping on the label and obscuring it or loosening the label.

_____ 9. Ask the patient to tilt his or her head to the side in the direction of the unaffected eye.

_____ 10. Before irrigating, cleanse the eyelids from the outer to the inner canthus.

_____ 11. Instruct the patient to keep both eyes open during the procedure.

_____ 12. Gently release the solution onto the eye at the inner canthus.

_____ 13. Direct the solution toward the cornea of the eye.

_____ 14. Do not allow the tip of the syringe to touch the eye because this can cause an injury.

_____ 15. Following the procedure, dry the eyelids with a gauze pad.

Video: Procedure 6-4: Performing an Eye Instillation

_____ 1. An eye instillation involves the dropping of a liquid into the lower conjunctival sac of the eye.

_____ 2. An eye instillation may be performed to treat infection, soothe irritation, dilate the pupil, or anesthetize the eye during examination or treatment.

_____ 3. Never place a medication in the eye unless it says _otic_ or _eye_ to avoid injury to the eye.

_____ 4. If the patient wears contact lenses, they can be left in for the procedure.

_____ 5. If the medication requires mixing, roll or shake the container well.

_____ 6. Ask the patient to look down to keep the dropper from touching the cornea and to keep the patient from blinking when the drops are instilled.

_____ 7. Invert the eye dropper container and hold the tip of the dropper approximately 2 inches above the eye sac.

_____ 8. Placing the drops directly on the eyeball can be uncomfortable for the patient.

_____ 9. Ask the patient to close his or her eyes gently and move the eyeballs to distribute the medication over the entire eye.

_____ 10. The abbreviation for a drop is dp.

Video: Procedure 6-5: Performing an Ear Irrigation

_____ 1. Ear irrigation is washing of the inner ear with a flowing solution.

_____ 2. Ear irrigations are performed to cleanse the external auditory canal to remove cerumen, discharge, or a foreign body.

_____ 3. Impacted cerumen can be softened by instilling warm saltwater into the ear.

_____ 4. Normal saline, also known as sodium chloride, typically is used to irrigate the ear.

_____ 5. Ear irrigation should never be performed if the tympanic membrane is perforated.

_____ 6. If the irrigating solution is too hot or too cold, it may stimulate the inner ear and make the patient dizzy.

_____ 7. Remove the cap of the irrigating solution container and place it on a flat surface with the open end facing downward to prevent contamination of the cap.

_____ 8. Pour the solution into the basin at a height of approximately 12 inches to reduce splashing.

_____ 9. The patient should be asked to tilt his or her head toward the affected ear to allow gravity to help the solution flow out of the ear and into the basin.

_____ 10. Expel air from the syringe to avoid forcing air into the patient's ear; this can be uncomfortable for the patient.

_____ 11. To straighten the ear canal of an adult or a child over the age of three, gently pull the ear downward and backward.

_____ 12. Make sure the tip of the syringe does not obstruct the canal to prevent patient discomfort and possible injury to the tympanic membrane.

_____ 13. Inject the irrigating solution directly onto the tympanic membrane.

_____ 14. The patient may experience a minimal amount of dizziness, fullness, and warmth as the ear solution comes in contact with the tympanic membrane.

_____ 15. After the procedure, ask the patient to lie with the affected side downward to allow any remaining solution to drain out.

Video: Procedure 6-6: Performing an Ear Instillation

_____ 1. An ear instillation involves the dropping of a liquid into the middle ear.

_____ 2. Ear instillations are performed to soften impacted cerumen, to combat infection with the use of antibiotic eardrops, and to relieve pain.

_____ 3. The medication label must bear the word _otic_ or _eardrops_, indicating it is for the ear.

_____ 4. Position the patient in a prone position.

_____ 5. Warm the eardrops to body temperature by placing the medication container in hot water.

_____ 6. If the drops are too cold or too warm, they may stimulate the inner ear and cause the patient to become dizzy.

_____ 7. If the medication requires mixing, shake the container well.

_____ 8. Tilt the patient's head in the direction of the unaffected ear to allow gravity to help the medication flow into the ear canal.

_____ 9. Straighten the external ear canal to permit the medication to reach all areas of the canal.

_____ 10. After the procedure, instruct the patient to keep his or her head tilted toward the unaffected side for 2 to 3 minutes to prevent the medication from running out of the ear.

PRACTICE FOR COMPETENCY

Eye Assessment and Procedures

Procedure 6-1: Distance Visual Acuity. Assess distance visual acuity using a Snellen eye chart, and record results in the chart provided. Circle any readings that indicate distance visual acuity above or below average.

Procedure 6-2: Color Vision. Assess color vision, and record results in the Ishihara charting grid provided. Circle any abnormal results.

Procedure 6-3: Eye Irrigation. Perform an eye irrigation, and record the procedure in the chart provided.

Procedure 6-4: Eye Instillation. Perform an eye instillation, and record the procedure in the chart provided.

Ear Procedures

Procedure 6-5: Ear Irrigation. Perform an ear irrigation, and record the procedure in the chart provided.

Procedure 6-6: Ear Instillation. Perform an ear instillation, and record the procedure in the chart provided.

CHART	
Date	

CHARTING GRID FOR THE ISHIHARA TEST

Plate No.	Normal Person	Results
1	12	
2	8	
3	5	
4	29	
5	74	
6	7	
7	45	
8	2	
9	X	
10	16	
11	Traceable	
Date:		
Evaluated by:		

CHARTING GRID FOR THE ISHIHARA TEST

Plate No.	Normal Person	Results
1	12	
2	8	
3	5	
4	29	
5	74	
6	7	
7	45	
8	2	
9	X	
10	16	
11	Traceable	
Date:		
Evaluated by:		

Procedure 6-1: Assessing Distance Visual Acuity—Snellen Chart

Name: _____ Date: _____

Evaluated by: _____ Score: _____

Performance Objective

Outcome:	Assess distance visual acuity.
Conditions:	Given the following: Snellen eye chart, eye occluder, and an antiseptic wipe.
Standards:	Time: 5 minutes. Student completed procedure in _____ minutes.
	Accuracy: Satisfactory score on the Performance Evaluation Checklist.

Performance Evaluation Checklist

Trial 1	Trial 2	Point Value	Performance Standards
		•	Sanitized hands.
		•	Assembled the equipment.
		•	Disinfected the eye occluder with an antiseptic wipe.
		•	Greeted the patient and introduced yourself.
		•	Identified the patient and explained the procedure.
		•	Determined whether the patient wears corrective lenses and instructed the patient to leave them on during the test.
		•	Positioned the patient 20 feet from the eye chart.
		•	Positioned the center of the eye chart at the patient's eye level.
		•	Instructed the patient to cover the left eye with the occluder and to keep the left eye open.
		▷	Stated how the occluder should be positioned if the patient wears glasses.
		▷	Explained why the patient's left eye should remain open.
		•	Instructed the patient not to squint during the test.
		▷	Explained why the patient should not squint during the test.
		•	Asked the patient to identify the 20/70 line, using the right eye.
		▷	Stated why the test should begin with a line that is above the 20/20 line.
		•	Proceeded down the chart if the patient identified the 20/70 line or proceeded up the chart if the patient was unable to identify the 20/70 line.
		•	Continued until the smallest line of letters that the patient could read was reached.
		•	Observed the patient for any unusual symptoms.
		•	Jotted down the numbers next to the smallest line read by the patient.
		•	Asked the patient to cover the right eye and to keep the right eye open.
		•	Measured visual acuity in the left eye.

Trial 1	Trial 2	Point Value	Performance Standards
		•	Jotted down the numbers next to the smallest line read by the patient.
		✳	The visual acuity measurements were identical to the evaluator's measurements.
		•	Charted the results correctly.
		•	Disinfected the occluder with an antiseptic wipe.
		•	Sanitized hands.
		✳	Completed the procedure within 5 minutes.
			Totals

CHART	
Date	

Evaluation of Student Performance

EVALUATION CRITERIA			COMMENTS
Symbol	**Category**	**Point Value**	
✳	Critical Step	16 points	
•	Essential Step	6 points	
▷	Theory Question	2 points	

Score calculation: 100 points

− _____ points missed

_____ Score

Satisfactory score: 85 or above

CAAHEP Competencies Achieved

Psychomotor (Skills)

☑ IV. 6. Prepare a patient for procedures and/or treatments.

Affective (Behavior)

☑ I. 2. Use language/verbal skills that enable patient's understanding.

☑ IV. 7. Demonstrate recognition of the patient's level of understanding in communications.

ABHES Competencies Achieved

☑ 8. cc. Communicate on the recipient's level of comprehension.

☑ 9. l. Prepare patient for examinations and treatments.

Procedure 6-2: Assessing Color Vision—Ishihara Test

Name: _____ Date: _____

Evaluated by: _____ Score: _____

Performance Objective

Outcome:	Assess color vision.
Conditions:	Given an Ishihara book of color plates and a cotton swab.
Standards:	Time: 10 minutes. Student completed procedure in _____ minutes.
	Accuracy: Satisfactory score on the Performance Evaluation Checklist.

Performance Evaluation Checklist

Trial 1	Trial 2	Point Value	Performance Standards
		•	Sanitized hands.
		•	Assembled the equipment.
		•	Conducted the test in a quiet room illuminated by natural daylight.
		▷	Stated why natural daylight should be used.
		•	Greeted the patient and introduced yourself.
		•	Identified the patient.
		•	Explained the procedure using the practice plate.
		▷	Stated the purpose of the practice plate.
		•	Held the first plate 30 inches from the patient at a right angle to the patient's line of vision.
		•	Instructed the patient to keep both eyes open.
		•	Told the patient that he or she would have 3 seconds to identify each plate.
		•	Asked the patient to identify the number on the plate.
		•	Asked the patient to trace plates with winding lines with a cotton swab.
		▷	Stated why a cotton swab should be used to make the tracing.
		•	Recorded the results after identification of each plate.
		•	Continued until the patient viewed all plates.
		•	Charted the results correctly.
		✷	The results were identical to the evaluator's results.
		•	Returned the Ishihara book to its proper place, storing it in a closed position.
		▷	Explained why the book should be stored in a closed position.
		✷	Completed the procedure within 10 minutes.
			Totals

Trial 1	Trial 2	Point Value	Performance Standards
			CHART
Date			

CHART		
Plate No.	**Normal Person**	**Results**
1	12	
2	8	
3	5	
4	29	
5	74	
6	7	
7	45	
8	2	
9	X	
10	16	
11	Traceable	
Date:		
Evaluated by:		

Evaluation of Student Performance

EVALUATION CRITERIA			COMMENTS
Symbol	**Category**	**Point Value**	
✶	Critical Step	16 points	
•	Essential Step	6 points	
▷	Theory Question	2 points	

Score calculation: 100 points

− _____ points missed

_____ Score

Satisfactory score: 85 or above

CAAHEP Competencies Achieved
Psychomotor (Skills)
☑ IV. 6. Prepare a patient for procedures and/or treatments.
Affective (Behavior)
☑ I. 2. Use language/verbal skills that enable patients' understanding.
☑ IV. 7. Demonstrate recognition of the patient's level of understanding in communications.

ABHES Competencies Achieved
☑ 8. cc. Communicate on the recipient's level of comprehension.
☑ 9. 1. Prepare patient for examinations and treatments.

Notes

e **Procedure 6-3: Performing an Eye Irrigation**

Name: _____ Date: _____

Evaluated by: _____ Score: _____

Performance Objective

Outcome:	Perform an eye irrigation.
Conditions:	Given the following: disposable (nonpowdered) gloves, irrigating solution, solution container, disposable rubber bulb syringe, basin, moisture-resistant towel, and sterile gauze pads.
Standards:	Time: 5 minutes. Student completed procedure in _____ minutes.
	Accuracy: Satisfactory score on the Performance Evaluation Checklist.

Performance Evaluation Checklist

Trial 1	Trial 2	Point Value	Performance Standards
		•	Sanitized hands.
		•	Assembled the equipment.
		•	Checked the solution label with the physician's instructions.
		•	Checked the expiration date of the solution.
		▷	Stated the reason for checking the expiration date.
		•	Warmed the irrigating solution to body temperature.
		▷	Explained why the solution should be at body temperature.
		•	Checked the label a second time, and poured the solution into a basin.
		•	Checked the label a third time before returning the container to storage.
		•	Greeted the patient and introduced yourself.
		•	Identified the patient and explained the procedure.
		•	Asked the patient to remove glasses or contact lenses.
		•	Positioned the patient in a lying or sitting position.
		•	Placed a moisture-resistant towel on the patient's shoulder.
		•	Positioned a basin tightly against the patient's cheek under the affected eye.
		•	Asked the patient to tilt head in the direction of the affected eye and hold the basin in place.
		▷	Explained why the patient's head is turned in the direction of the affected eye.
		•	Applied nonpowdered gloves.
		▷	Stated why nonpowdered gloves should be used.
		•	Cleansed the eyelids from inner to outer canthus.
		▷	Stated why eyelids are cleansed.

Trial 1	Trial 2	Point Value	Performance Standards
		•	Filled irrigating syringe.
		•	Instructed the patient to keep both eyes open and to look at a focal point.
		▷	Stated the reason for looking at a focal point.
		•	Separated the eyelids.
		•	Held the tip of the syringe 1 inch above the eye at the inner canthus.
		•	Allowed solution to flow over the eye at a moderate rate from the inner canthus to the outer canthus and directed solution to the lower conjunctiva.
		▷	Explained why the solution should be directed toward the lower conjunctiva.
		•	Did not allow syringe to touch the eye.
		•	Refilled the syringe and continued irrigating until the desired results were obtained or all the solution was used.
		•	Dried the eyelids with a gauze pad from the inner to outer canthus.
		•	Removed gloves and sanitized hands.
		•	Charted the procedure correctly.
		•	Returned the equipment.
		✶	Completed the procedure within 5 minutes.
			Totals
CHART			
Date			

Evaluation of Student Performance

EVALUATION CRITERIA			COMMENTS
Symbol	**Category**	**Point Value**	
✶	Critical Step	16 points	
•	Essential Step	6 points	
▷	Theory Question	2 points	

Score calculation: 100 points

− _____ points missed

_____ Score

Satisfactory score: 85 or above

CAAHEP Competencies Achieved
Psychomotor (Skills)
☑ II. 1. Prepare proper dosages of medication for administration.
☑ IV. 6. Prepare a patient for procedures and/or treatments.
Affective (Behavior)
☑ II. 1. Verify ordered doses/dosages prior to administration.
☑ IV. 5. Demonstrate sensitivity appropriate to the message being delivered.

ABHES Competencies Achieved
☑ 8. bb. Are impartial and show empathy when dealing with patients.
☑ 9. d. Recognize and understand various treatment protocols.
☑ 9. l. Prepare patient for examinations and treatments.

Notes

Procedure 6-4: Performing an Eye Instillation

Name: _____   Date: _____

Evaluated by: _____   Score: _____

Performance Objective

Outcome:	Perform an eye instillation.
Conditions:	Given the following: disposable (nonpowdered) gloves, ophthalmic medication, tissues, and gauze pads.
Standards:	Time: 5 minutes. Student completed procedure in _____ minutes.
	Accuracy: Satisfactory score on the Performance Evaluation Checklist.

Performance Evaluation Checklist

Trial 1	Trial 2	Point Value	Performance Standards
		•	Sanitized hands.
		•	Assembled the equipment.
		•	Checked the drug label when removing it from storage.
		▷	Stated what word must appear on the medication label.
		•	Checked the drug label and dosage against the physician's instructions.
		•	Checked the expiration date of the medication.
		•	Greeted the patient and introduced yourself.
		•	Identified the patient and explained the procedure.
		•	Positioned the patient in a sitting or supine position.
		•	Applied nonpowdered gloves.
		•	Prepared the medication.
		•	Checked the drug label and removed the cap.
		•	Asked the patient to look up and exposed the lower conjunctival sac.
		▷	Explained the reason for asking patient to look up.
		•	Drew the skin of the cheek downward and exposed the conjunctival sac.
		•	Inserted the medication correctly.
		▷	Explained how to instill eyedrops and ointment.
		•	Instructed the patient to close his or her eyes gently and move the eyeballs.
		▷	Stated the reason for closing the eyes and moving the eyeballs.
		•	Told the patient that the instillation may temporarily blur vision.
		•	Dried the eyelids with a gauze pad from the inner to outer canthus.

Trial 1	Trial 2	Point Value	Performance Standards
		•	Removed gloves and sanitized hands.
		•	Charted the procedure correctly.
		•	Returned the equipment.
		✳	Completed the procedure within 5 minutes.
			Totals

CHART	
Date	

Evaluation of Student Performance

EVALUATION CRITERIA			COMMENTS
Symbol	Category	Point Value	
✳	Critical Step	16 points	
•	Essential Step	6 points	
▷	Theory Question	2 points	

Score calculation: 100 points

− _____ points missed

_____ Score

Satisfactory score: 85 or above

CAAHEP Competencies Achieved

Psychomotor (Skills)

☑ II. 1. Prepare proper dosages of medication for administration.

☑ IV. 6. Prepare a patient for procedures and/or treatments.

Affective (Behavior)

☑ II. 1. Verify ordered doses/dosages prior to administration.

☑ IV. 5. Demonstrate sensitivity appropriate to the message being delivered.

ABHES Competencies Achieved

☑ 8. bb. Are impartial and show empathy when dealing with patients.

☑ 9. d. Recognize and understand various treatment protocols.

☑ 9. l. Prepare patient for examinations and treatments.

EVALUATION OF COMPETENCY

e Procedure 6-5: Performing an Ear Irrigation

Name: _____   Date: _____

Evaluated by: _____   Score: _____

Performance Objective

Outcome:	Perform an ear irrigation.
Conditions:	Given the following: disposable gloves, irrigating solution, solution container, irrigating syringe, ear basin, moisture-resistant towel, gauze pads, and ear wick.
Standards:	Time: 10 minutes. Student completed procedure in _____ minutes.
	Accuracy: Satisfactory score on the Performance Evaluation Checklist.

Performance Evaluation Checklist

Trial 1	Trial 2	Point Value	Performance Standards
		•	Sanitized hands.
		•	Assembled the equipment.
		•	Checked the label of the irrigating solution with the physician's instructions.
		•	Checked the expiration date of the solution.
		•	Warmed the irrigating solution to body temperature.
		▷	Stated the reason for warming the irrigating solution.
		•	Checked the label a second time, and poured the solution into a basin.
		•	Checked the label a third time before returning the container to storage.
		•	Greeted the patient and introduced yourself.
		•	Identified the patient and explained the procedure.
		•	Positioned the patient in a sitting position.
		•	Placed a towel on the patient's shoulder under the ear to be irrigated.
		•	Positioned a basin under the affected ear and asked the patient to hold it in place.
		•	Asked the patient to tilt his or her head toward the affected ear.
		▷	Explained why the head should be tilted toward the affected ear.
		•	Applied gloves.
		•	Cleansed the outer ear.
		▷	Explained why the outer ear should be cleansed.
		•	Filled the irrigating syringe.
		•	Expelled air from the syringe.

Trial 1	Trial 2	Point Value	Performance Standards
		▷	Explained why air should be expelled from the syringe.
		•	Properly straightened the ear canal.
		▷	Stated why the ear canal must be straightened.
		•	Inserted the syringe tip into the ear.
		•	Did not insert the syringe too deeply.
		•	Made sure that the tip of the syringe did not obstruct the canal opening.
		▷	Stated why the canal should not be obstructed.
		•	Injected the irrigating solution toward the roof of the ear canal.
		▷	Stated why solution should be injected toward the roof of the canal.
		•	Refilled the syringe and continued irrigating until the desired results were obtained or all the solution was used.
		•	Observed the returning solution to note the material present and the amount.
		•	Dried the outside of the ear with a gauze pad.
		•	Informed the patient that the ear will feel sensitive.
		•	Instructed the patient to lie on the affected side on treatment table.
		▷	Explained why the patient should lie on the affected side.
		•	Inserted a cotton wick loosely in the ear canal for 15 minutes.
		▷	Stated the purpose of the cotton wick.
		•	Removed gloves and sanitized hands.
		•	Charted the procedure correctly.
		•	Returned the equipment.
		✳	Completed the procedure within 10 minutes.
			Totals
CHART			
Date			

Evaluation of Student Performance

EVALUATION CRITERIA			COMMENTS
Symbol	**Category**	**Point Value**	
✱	Critical Step	16 points	
•	Essential Step	6 points	
▷	Theory Question	2 points	

Score calculation: 100 points

$-$ _____ points missed

_____ Score

Satisfactory score: 85 or above

CAAHEP Competencies Achieved

Psychomotor (Skills)

☑ II. 1. Prepare proper dosages of medication for administration.

☑ IV. 6. Prepare a patient for procedures and/or treatments.

Affective (Behavior)

☑ II. 1. Verify ordered doses/dosages prior to administration.

☑ IV. 5. Demonstrate sensitivity appropriate to the message being delivered.

ABHES Competencies Achieved

☑ 8. bb. Are impartial and show empathy when dealing with patients.

☑ 9. d. Recognize and understand various treatment protocols.

☑ 9. l. Prepare patient for examinations and treatments.

Notes

Procedure 6-6: Performing an Ear Instillation

Name: _____ Date: _____

Evaluated by: _____ Score: _____

Performance Objective

Outcome:	Perform an ear instillation.
Conditions:	Given the following: disposable gloves, otic medication, and gauze pad.
Standards:	Time: 5 minutes. Student completed procedure in _____ minutes.
	Accuracy: Satisfactory score on the Performance Evaluation Checklist.

Performance Evaluation Checklist

Trial 1	Trial 2	Point Value	Performance Standards
		•	Sanitized hands.
		•	Assembled the equipment.
		•	Checked the drug label when removing the medication from storage.
		▷	Stated what word must appear on the medication label.
		•	Checked the drug label and dosage against the physician's instructions.
		•	Checked the expiration date of the medication.
		▷	Explained what may occur if the medication is outdated.
		•	Greeted the patient and introduced yourself.
		•	Identified the patient and explained the procedure.
		•	Positioned the patient in a sitting position.
		•	Warmed the eardrops with your hands.
		•	Applied gloves.
		•	Mixed the medication if required, by shaking the container.
		•	Checked the drug label and removed the cap.
		•	Asked the patient to tilt the head in the direction of the unaffected ear.
		•	Properly straightened the ear canal.
		▷	Stated the reason for straightening the canal.
		•	Placed tip of dropper at the opening of the ear canal and inserted the proper amount of medication.
		•	Instructed the patient to lie on the unaffected side for 2 to 3 minutes.
		▷	Explained why the patient should lie on the unaffected side.

Trial 1	Trial 2	Point Value	Performance Standards
		•	Placed a moistened cotton wick loosely in the ear canal for 15 minutes.
		▷	Stated the reason for moistening the wick.
		•	Removed gloves and sanitized hands.
		•	Charted the procedure correctly.
		•	Returned the equipment.
		✳	Completed the procedure within 5 minutes.
			Totals
CHART			
Date			

Evaluation of Student Performance

EVALUATION CRITERIA			COMMENTS
Symbol	**Category**	**Point Value**	
✳	Critical Step	16 points	
•	Essential Step	6 points	
▷	Theory Question	2 points	

Score calculation: 100 points

− _____ points missed

_____ Score

Satisfactory score: 85 or above

CAAHEP Competencies Achieved

Psychomotor (Skills)

☑ II. 1. Prepare proper dosages of medication for administration.

☑ IV. 6. Prepare a patient for procedures and/or treatments.

Affective (Behavior)

☑ II. 1. Verify ordered doses/dosages prior to administration.

☑ IV. 5. Demonstrate sensitivity appropriate to the message being delivered.

ABHES Competencies Achieved

☑ 8. bb. Are impartial and show empathy when dealing with patients.

☑ 9. d. Recognize and understand various treatment protocols.

☑ 9. l. Prepare patient for examinations and treatments.

---

7 Physical Agents to Promote Tissue Healing

CHAPTER ASSIGNMENTS

√ After Completing	Date Due	Textbook Pages	TEXTBOOK ASSIGNMENTS	Possible Points	Points You Earned
		240–266	Read Chapter 7: Physical Agents to Promote Tissue Healing		
		243 264	Read Case Study 1 Case Study 1 questions	5	
		255 264	Read Case Study 2 Case Study 2 questions	5	
		258 264	Read Case Study 3 Case Study 3 questions	5	
			Total points		

√ After Completing	Date Due	Study Guide Pages	STUDY GUIDE ASSIGNMENTS (CTA = Critical Thinking Activity)	Possible Points	Points You Earned
		271	Pretest	10	
		272	Term Key Term Assessment	15	
		272–275	Evaluation of Learning questions	28	
		276	CTA A: Dear Gabby	10	
		276–277	CTA B: Fractures and Sprains	12	
		277–279	CTA C: Cast Care	20	
		281	CTA D: Crutch Guidelines	8	
		282	CTA E: Accessibility for Physical Disabilities	7	
		283	CTA F: Crossword Puzzle	26	
		284–286	CTA G: Bone and Joint Conditions	40	
			Evolve Site: Chapter 7 Animations (2 points each)	10	
			Evolve Site: Chapter 7 Quiz Show (Record points earned)		

√ After Completing	Date Due	Study Guide Pages	STUDY GUIDE ASSIGNMENTS (CTA = Critical Thinking Activity)	Possible Points	Points You Earned
			ⓔ Evolve Site: Chapter 7 Nutrition Nugget: Fuel for Activity	10	
			ⓔ Evolve Site: Apply Your Knowledge questions	10	
		287–289	ⓔ Video Evaluation	63	
		271	🗎 Posttest	10	
			ADDITIONAL ASSIGNMENTS		
			Total points		

√ When Assigned by Your Instructor	Study Guide Pages	Practices Required	LABORATORY ASSIGNMENTS (Procedure Number and Name)	Score*
	291–292	3	Practice for Competency 7-1: Applying a Heating Pad Textbook reference: pp. 244–245	
	293–294		Evaluation of Competency 7-1: Applying a Heating Pad	*
	291–292	3	Practice for Competency 7-2: Applying a Hot Soak Textbook reference: pp. 245–246	
	295–296		Evaluation of Competency 7-2: Applying a Hot Soak	*
	291–292	3	Practice for Competency 7-3: Applying a Hot Compress Textbook reference: pp. 246–247	
	297–298		Evaluation of Competency 7-3: Applying a Hot Compress	*
	291–292	3	Practice for Competency 7-4: Applying an Ice Bag Textbook reference: pp. 247–248	
	299–300		Evaluation of Competency 7-4: Applying an Ice Bag	*
	291–292	3	Practice for Competency 7-5: Applying a Cold Compress Textbook reference: pp. 248–249	
	301–302		Evaluation of Competency 7-5: Applying a Cold Compress	*
	291–292	3	Practice for Competency 7-6: Applying a Chemical Pack Textbook reference: pp. 249–250	
	303–304		Evaluation of Competency 7-6: Applying a Chemical Pack	*
	291–292	3	Practice for Competency 7-7: Measuring for Axillary Crutches Textbook reference: p. 259	
	305–306		Evaluation of Competency 7-7: Measuring for Axillary Crutches	*
	291–292	3 × for each gait	Practice for Competency 7-8: Instructing a Patient in Crutch Gaits Textbook reference: pp. 260–262	
	307–309		Evaluation of Competency 7-8: Instructing a Patient in Crutch Gaits	*

√ When Assigned by Your Instructor	Study Guide Pages	Practices Required	LABORATORY ASSIGNMENTS (Procedure Number and Name)	Score*
	291–292	Cane: 3 Walker: 3	Practice for Competency 7-9 and 7-10: Instructing a Patient in the Use of a Cane and Walker Textbook reference: p. 263	
	311–312		Evaluation of Competency 7-9 and 7-10: Instructing a Patient in the Use of a Cane and Walker	*
			ADDITIONAL ASSIGNMENTS	

Name: _____ Date: _____

? PRETEST

True or False

_____ 1. A hot compress is an example of moist heat.

_____ 2. Erythema is redness of the skin caused by dilation of superficial blood vessels.

_____ 3. The local application of cold may be used to relieve muscle spasms.

_____ 4. Chemical cold packs should be stored in the refrigerator.

_____ 5. An orthodontist is a physician who specializes in the diagnosis and treatment of disorders of the musculoskeletal system.

_____ 6. The most frequent reason for applying a cast is to aid in the nonsurgical correction of a deformity.

_____ 7. Numbness of the fingers or toes may indicate that a cast is too tight.

_____ 8. A coat hanger can be used to scratch under a cast if itching occurs.

_____ 9. Ambulation refers to the inability to walk.

_____ 10. A patient using crutches should be instructed to support his or her weight against the axilla.

? POSTTEST

True or False

_____ 1. The recommended time for the application of heat is 15 to 30 minutes.

_____ 2. The local application of heat results in constriction of blood vessels in the area to which it is applied.

_____ 3. The most frequent cause of low back pain is poor posture.

_____ 4. An ice bag should be filled with large pieces of ice.

_____ 5. If axillary crutches have been fitted properly, the elbow will be flexed at an angle of 30 degrees.

_____ 6. A wet cast can cause a pressure area to occur.

_____ 7. The purpose of cast padding is to prevent pressure areas.

_____ 8. It usually takes 10 to 12 weeks for a fracture to heal.

_____ 9. Incorrectly fitted crutches may cause crutch palsy.

_____ 10. A cane should be held on the strong side of the body.

Chapter **7** **Physical Agents to Promote Tissue Healing**

Directions: Match each medical term (numbers) with its definition (letters).

_____ 1. Ambulation

_____ 2. Brace

_____ 3. Compress

_____ 4. Edema

_____ 5. Erythema

_____ 6. Exudate

_____ 7. Long arm cast

_____ 8. Maceration

_____ 9. Orthopedist

_____ 10. Short leg cast

_____ 11. Soak

_____ 12. Splint

_____ 13. Sprain

_____ 14. Strain

_____ 15. Suppuration

A. A discharge produced by the body's tissues
B. An overstretching of a muscle caused by trauma
C. A soft, moist, absorbent cloth that is folded in several layers and applied to a part of the body in the local application of heat or cold
D. Walking or moving from one place to another
E. The direct immersion of a body part in water or a medicated solution
F. The retention of fluid in the tissues, resulting in swelling
G. An orthopedic device used to support and hold a part of the body in the correct position to allow functioning and healing
H. A cast that extends from the axilla to the fingers
I. Reddening of the skin caused by dilation of superficial blood vessels in the skin
J. Trauma to a joint that causes injury to the ligaments
K. The process of pus formation
L. A physician who specializes in the diagnosis and treatment of disorders of the musculoskeletal system
M. The softening and breaking down of the skin as a result of prolonged exposure to moisture
N. A cast that begins just below the knee and extends to the toes
O. An orthopedic device used to support and immobilize a part of the body

EVALUATION OF LEARNING

Directions: Fill in each blank with the correct answer.

1. State whether the following is an example of dry heat, moist heat, dry cold, or moist cold.

a. Hot compress

_____

b. Ice bag

_____

c. Heating pad

_____

d. Chemical hot pack

_____

e. Cold compress

_____

2. List three factors that must be taken into consideration when applying heat or cold.

_____

_____

3. How does the local application of heat to an affected area for a short period of time influence the following?

    a. The diameter of the blood vessels in the affected area

    _____

    b. The blood supply to the affected area

    _____

    c. Tissue metabolism in the affected area

    _____

4. What happens to the diameter of blood vessels if heat is applied for a prolonged period (more than 1 hour)?

_____

_____

5. List three reasons for applying heat locally.

_____

_____

_____

6. How does the local application of cold for a short period to an affected area influence the following?

    a. The diameter of the blood vessels in the affected area

    _____

    _____

    b. The blood supply to the affected area

    _____

    _____

    c. Tissue metabolism in the affected area

    _____

    _____

7. List two reasons for applying cold locally.

_____

_____

8. What are three reasons for applying a cast?

_____

_____

_____

9. What causes a pressure area?

_____

_____

10. What are the symptoms of a pressure area?

_____

11. What are the complications of a pressure ulcer?

_____

_____

12. What is the purpose of covering the body part with a stockinette before applying a cast?

_____

_____

13. What is the purpose of applying cast padding during cast application?

_____

_____

14. Why should each of the following precautions be taken when applying a synthetic cast?

   a. Removing synthetic casting particles using an alcohol swab

   _____

   b. Checking the circulation, sensation, and movement of the extremity

   _____

15. Why is it important to dry a synthetic cast as soon as possible after it gets wet?

_____

16. What symptoms may indicate that a cast is too tight and an infection is developing?

_____

17. How is a cast removed?

_____

_____

18. What will the affected extremity look like after a cast has been removed?

_____

19. List two examples of conditions for which a splint may be applied.

_____

_____

20. List one example of a condition for which a brace may be applied.

_____

_____

21. What factors does the physician take into consideration when prescribing an ambulatory assistive device?

_____

_____

22. Describe one advantage of the forearm crutch.

_____

23. What may occur if axillary crutches are not fitted properly?

_____

_____

24. List eight guidelines that must be followed during crutch use to ensure safety.

_____

_____

_____

_____

_____

_____

25. List one use of each of the following crutch gaits:

    a. Four-point gait _____

    b. Three-point gait _____

    c. Swing-to gait _____

26. List and describe the three types of canes.

_____

_____

27. List two reasons for prescribing a cane.

_____

28. List two reasons for prescribing a walker.

_____

A. Dear Gabby

Gabby was called out of town unexpectedly and wants you to fill in for her. In the space provided, respond to the following letter.

Dear Gabby:

I am 15 years old and in the tenth grade. I need your help. I have a backpack; my dad weighed it and said it was 40 pounds. I only weigh 105 pounds. My back and neck hurt from lugging it around. I have to walk almost one-half mile to the bus stop. I do not have time to use my locker between classes because it is down a flight of stairs and at the end of the hall. Once, when I started using my locker, my science teacher got mad at me because I was late getting to class. Gabby, what should I do?

Signed, Pain in the Neck

_____

_____

_____

_____

_____

_____

_____

_____

_____

_____

B. Fractures and Sprains

Complete an interactive tutorial on fractures and sprains by following these directions: Go to www.nlm.nih.gov/medlineplus/fractures.html. Under *Start Here*, click on Fractures and Sprains Interactive Tutorial. To start the tutorial, click on Go to Module. Answer the following questions related to the tutorial:

1. What are the names of the bones in the lower leg?

_____

_____

2. What are the names of the bones that join the wrist to the fingers?

_____

_____

3. What are the names of the bones that join the ankle to the toes?

_____

_____

4. How many phalanges does each finger have? How many does the thumb have?

_____

_____

5. What holds bones together?

_____

_____

6. What is a pneumatic brace?

_____

_____

7. How can itching be relieved when wearing a cast?

_____

_____

8. What is atrophy and how does it occur?

_____

_____

9. What complications can occur from a cast or splint?

_____

_____

10. What may cause a cast to become loose? What should the patient do if this occurs?

_____

_____

11. What symptoms are present when a blood clot occurs in the leg?

_____

_____

12. What complication can occur if a blood clot in the leg dislodges?

_____

_____

C. Cast Care

1. You are employed by a pediatric orthopedic surgeon. She is concerned because many of her school-aged patients do not follow proper guidelines for the care of their fiberglass casts, even with their parents' constant reminders. She asks you to develop a creative and colorful instruction sheet in the shape of a cast that presents cast care instructions at a level that can be understood by this age group (6 to 12 years old). Use the illustration of the cast on page 279 to design your instruction sheet.

2. After developing your instruction sheet, get into a group of three or four students, and share your sheets. Have the group decide whether the instructions on each sheet are appropriate for a school-aged child and whether the sheet would be visually appealing to this age group.

Notes

C. Instruction Sheet for Cast Care

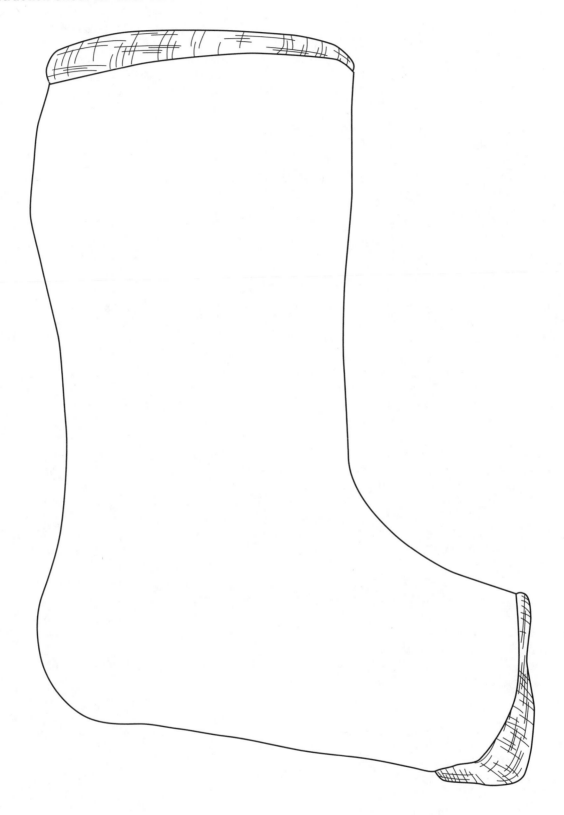

Notes

D. Crutch Guidelines

Each of the following patients is wearing a long leg cast because of a broken tibia and is using wooden axillary crutches to ambulate. Evaluate the crutch technique being practiced by each patient. Write **C** if the technique is correct and **I** if the technique is incorrect. If the technique is correct, explain why it should be performed this way. If incorrect, indicate what may happen from performing the technique in this manner.

1. Andy Morris wears Nike sports shoes when ambulating with his crutches.

   _____

   _____

2. Juliet Wright does not stand up straight when using her crutches.

   _____

   _____

3. Miguel Saldivia puts his weight on the axilla when getting around on his crutches.

   _____

   _____

4. Lindy Campbell has a lot of decorative throw rugs in her house, and she does not want to remove them.

   _____

   _____

5. Andrew Spence likes to move quickly on his crutches so he advances them forward about 20 inches with each step when using the swing-through gait.

   _____

   _____

6. Hanna Romes has tingling in her hands but thinks it is just part of what happens when one uses crutches.

   _____

   _____

7. Tamra Hetrick pads both the shoulder rests and the handgrips of her crutches.

   _____

   _____

8. Erica Anderson's crutch tips get wet but she does not take the time to dry them before going into a shopping mall.

   _____

   _____

E. Accessibility for Physical Disabilities

Next to each of the following facilities, list the features you have observed that facilitate accessibility of individuals with a physical disability.

1. Schools

_____

_____

2. Grocery stores

_____

_____

3. Shopping malls

_____

_____

4. Movie theaters

_____

_____

5. Restaurants

_____

_____

6. Doctors' offices

_____

_____

7. Community parks

_____

_____

F. Crossword Puzzle: Physical Agents to Promote Tissue Healing

Directions: Complete the crossword puzzle using the clues presented below.

Across

1 Transfers weight from legs to arms
4 Cold blood vessels do this
6 Removable immobilizer
9 Popular synthetic cast
10 Warm blood vessels do this
11 Prevents pressure areas
16 Examples: standard, tripod, or quad
17 Takes 4 to 6 weeks for fracture to do this
20 Discharge
21 Purpose of a cast
23 Needed after knee replacement
24 Bone doctor
25 Cuts cast in half

Down

2 "Too long" crutches may cause this
3 Soft and broken down skin
5 Maximum minutes for heat application
6 Elevate cast to prevent this
7 Do not bend here to lift!
8 Prevents LBP
12 Cast is rubbing against the skin
13 Red skin
14 Pus formation
15 Located between skin and cast padding
18 Walking
19 Blow-dry a cast on this setting
22 Holds body part in correct position

G. Bone and Joint Conditions

1. It is National Bone and Joint Week. The mayor has asked you and your classmates to develop informative, creative, and colorful brochures for the community about bone and joint conditions. Choose a condition below and design a brochure using the blank Frequently Asked Questions (FAQ) brochure provided on the following page. Each student in the class should select a different topic. On a separate sheet of paper, write three true/false questions relating to the information in your brochure.

2. Present your brochure to the class. After all the brochures have been presented, each student should ask the three questions to the entire class to see how well the class understands bone and joint conditions. (*Note:* You can take notes during the presentations and refer to them when answering the questions.)

   1. Bursitis

   2. Congenital hip dysplasia

   3. Epicondylitis

   4. Fibromyalgia

   5. Gout

   6. Hammer toe

   7. Herniated disk

   8. Juvenile rheumatoid arthritis

   9. Knee-replacement surgery

   10. Kyphosis

   11. Osteoarthritis

   12. Osteomyelitis

   13. Osteoporosis

   14. Paget's disease

   15. Rheumatoid arthritis

   16. Scoliosis

   17. Sprain

   18. Strain

   19. Tendinitis

FAQ
ON:

Q:
A:

Q:
A:

Q:
A:

Q:
A:

Q:

A:

Q:

A:

Illustration

Q:

A:

Q:

A:

Name: _____

Directions:
a. Watch the indicated videos.
b. Mark each true statement with a T and each false statement with an F. For each false statement, change the wording of the question so that it becomes a true statement.

Video: Procedure 7-1: Applying a Heating Pad

_____ 1. Heat may be used to treat low back pain, arthritis, menstrual cramps, and localized abscesses.

_____ 2. When heat is applied locally to a body part, the blood vessels in that area dilate.

_____ 3. Hypothermia is reddening of the skin caused by dilation of superficial blood vessels.

_____ 4. Prolonged heat for longer than 1 hour can reverse the healing process.

_____ 5. A heating pad is placed in a protective covering to provide comfort for the patient and absorb perspiration.

_____ 6. When applying a heating pad, the selector switch is usually set on a high setting.

_____ 7. The patient should be instructed to lie on the heating pad.

_____ 8. The patient should be checked periodically for signs of an increase or decrease in redness or swelling.

Video: Procedure 7-2: Applying a Hot Soak

_____ 1. The soaking solution should be warmed to 105° F to 110° F.

_____ 2. The purposes of a hot soak are to relieve pain and promote healing.

_____ 3. The patient's body part should be rapidly immersed into the solution.

_____ 4. A hot soak should be applied for 45 to 60 minutes.

_____ 5. After the procedure, completely and gently dry the affected part.

Video: Procedure 7-3: Applying a Hot Compress

_____ 1. Check the temperature of the solution with the bath thermometer to make sure it is at room temperature.

_____ 2. Wring the compress to rid it of excess moisture until it is wet but not dripping.

_____ 3. Apply the compress lightly at first to the affected site to allow the patient gradually to become used to the heat.

_____ 4. Repeat the application of the compress every 10 to 12 minutes for the duration of the time specified by the physician.

_____ 5. Check the patient's skin periodically for signs of an increase or decrease in redness or swelling.

Video: Procedure 7-4: Applying an Ice Bag

_____ 1. Cold can reduce bleeding, swelling, and pain.

_____ 2. When cold is applied locally to a body part, the blood vessels in that area constrict.

_____ 3. The application of cold causes the skin to become cool and pale.

_____ 4. Applying cold directly to the skin can result in a skin burn.

_____ 5. Applying of cold for more than 20 minutes can have a reverse, secondary effect.

_____ 6. The ice bag should be filled completely full with small pieces of ice.

_____ 7. The application of ice is usually uncomfortable, but most patients accept it if they realize the benefits they can derive from it.

Video: Procedure 7-5: Applying a Cold Compress

_____ 1. Large pieces of ice are used for a cold compress to prevent them from sticking to the compress and slowing the rate at which they melt in the water.

_____ 2. After applying a cold compress, it can be covered with an ice bag to keep it cold.

_____ 3. Repeat the application of the cold compress every 2 to 3 minutes for the duration of the time specified by the physician.

_____ 4. Add ice to the basin, if needed, to keep the solution cold.

Video: Procedure 7-6: Applying a Chemical Cold and Hot Pack

_____ 1. A chemical pack is activated by applying pressure to the pack to break an inner bag.

_____ 2. Shake the chemical pack vigorously to mix the contents.

_____ 3. Chemical packs do not need to be covered with a protective covering.

_____ 4. Discard the chemical pack in a biohazard waste container.

Video: Procedure 7-7: Measuring for Axillary Crutches

_____ 1. Crutches remove weight from the arms and transfer it to the legs.

_____ 2. Incorrectly fitted crutches increase the patient's risk of developing back pain, nerve damage, and injuries to the axilla and palms of the hands.

_____ 3. The crutches should be adjusted so that the crutch length is approximately 4 to 6 inches below the axilla.

_____ 4. Tubular aluminum crutches are adjusted by pressing spring-loaded push-buttons.

_____ 5. The handgrips on the crutches should be adjusted so that the patient's elbow is flexed to an angle of approximately 30 degrees.

_____ 6. If the crutches are measured correctly, the medical assistant should be able to insert two fingers between the top of the crutches and the axilla when the patient is standing erect with the crutches under his or her arms.

Chapter **7** **Physical Agents to Promote Tissue Healing**

Video: Procedure 7-8: Instructing the Patient in Crutch Gaits

_____ 1. The type of gait the patient uses depends on the patient's height and weight.

_____ 2. Patients can reduce their fatigue by learning more than one crutch gait.

_____ 3. A faster gait is useful in crowded spaces.

_____ 4. The tripod position provides a wide base of support and enhances stability and balance.

_____ 5. The four-point gait is the most stable and safest of the crutch gaits.

_____ 6. The four-point gait is used by patients with a sprained ankle.

_____ 7. The two-point gait is slower than the four-point gait.

_____ 8. To use the two-point gait, the patient must be capable of partial weight bearing on each foot and have good muscular coordination.

_____ 9. The three-point gait is used by patients who cannot bear weight on one leg but can support full weight on the unaffected leg.

_____ 10. The three-point gait is used by patients with a leg fracture.

_____ 11. The patient must have good muscular coordination and strength to use the three-point gait.

_____ 12. The swing gaits are used by patients with severe upper extremity disabilities.

Video: Procedure 7-9: Instructing a Patient in the Use of a Cane

_____ 1. Canes are used by patients who have weakness on one side of the body.

_____ 2. Patients with joint disabilities or defects of the neuromuscular system may require the use of a cane.

_____ 3. The standard cane provides the most amount of support.

_____ 4. The tripod cane has three legs, and the quad cane has four legs.

_____ 5. A cane is held on the side of the body that is on the same the side that needs support.

_____ 6. The cane handle should be approximately level with the greater trochanter.

_____ 7. The elbow should be flexed at a 25- to 30-degree angle.

_____ 8. The patient should stand erect and lean on the cane.

Video: Procedure 7-10: Instructing the Patient in the Use of a Walker

_____ 1. Walkers are most often used by geriatric patients who have weakness or balance problems.

_____ 2. Patients who have had knee or hip joint replacement surgery often use a walker following the surgery.

_____ 3. Walkers can be difficult to maneuver and limit how fast the patient can move.

_____ 4. The walker should extend from the ground to approximately the level of the patient's waist.

Chapter **7 Physical Agents to Promote Tissue Healing**

Notes

Local Application of Heat and Cold

Procedures 7-1, 7-2, and 7-3: Application of Heat. Apply the following heat treatments, and record the procedure in the chart provided: heating pad, hot soak, hot compress, and chemical hot pack.

Procedures 7-4, 7-5, and 7-6: Application of Cold. Apply the following cold treatments, and record the results in the chart provided: ice bag, cold compress, and chemical cold pack.

Ambulatory Aids

Procedure 7-7: Axillary Crutch Measurement. Measure an individual for axillary crutches, and record the procedure in the chart provided.

Procedure 7-8: Crutch Gaits. Instruct an individual in mastering the following crutch gaits: four-point, two-point, three-point, swing-to, and swing-through gaits. Record the procedure in the chart provided.

Procedure 7-9: Cane. Instruct an individual in the use of a cane, and record the procedure in the chart provided.

Procedure 7-10: Walker. Instruct an individual in the use of a walker, and record the procedure in the chart provided.

CHART	
Date	

CHART	
Date	

Chapter **7 Physical Agents to Promote Tissue Healing**

Procedure 7-1: Applying a Heating Pad

Name: _____ Date: _____

Evaluated by: _____ Score: _____

Performance Objective

Outcome:	Apply a heating pad.
Conditions:	Given a heating pad with a protective covering.
Standards:	Time: 5 minutes. Student completed procedure in _____ minutes.
	Accuracy: Satisfactory score on the Performance Evaluation Checklist.

Performance Evaluation Checklist

Trial 1	Trial 2	Point Value	Performance Standards
		•	Sanitized hands.
		•	Assembled the equipment.
		•	Greeted the patient and introduced yourself.
		•	Identified the patient and explained the procedure.
		•	Placed the heating pad in a protective covering.
		•	Connected the plug to an electrical outlet and set the selector switch to the proper setting.
		•	Placed the heating pad on the patient's affected body area and asked how the temperature felt.
		•	Instructed the patient not to lie on the pad or turn the temperature setting higher.
		▷	Stated why the patient should be instructed not to lie on the heating pad.
		▷	Explained why the patient may want to increase the temperature.
		•	Checked the patient's skin periodically.
		•	Administered treatment for the proper length of time as designated by the physician.
		•	Sanitized hands.
		•	Charted the procedure correctly.
		•	Properly cared for and returned the equipment to its storage place.
		✶	Completed the procedure within 5 minutes.
		Totals	

EVALUATION CRITERIA			COMMENTS
Symbol	**Category**	**Point Value**	
✳	Critical Step	16 points	
•	Essential Step	6 points	
▷	Theory Question	2 points	

Score calculation: 100 points

     − _____ points missed

       _____ Score

Satisfactory score: 85 or above

CAAHEP Competencies Achieved

Psychomotor (Skills)

☑ IV. 2. Report relevant information to others succinctly and accurately.

☑ IV. 6. Prepare a patient for procedures and/or treatments.

Affective (Behavior)

☑ I. 1. Apply critical thinking skills in performing patient assessment and care.

ABHES Competencies Achieved

☑ 8. cc. Communicate on the recipient's level of comprehension.

☑ 9. d. Recognize and understand various treatment protocols.

☑ 9. l. Prepare patient for examinations and treatments.

Procedure 7-2: Applying a Hot Soak

Name: _____ Date: _____

Evaluated by: _____ Score: _____

Performance Objective

Outcome:	Apply a hot soak.
Conditions:	Given the following: soaking solution, bath thermometer, basin, and bath towels.
Standards:	Time: 10 minutes. Student completed procedure in _____ minutes.
	Accuracy: Satisfactory score on the Performance Evaluation Checklist.

Performance Evaluation Checklist

Trial 1	Trial 2	Point Value	Performance Standards
		•	Sanitized hands.
		•	Assembled the equipment.
		•	Checked the label on the solution container.
		•	Warmed the soaking solution.
		•	Greeted the patient and introduced yourself.
		•	Identified the patient and explained the procedure.
		•	Filled a basin one-half to two-thirds full with the warmed soaking solution.
		•	Checked the temperature of the solution with a bath thermometer.
		▷	Stated the safe temperature range that should be used for an adult patient (105° F to 110° F).
		•	Assisted the patient in a comfortable position and padded the side of the basin with a towel.
		•	Slowly and gradually immersed the affected body part into the solution and asked the patient how the temperature felt.
		•	Kept the solution at a constant temperature by removing cooler solution and adding hot solution.
		•	Placed a hand between the patient and the solution when adding more solution.
		•	Stirred the solution with your hand while pouring it.
		•	Checked the patient's skin periodically.
		•	Applied hot soak for the proper length of time as designated by the physician.
		•	Completely dried the affected part.
		•	Sanitized hands.
		•	Charted the procedure correctly.

Trial 1	Trial 2	Point Value	Performance Standards
		•	Properly cared for and returned the equipment to its storage place.
		✳	Completed the procedure within 10 minutes.
			Totals
CHART			
Date			

Evaluation of Student Performance

EVALUATION CRITERIA			COMMENTS
Symbol	**Category**	**Point Value**	
✳	Critical Step	16 points	
•	Essential Step	6 points	
▷	Theory Question	2 points	

Score calculation: 100 points

— _____ points missed

_____ Score

Satisfactory score: 85 or above

CAAHEP Competencies Achieved

Psychomotor (Skills)

☑ IV. 2. Report relevant information to others succinctly and accurately.

☑ IV. 6. Prepare a patient for procedures and/or treatments.

Affective (Behavior)

☑ I. 1. Apply critical thinking skills in performing patient assessment and care.

ABHES Competencies Achieved

☑ 8. cc. Communicate on the recipient's level of comprehension.

☑ 9. d. Recognize and understand various treatment protocols.

☑ 9. l. Prepare patient for examinations and treatments.

Procedure 7-3: Applying a Hot Compress

Name: _____ Date: _____

Evaluated by: _____ Score: _____

Performance Objective

Outcome:	Apply a hot compress.
Conditions:	Given the following: solution for the compresses, bath thermometer, basin, washcloths, and a towel.
Standards:	Time: 10 minutes. Student completed procedure in _____ minutes.
	Accuracy: Satisfactory score on the Performance Evaluation Checklist.

Performance Evaluation Checklist

Trial 1	Trial 2	Point Value	Performance Standards
		•	Sanitized hands.
		•	Assembled the equipment.
		•	Checked the label on the solution container.
		•	Warmed the soaking solution.
		•	Greeted the patient and introduced yourself.
		•	Identified the patient and explained the procedure.
		•	Filled the basin half full with the warmed solution.
		•	Checked the temperature of the solution with a bath thermometer.
		▷	Stated the safe temperature range that should be used for an adult patient (105° F to 110° F).
		•	Completely immersed the compress in the solution.
		•	Squeezed excess solution from the compress.
		•	Applied the compress to the affected body part and asked the patient how the temperature felt.
		•	Placed additional compresses in the solution.
		•	Repeated the application every 2 to 3 minutes for the duration of time specified by the physician.
		•	Checked the patient's skin periodically.
		•	Checked the temperature of the solution periodically, removed cooler fluid, and added hot fluid if needed.
		•	Administered treatment for the proper length of time as designated by a physician.
		•	Thoroughly dried the affected part.
		•	Sanitized hands.

Trial 1	Trial 2	Point Value	Performance Standards
		•	Charted the procedure correctly.
		•	Properly cared for and returned the equipment to its storage place.
		✱	Completed the procedure within 10 minutes.
			Totals

	CHART
Date	

Evaluation of Student Performance

EVALUATION CRITERIA			COMMENTS
Symbol	**Category**	**Point Value**	
✱	Critical Step	16 points	
•	Essential Step	6 points	
▷	Theory Question	2 points	

Score calculation: 100 points

— _____ points missed

_____ Score

Satisfactory score: 85 or above

CAAHEP Competencies Achieved

Psychomotor (Skills)

☑ IV. 2. Report relevant information to others succinctly and accurately.

☑ IV. 6. Prepare a patient for procedures and/or treatments.

Affective (Behavior)

☑ I. 1. Apply critical thinking skills in performing patient assessment and care.

ABHES Competencies Achieved

☑ 8. cc. Communicate on the recipient's level of comprehension.

☑ 9. d. Recognize and understand various treatment protocols.

☑ 9. l. Prepare patient for examinations and treatments.

Procedure 7-4: Applying an Ice Bag

Name: _____ Date: _____

Evaluated by: _____ Score: _____

Performance Objective

Outcome:	Apply an ice bag.
Conditions:	Given the following: ice bag and protective covering, and small pieces of ice.
Standards:	Time: 10 minutes. Student completed procedure in _____ minutes.
	Accuracy: Satisfactory score on the Performance Evaluation Checklist.

Performance Evaluation Checklist

Trial 1	Trial 2	Point Value	Performance Standards
		•	Sanitized hands.
		•	Assembled the equipment.
		•	Greeted the patient and introduced yourself.
		•	Identified the patient and explained the procedure.
		•	Checked the ice bag for leakage.
		•	Filled the bag one-half to two-thirds full with small pieces of ice.
		▷	Explained why small pieces of ice are used.
		•	Expelled air from the bag.
		▷	Explained the reason for expelling air from the bag.
		•	Placed the bag in a protective covering.
		▷	Stated the purpose of placing the bag in a protective covering.
		•	Placed the bag on the affected body area and asked patient how the temperature felt.
		•	Checked the patient's skin periodically.
		▷	Listed skin changes that would warrant removal of the bag.
		•	Refilled the bag with ice and changed the protective covering when needed.
		•	Administered treatment for the proper length of time as designated by the physician.
		•	Sanitized hands.
		•	Charted the procedure correctly.
		•	Properly cared for and returned the equipment to its storage place.
		✶	Completed the procedure within 10 minutes.
			Totals

CHART	
Date	

Evaluation of Student Performance

EVALUATION CRITERIA			COMMENTS
Symbol	Category	Point Value	
✳	Critical Step	16 points	
•	Essential Step	6 points	
▷	Theory Question	2 points	
Score calculation: 100 points			
− _____ points missed			
_____ Score			
Satisfactory score: 85 or above			

CAAHEP Competencies Achieved

Psychomotor (Skills)

☑ IV. 2. Report relevant information to others succinctly and accurately.

☑ IV. 6. Prepare a patient for procedures and/or treatments.

Affective (Behavior)

☑ I. 1. Apply critical thinking skills in performing patient assessment and care.

ABHES Competencies Achieved

☑ 8. cc. Communicate on the recipient's level of comprehension.

☑ 9. d. Recognize and understand various treatment protocols.

☑ 9. l. Prepare patient for examinations and treatments.

Procedure 7-5: Applying a Cold Compress

Name: _____   Date: _____

Evaluated by: _____   Score: _____

Performance Objective

Outcome:	Apply a cold compress.
Conditions:	Given the following: ice cubes, a basin, and washcloths.
Standards:	Time: 10 minutes. Student completed procedure in _____ minutes.
	Accuracy: Satisfactory score on the Performance Evaluation Checklist.

Performance Evaluation Checklist

Trial 1	Trial 2	Point Value	Performance Standards
		•	Sanitized hands.
		•	Assembled the equipment.
		•	Checked the label on the solution.
		•	Greeted the patient and introduced yourself.
		•	Identified the patient and explained the procedure.
		•	Placed large ice cubes in the basin and added the solution until the basin is half full.
		▷	Explained why larger pieces of ice are used.
		•	Completely immersed the compress in the solution.
		•	Squeezed excess solution from the compress.
		•	Applied the compress to the affected body part and asked the patient how the temperature felt.
		•	Placed additional compresses in the solution.
		•	Repeated the application every 2 to 3 minutes for the duration of time specified by the physician.
		•	Checked the patient's skin periodically.
		•	Added ice if needed to keep the solution cold.
		•	Administered treatment for the proper length of time as designated by the physician.
		•	Thoroughly dried the affected part.
		•	Sanitized hands.
		•	Charted the procedure correctly.
		•	Properly cared for and returned the equipment to its storage place.
		✶	Completed the procedure within 10 minutes.
			Totals

CHART	
Date	

Evaluation of Student Performance

EVALUATION CRITERIA			COMMENTS
Symbol	**Category**	**Point Value**	
✻	Critical Step	16 points	
•	Essential Step	6 points	
▷	Theory Question	2 points	

Score calculation: 100 points

− _____ points missed

_____ Score

Satisfactory score: 85 or above

CAAHEP Competencies Achieved

Psychomotor (Skills)

☑ IV. 2. Report relevant information to others succinctly and accurately.

☑ IV. 6. Prepare a patient for procedures and/or treatments.

Affective (Behavior)

☑ I. 1. Apply critical thinking skills in performing patient assessment and care.

ABHES Competencies Achieved

☑ 8. cc. Communicate on the recipient's level of comprehension.

☑ 9. d. Recognize and understand various treatment protocols.

☑ 9. l. Prepare patient for examinations and treatments.

Procedure 7-6: Applying a Chemical Pack

Name: _____   Date: _____

Evaluated by: _____   Score: _____

Performance Objective

Outcome:	Apply a chemical cold and hot pack.
Conditions:	Given a chemical cold and hot pack.
Standards:	Time: 5 minutes. Student completed procedure in _____ minutes.
	Accuracy: Satisfactory score on the Performance Evaluation Checklist.

Performance Evaluation Checklist

Trial 1	Trial 2	Point Value	Performance Standards
		•	Sanitized hands.
		•	Assembled the equipment.
		•	Greeted the patient and introduced yourself.
		•	Identified the patient and explained the procedure.
		•	Shook the crystals to the bottom of the bag.
		•	Squeezed the bag firmly to break the inner water bag.
		•	Shook the bag vigorously to mix the contents.
		•	Covered the bag with a protective covering.
		•	Applied the bag to the affected area.
		•	Checked the patient's skin periodically.
		•	Administered treatment for the proper length of time.
		•	Discarded the bag in an appropriate receptacle.
		•	Sanitized hands.
		•	Charted the procedure correctly.
		✶	Completed the procedure within 5 minutes.
			Totals

EVALUATION CRITERIA			COMMENTS
Symbol	**Category**	**Point Value**	
*	Critical Step	16 points	
•	Essential Step	6 points	
▷	Theory Question	2 points	

Score calculation: 100 points

                            −_____ points missed
                            _____ Score

Satisfactory score: 85 or above

CAAHEP Competencies Achieved

Psychomotor (Skills)

☑ IV. 2. Report relevant information to others succinctly and accurately.

☑ IV. 6. Prepare a patient for procedures and/or treatments.

Affective (Behavior)

☑ I. 1. Apply critical thinking skills in performing patient assessment and care.

ABHES Competencies Achieved

☑ 8. cc. Communicate on the recipient's level of comprehension.

☑ 9. d. Recognize and understand various treatment protocols.

☑ 9. l. Prepare patient for examinations and treatments.

Procedure 7-7: Measuring for Axillary Crutches

Name: _____ Date: _____

Evaluated by: _____ Score: _____

Performance Objective

Outcome:	Measure an individual for axillary crutches.
Conditions:	Given the following: axillary crutches and a tape measure.
Standards:	Time: 10 minutes. Student completed procedure in _____ minutes.
	Accuracy: Satisfactory score on the Performance Evaluation Checklist.

Performance Evaluation Checklist

Trial 1	Trial 2	Point Value	Performance Standards
		•	Asked the patient to stand erect.
		•	Positioned the crutches with the tips at a distance of 2 inches in front of, and 4 to 6 inches to the side of, each foot.
		•	Adjusted crutch length so that the shoulder rests were approximately 1 1/2 to 2 inches below the axilla.
		•	Asked the patient to support his or her weight by the handgrips.
		•	Adjusted the handgrips so that patient's elbow was flexed approximately 30 degrees.
		•	Checked the fit of the crutches by placing two fingers between the top of the crutch and the patient's axilla.
		•	Charted the procedure correctly.
		✳	Completed the procedure within 10 minutes.
			Totals
		CHART	
Date			

EVALUATION CRITERIA			COMMENTS
Symbol	**Category**	**Point Value**	
∗	Critical Step	16 points	
•	Essential Step	6 points	
▷	Theory Question	2 points	

Score calculation: 100 points

− _____ points missed

_____ Score

Satisfactory score: 85 or above

CAAHEP Competencies Achieved

Psychomotor (Skills)

☑ IV. 6. Prepare a patient for procedures and/or treatments.

Affective (Behavior)

☑ I. 1. Apply critical thinking skills in performing patient assessment and care.

ABHES Competencies Achieved

☑ 5. b. Identify and respond appropriately when working/caring for patients with special needs.

Procedure 7-8: Instructing a Patient in Crutch Gaits

Name: _____   Date: _____

Evaluated by: _____   Score: _____

Performance Objective

Outcome:	Instruct an individual in the following crutch gaits: four-point, two-point, three-point, swing-to, and swing-through gaits.
Conditions:	Given axillary crutches.
Standards:	Time: 15 minutes. Student completed procedure in _____ minutes.
	Accuracy: Satisfactory score on the Performance Evaluation Checklist.

Performance Evaluation Checklist

Trial 1	Trial 2	Point Value	Performance Standards
			Tripod Position
			Instructed the patient:
		•	Stand erect and face straight ahead.
		•	Place the tips of crutches 4 to 6 inches in front of, and 4 to 6 inches to side of, each foot.
		▷	Stated one use of the tripod position.
			Four-Point Gait
			Instructed the patient:
		•	Begin in the tripod position.
		•	Move the right crutch forward.
		•	Move the left foot forward to the level of the left crutch.
		•	Move the left crutch forward.
		•	Move the right foot forward to the level of the right crutch.
		•	Repeat the above sequence.
		▷	Stated one use of the four-point gait.
			Two-Point Gait
			Instructed the patient:
		•	Begin in the tripod position.
		•	Move the left crutch and the right foot forward at the same time.
		•	Move the right crutch and left foot forward at the same time.
		•	Repeat the above sequence.

Trial 1	Trial 2	Point Value	Performance Standards
		▷	Stated one use of the two-point gait.
			Three-Point Gait
			Instructed the patient:
		•	Begin in the tripod position.
		•	Move both crutches and the affected leg forward.
		•	Move the unaffected leg forward while balancing weight on both crutches.
		•	Repeat the above sequence.
		▷	Stated two uses of the three-point gait.
			Swing-To Gait
			Instructed the patient:
		•	Begin in the tripod position.
		•	Move both crutches forward together.
		•	Lift and swing body to the crutches.
		•	Repeat the above sequence.
		▷	Stated one use of the swing-to gait.
			Swing-Through Gait
			Instructed the patient:
		•	Begin in the tripod position.
		•	Move both crutches forward together.
		•	Lift and swing body past the crutches.
		•	Repeat the above sequence.
		▷	Stated one use of the swing-through gait.
		✶	Completed the procedure within 15 minutes.
			Totals

Evaluation of Student Performance

EVALUATION CRITERIA			COMMENTS
Symbol	**Category**	**Point Value**	
✶	Critical Step	16 points	
•	Essential Step	6 points	
▷	Theory Question	2 points	

Score calculation: 100 points

− _____ points missed

_____ Score

Satisfactory score: 85 or above

CAAHEP Competencies Achieved

Psychomotor (Skills)

☑ IV. 5. Instruct patients according to their needs to promote health maintenance and disease prevention.

☑ IV. 6. Prepare a patient for procedures and/or treatments.

Affective (Behavior)

☑ I. 2. Use language/verbal skills that enable patients' understanding.

☑ IV. 6. Demonstrate awareness of how an individual's personal appearance affects anticipated responses.

ABHES Competencies Achieved

☑ 9. q. Instruct patients with special needs.

Notes

EVALUATION OF COMPETENCY

Procedures 7-9 and 7-10: Instructing a Patient in Use of a Cane and Walker

Name: _____   Date: _____

Evaluated by: _____   Score: _____

Performance Objective

Outcome:	Instruct an individual in the use of a cane and walker.
Conditions:	Given the following: a cane and a walker.
Standards:	Time: 10 minutes. Student completed procedure in _____ minutes.
	Accuracy: Satisfactory score on the Performance Evaluation Checklist.

Performance Evaluation Checklist

Trial 1	Trial 2	Point Value	Performance Standards
			Cane
			Instructed the patient:
		•	Hold the cane on the strong side of body.
		•	Place the tip of the cane 4 to 6 inches to the side of foot.
		•	Move the cane forward approximately 12 inches.
		•	Move the affected leg forward to the level of the cane.
		•	Move the strong leg forward and ahead of the cane and weak leg.
		•	Repeat the above sequence.
		▷	Stated one condition for which a cane is used.
			Walker
			Instructed the patient:
		•	Pick up the walker and move it forward approximately 6 inches.
		•	Move the right foot and then the left foot up to the walker.
		•	Repeat the above sequence.
		▷	Stated one condition for which a walker is used.
		✶	Completed the procedure within 10 minutes.
			Totals

Evaluation of Student Performance

EVALUATION CRITERIA			COMMENTS
Symbol	**Category**	**Point Value**	
✳	Critical Step	16 points	
•	Essential Step	6 points	
▷	Theory Question	2 points	

Score calculation: 100 points

− _____ points missed

____ Score

Satisfactory score: 85 or above

CAAHEP Competencies Achieved

Psychomotor (Skills)

☑ IV. 5. Instruct patients according to their needs to promote health maintenance and disease prevention.

☑ IV. 6. Prepare a patient for procedures and/or treatments.

Affective (Behavior)

☑ I. 2. Use language/verbal skills that enable patients' understanding.

☑ IV. 6. Demonstrate awareness of how an individual's personal appearance affects anticipated responses.

ABHES Competencies Achieved

☑ 9. q. Instruct patients with special needs.

8 The Gynecologic Examination and Prenatal Care

√ After Completing	Date Due	Textbook Pages	TEXTBOOK ASSIGNMENTS	Possible Points	Points You Earned
		267–318	Read Chapter 8: The Gynecologic Examination and Prenatal Care		
		270 311	Read Case Study 1 Case Study 1 questions	5	
		289 311–312	Read Case Study 2 Case Study 2 questions	5	
		298 312	Read Case Study 3 Case Study 3 questions	5	
		302 312	Read Case Study 4 Case Study 4 questions	5	
			Total points		

√ After Completing	Date Due	Study Guide Pages	STUDY GUIDE ASSIGNMENTS (CTA = Critical Thinking Activity)	Possible Points	Points You Earned
		317	Pretest	10	
		318–319 320	Term Key Term Assessment A. Definitions B. Word Parts (Add 1 point for each medical term)	54 23	
		321–328	Evaluation of Learning questions	56	
		329	CTA A: Breast Cancer (5 points/question)	15	
			Evolve Site: Chapter 8 What's on Your Tray?: Tray Set-up (Record points earned)		
		330–334	CTA B: Methods of Contraception (3 points/each method)	45	
		335–340	CTA C: Herpesvirus and Human Papillomavirus (40 points/brochure)	80	

√ After Completing	Date Due	Study Guide Pages	STUDY GUIDE ASSIGNMENTS (CTA = Critical Thinking Activity)	Possible Points	Points You Earned
		341	CTA D: Signs and Symptoms of Pregnancy	16	
		341–342	CTA E: Calculation of the Expected Date of Delivery	5	
		342	CTA F: Recording Gravidity and Parity	4	
		342–343	CTA G: Nutrition During Pregnancy	8	
		344–345	CTA H: Minor Discomforts of Pregnancy	10	
		345	CTA I: Health Promotion During Pregnancy	7	
		346	CTA J: Breast-Feeding	8	
		346	CTA K: Prenatal Ultrasound	5	
		347	CTA L: Crossword Puzzle	29	
			Evolve Site: Chapter 8 Road to Recovery Game OB/GYN Terminology (Record points earned)		
			Evolve Site: Chapter 8 Animations (2 points each)	24	
			Evolve Site: Chapter 8 Nutrition Nugget: Fetal Alcohol Syndrome	10	
			Evolve Site: Apply Your Knowledge questions	15	
		349–351	Video Evaluation	48	
		317	Posttest	10	
			ADDITIONAL ASSIGNMENTS		
			Total points		

√ When Assigned by Your Instructor	Study Guide Pages	Practices Required	LABORATORY ASSIGNMENTS (Procedure Number and Name)	Score*
	353–354	5	*e* Practice for Competency 8-1: Breast Self-Examination Instructions Textbook reference: pp. 279–281	
	363–366		Evaluation of Competency 8-1: Breast Self-Examination Instructions	*
	355–356	5	*e* Practice for Competency 8-2: Assisting with a Gynecological Examination Textbook reference: pp. 281–285	
	367–370		Evaluation of Competency 8-2: Assisting with a Gynecological Examination	*
	357–362	5	*e* Practice for Competency 8-3: Assisting with a Return Prenatal Examination Textbook reference: pp. 307–309	
	371–374		Evaluation of Competency 8-3: Assisting with a Return Prenatal Examination	*
			ADDITIONAL ASSIGNMENTS	

Notes

Name: _____ Date: _____

True or False

_____ 1. A complete gynecologic examination consists of a breast examination and a pelvic examination.

_____ 2. The American College of Obstetricians and Gynecologists recommends that a woman perform a breast self-examination weekly.

_____ 3. The purpose of the Pap test is for the early detection of cervical cancer.

_____ 4. The patient should be instructed to douche before having a Pap test.

_____ 5. Trichomoniasis produces a profuse, frothy vaginal discharge.

_____ 6. Another name for candidiasis is a yeast infection.

_____ 7. Prenatal refers to the care of the pregnant woman before delivery of the infant.

_____ 8. During each return prenatal visit, the mother's urine is tested for glucose and protein.

_____ 9. The normal range for the fetal pulse rate is between 120 and 160 beats per minute.

_____ 10. Amniocentesis can be used to diagnose certain genetically transmitted conditions.

? POSTTEST

True or False

_____ 1. The patient position for a breast examination is the lithotomy position.

_____ 2. Most breast lumps are discovered by the physician.

_____ 3. Trichomoniasis is caused by a virus.

_____ 4. Chlamydia often occurs in association with syphilis.

_____ 5. In the absence of complications, the first prenatal visit should be scheduled after a woman misses her first period.

_____ 6. True labor pains are referred to as Braxton Hicks contractions.

_____ 7. The purpose of measuring fundal height is to determine the degree of cervical dilation and effacement.

_____ 8. The fetal heart tones can first be detected between 4 and 6 weeks of gestation using a Doppler fetal pulse detector.

_____ 9. The mother must fast for 12 hours before having an obstetric ultrasound scan.

_____ 10. The perineum is the period of time in which the body systems are returning to their prepregnant state.

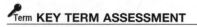

A. Definitions

Gynecologic Examination

Directions: Match each medical term (numbers) with its definition (letters).

_____ 1. Adnexal

_____ 2. Amenorrhea

_____ 3. Atypical

_____ 4. Cervix

_____ 5. Colposcopy

_____ 6. Cytology

_____ 7. Dysmenorrhea

_____ 8. Dyspareunia

_____ 9. Dysplasia

_____ 10. Endocervix

_____ 11. External os

_____ 12. Gynecology

_____ 13. Internal os

_____ 14. Menopause

_____ 15. Menorrhagia

_____ 16. Metrorrhagia

_____ 17. Perimenopause

_____ 18. Perineum

_____ 19. Risk factor

_____ 20. Vulva

A. The opening of the cervical canal of the uterus into the vagina
B. The mucous membrane lining the cervical canal
C. Deviation from the normal
D. The external region between the vaginal orifice and the anus in a female and between the scrotum and the anus in a male
E. Adjacent
F. The absence or cessation of the menstrual period
G. The region of the female external genital organs
H. The science that deals with the study of cells, including their origin, structure, function, and pathology
I. The branch of medicine that deals with the diseases of the reproductive organs of women
J. The internal opening of the cervical canal into the uterus
K. Anything that increases an individual's chance of developing a disease
L. The growth of abnormal cells
M. Before the onset of menopause, the phase during which the woman with regular periods changes to irregular cycles and increased periods of amenorrhea
N. Pain in the vagina or pelvis experienced by a woman during sexual intercourse
O. Examination of the cervix using a lighted instrument with a magnifying lens
P. Bleeding between menstrual periods
Q. Excessive bleeding during a menstrual period
R. The lower narrow end of the uterus that opens into the vagina
S. Pain associated with the menstrual period
T. The permanent cessation of menstruation

Prenatal Care

Directions: Match each medical term (numbers) with its definition (letters).

_____ 1. Abortion

_____ 2. Braxton Hicks contractions

_____ 3. Dilation (of the cervix)

_____ 4. EDD

_____ 5. Effacement

A. A woman who has completed two or more pregnancies to the age of viability, regardless of whether they ended in live infants or stillbirths
B. The entrance of the fetal head or the presenting part into the pelvic inlet
C. Before birth
D. Three months, or one third, of the gestational period of pregnancy

_____ 6. Embryo

_____ 7. Engagement

_____ 8. Fetal heart rate

_____ 9. Fetal heart tones

_____ 10. Fetus

_____ 11. Fundus

_____ 12. Gestation

_____ 13. Gestational age

_____ 14. Gravidity

_____ 15. Infant

_____ 16. Lochia

_____ 17. Multigravida

_____ 18. Multipara

_____ 19. Nullipara

_____ 20. Obstetrics

_____ 21. Parity

_____ 22. Position

_____ 23. Postpartum

_____ 24. Preeclampsia

_____ 25. Prenatal

_____ 26. Presentation

_____ 27. Preterm birth

_____ 28. Primigravida

_____ 29. Primipara

_____ 30. Puerperium

_____ 31. Quickening

_____ 32. Term birth

_____ 33. Toxemia

_____ 34. Trimester

E. The condition of having borne offspring regardless of the outcome

F. The period, usually 4 to 6 weeks, after delivery, in which the uterus and the body systems are returning to normal

G. The termination of the pregnancy before the fetus reached the age of viability (20 weeks)

H. The dome-shaped upper portion of the uterus between the fallopian tubes

I. The number of times per minute the fetal heart beats

J. The first movements of the fetus in utero as felt by the mother

K. The child in utero, from the third month after conception to birth

L. A woman who has been pregnant more than once

M. Projected birth date of the infant

N. A woman who has carried a pregnancy to fetal viability for the first time, regardless of whether the infant was stillborn or alive at birth

O. The stretching of the external os from an opening a few millimeters wide to an opening large enough to allow the passage of an infant (approximately 10 cm)

P. The period of intrauterine development from conception to birth

Q. A discharge from the uterus after delivery consisting of blood, tissue, white blood cells, and some bacteria

R. The thinning and shortening of the cervical canal from its normal length of 1 to 2 cm to a structure with paper-thin edges in which there is no canal at all

S. The total number of pregnancies a woman has had regardless of duration, including a current pregnancy

T. A woman who has not carried a pregnancy to the point of viability (20 weeks of gestation)

U. The branch of medicine concerned with the care of the woman during pregnancy, childbirth, and the postpartal period

V. A woman who is pregnant for the first time

W. Occurring after childbirth

X. Intermittent and irregular painless uterine contractions that occur throughout pregnancy

Y. The relation of the presenting part of the fetus to the maternal pelvis

Z. The sounds of the heartbeat of the fetus heard through the mother's abdominal wall

AA. A child from birth to 12 months of age

BB. The child in utero from the time of conception to the beginning of the first trimester

CC. The age of the fetus between conception and birth

DD. A major complication of pregnancy characterized by increasing hypertension, albuminuria, and edema

EE. Indication of the part of the fetus that is closest to the cervix and will be delivered first

FF. Delivery occurring between 20 and 37 weeks, regardless of whether the child was born alive or stillborn

GG. Delivery occurring after 37 weeks, regardless of whether the child was born alive or stillborn

HH. A condition occurring in pregnant women that includes preeclampsia and eclampsia

B. Word Parts

Directions: Indicate the meaning of each word part in the space provided. List as many medical terms as possible that incorporate the word part in the space provided.

Word Part	Meaning of Word Part	Medical Terms That Incorporate Word Part
1. a-		
2. men/o		
3. -orrhea		
4. colp/o		
5. -scopy		
6. cyt/o		
7. -ology		
8. dys-		
9. plasia		
10. ecto-		
11. endo-		
12. gravid/o		
13. gynec/o		
14. multi-		
15. par/o		
16. nulli-		
17. peri-		
18. post-		
19. pre-		
20. nat/o		
21. -al		
22. prim/i		
23. tri-		

Gynecologic Examination

Directions: Fill in each blank with the correct answer.

1. What is the purpose of the gynecologic examination?

   _____

   _____

   _____

2. What is the purpose of performing a breast examination?

   _____

   _____

   _____

3. How often should a woman perform a breast self-examination at home? When should it be performed in relation to the menstrual cycle and why?

   _____

   _____

   _____

4. What are the components of the pelvic examination?

   _____

   _____

5. What position is generally used for the pelvic examination?

   _____

6. How can the medical assistant help the patient to relax during the pelvic examination?

   _____

   _____

7. What is the function of a vaginal speculum?

   _____

   _____

8. What is the purpose of performing a visual examination of the vagina and the cervix?

   _____

   _____

9. What are three examples of vaginal infections that produce a discharge?

   _____

   _____

10. What is the purpose of performing a Pap test?

_____

_____

11. What causes most cervical cancers?

_____

12. Describe the schedule for having a Pap test recommended by the American Cancer Society.

_____

_____

_____

13. Why should the medical assistant instruct the patient not to douche or insert vaginal medications for 2 days before coming to the medical office to have a Pap test?

_____

_____

_____

_____

14. What are the three types of specimens that may be obtained for a Pap test? Where is each collected?

_____

_____

_____

15. Why must the slides be fixed immediately after collection of a specimen for the direct-smear Pap test method?

_____

_____

_____

16. What are the advantages of using the liquid-based Pap test method?

_____

_____

_____

_____

17. List three conditions that the maturation index can help to evaluate.

_____

_____

_____

18. Why is the Bethesda system recommended for reporting the results of the Pap test?

_____

_____

_____

19. Describe the information included in each of the following categories of a cytology report:

   a. Specimen type

_____

_____

   b. Satisfactory for evaluation

_____

_____

   c. Unsatisfactory for evaluation

_____

_____

   d. Negative for intraepithelial lesion or malignancy

_____

_____

   e. Epithelial cell abnormality

_____

_____

   f. Interpretation or result

_____

_____

   g. Automated review

_____

_____

   h. Ancillary testing

_____

_____

20. What is the purpose of performing the bimanual pelvic examination?

_____

_____

_____

21. What is the purpose of the rectal-vaginal examination?

_____

_____

22. Describe the laboratory procedure that can be used to identify *Trichomonas vaginalis* in the medical office.

_____

_____

_____

23. What medication is used to treat trichomoniasis? Why must the patient's sexual partner also be treated?

_____

_____

24. Describe the laboratory procedure that can be used to identify *Candida albicans* in the medical office.

_____

_____

_____

25. What medications are used to treat candidiasis?

_____

_____

26. What are the symptoms of PID? What complications can occur from PID?

_____

_____

27. How are chlamydial and gonorrheal infections usually diagnosed?

_____

_____

28. List the symptoms of each of the following sexually transmitted diseases:

a. Trichomoniasis in the female

_____

_____

_____

_____

b. Candidiasis in the female

_____

_____

_____

_____

c. Chlamydia

   i. Female:

_____

_____

   ii. Male:

_____

_____

d. Gonorrhea

   i. Female:

_____

_____

   ii. Male:

_____

_____

Prenatal Care

Directions: Fill in each blank with the correct answer.

1. List the three categories of medical office visits for provision of prenatal and postnatal care to the pregnant woman.

_____

_____

_____

2. List the four components of the first prenatal visit.

_____

_____

_____

_____

3. What is the purpose of the prenatal record?

_____

_____

4. List two types of information included in the past medical history (of the prenatal record).

_____

_____

_____

5. List three types of information included in the present pregnancy history.

_____

_____

_____

6. What are the warning signs of a spontaneous abortion?

_____

_____

7. What is the purpose of the interval prenatal history?

_____

_____

8. Explain the importance of performing a physical examination on the prenatal patient.

_____

_____

_____

9. List the procedures usually included in the initial prenatal examination, and next to each procedure, list the purpose for performing each.

_____

_____

_____

_____

_____

_____

_____

_____

10. What is the importance of making sure a pregnant woman does not have gonorrhea before delivery of the infant?

_____

_____

11. Why is a pregnant woman tested for group B streptococcus (GBS)? When is the woman tested for GBS?

_____

_____

12. What is the purpose of performing a hemoglobin and hematocrit evaluation on a prenatal patient?

_____

_____

13. What is the importance of assessing the Rh factor and ABO blood type of a pregnant woman?

_____

_____

14. What is the purpose of performing a glucose challenge test on a pregnant woman?

_____

_____

15. What is the purpose of performing a rubella titer test on a pregnant woman?

_____

_____

16. Why does the CDC recommend that pregnant women have a blood test to screen for exposure to the hepatitis B virus?

_____

_____

17. What is the purpose of the return prenatal visit? List the usual schedule for return prenatal visits.

_____

_____

_____

18. What tests are performed on the patient's urine specimen at each return visit, and why is each performed?

_____

_____

_____

_____

19. List two purposes of measuring the fundal height.

_____

_____

20. What is the normal range for the fetal heart rate?

_____

21. What is the purpose of performing a vaginal examination as the patient nears term?

_____

_____

22. What is the purpose of performing each of the following special tests and procedures?

a. Multiple marker test

_____

b. Obstetric ultrasound scan

_____

c. Amniocentesis

_____

d. Fetal heart rate monitoring

_____

23. What type of patient preparation is required for transabdominal ultrasound scan?

_____

_____

24. What conditions may warrant performing an amniocentesis?

_____

_____

_____

25. What is the difference between the following fetal heart rate monitoring tests: nonstress test and contraction stress test?

_____

_____

_____

26. What occurs during the puerperium?

_____

_____

27. Explain the changes in the lochia that should normally occur during the puerperium.

_____

_____

_____

_____

28. List the procedures generally included in the 6-week postpartum examination.

_____

_____

_____

_____

A. Breast Cancer

Select three of the following questions that interest you the most. Using the following Internet sites, answer these questions in the space provided.

National Cancer Institute: www.cancer.gov

American Cancer Society: www.cancer.org

Cancer Center: www.cancercenter.com

1. Can a male develop breast cancer? Elaborate on your answer.
2. How does tamoxifen work in treating breast cancer?
3. What are the pros and cons of being tested for the breast cancer gene?
4. What methods are used to reconstruct the breast after a mastectomy?
5. What new diagnostic methods are being explored to detect breast cancer?
6. What complementary and alternative therapies are being used in the treatment of breast cancer?

Question # _____

_____

_____

_____

_____

_____

Question # _____

_____

_____

_____

_____

_____

Question # _____

_____

_____

_____

_____

_____

_____

B. Methods of Contraception

Patients coming to the medical office for gynecologic examinations frequently ask the medical assistant questions regarding methods of contraception. The medical assistant should have knowledge of the various types of contraceptives, how they work to prevent pregnancy, and the advantages and disadvantages of each. A list of common contraceptive methods is provided. List the information requested for each in the spaces provided. The contraceptive Internet sites listed under "On the Web" at the end of Chapter 8 in your textbook can be used to complete this activity.

Contraceptive Method	Mode of Action	Advantages	Disadvantages
Oral contraceptives			
Contraceptive injections			
Contraceptive patch			

Contraceptive Method	Mode of Action	Advantages	Disadvantages
Birth control implant			
Male condom			
Female condom			

Contraceptive Method	Mode of Action	Advantages	Disadvantages
Spermicide			
Diaphragm			
Cervical cap			

Contraceptive Method	Mode of Action	Advantages	Disadvantages
Vaginal sponge			
Vaginal ring			
Intrauterine device (IUD)			

Contraceptive Method	Mode of Action	Advantages	Disadvantages
Fertility awareness-based method			
Surgical sterilization			
Emergency contraception			

C. Herpesvirus and Human Papillomavirus

You are working for an obstetrics and gynecology (OB/GYN) office. Your physician is concerned about the increase in the number of patients contracting herpesvirus and human papillomavirus (HPV) infections. He asks you to design a colorful, creative, and informative brochure on herpesvirus and HPV infections by using the brochures provided on the following pages. These brochures will be published and placed in the waiting room to educate patients about these sexually transmitted diseases (STDs). The STD Internet sites listed under "On the Web" at the end of Chapter 8 in your textbook can be used to complete this activity.

Notes

HERPES

How common is herpes?

How can herpes be prevented?

What is herpes?

How do you get herpes?

How is herpes diagnosed?

What are the symptoms?

What causes herpes to recur?

How is herpes treated?

Chapter **8** **The Gynecologic Examination and Prenatal Care**

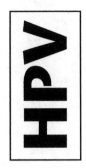

HPV

How common is HPV?

What are the complications of HPV?

What is HPV?

What are the symptoms?

How do you get HPV?

How is HPV diagnosed?

How is HPV tested?

How can HPV be prevented?

Chapter **8** **The Gynecologic Examination and Prenatal Care**

D. Signs and Symptoms of Pregnancy

Listed here are common signs and symptoms of pregnancy. Define each of them and, if possible, explain what causes the sign or symptom to occur. The pregnancy and childbirth Internet sites listed under "On the Web" at the end of Chapter 8 in your textbook can be used to obtain information to complete this activity.

1. Amenorrhea

_____

_____

2. Fatigue

_____

_____

3. Urinary frequency

_____

4. Quickening

_____

_____

5. Goodell's sign

_____

6. Hegar's sign

_____

_____

7. Braxton Hicks contractions

_____

_____

8. Skin changes: striae gravidarum, chloasma, linea nigra

_____

_____

_____

_____

E. Calculation of the Expected Date of Delivery

Calculate the expected date of delivery (EDD) for the following patients using Nägele's rule. The first day of each patient's last menstrual period (LMP) is listed.

1. February 10, 2015 _____

2. April 28, 2015 _____

3. July 20, 2015 _____

Chapter **8** The Gynecologic Examination and Prenatal Care

4. October 2, 2015 _____

5. December 22, 2015 _____

F. Recording Gravidity and Parity

The following patients are in your medical office for their first prenatal visit. In the space provided, record the following information in terms of gravidity and parity.

1. Melissa Turner is pregnant for the third time. Her first pregnancy resulted in the birth of a baby boy, now alive and well. She lost her second pregnancy at 16 weeks' gestation.

   G: _____   T: _____   P: _____   A: _____   L: _____

2. Amanda Schuster is pregnant for the third time. Her first pregnancy resulted in the birth of twin girls, now alive and well. Her second pregnancy resulted in the birth of a baby girl, now alive and well.

   G: _____   T: _____   P: _____   A: _____   L: _____

3. Leah Morrow is pregnant for the fourth time. She lost her first pregnancy at 2 month's gestation. Her second pregnancy was carried to term but resulted in the birth of a stillborn. Her third pregnancy resulted in the birth of a baby girl, now alive and well.

   G: _____   T: _____   P: _____   A: _____   L: _____

4. Rose Samson is pregnant for the fifth time. She carried her first pregnancy to 24 weeks and delivered a stillborn baby. Her second pregnancy resulted in the birth of a baby girl, now alive and well. She lost her third pregnancy at 12 weeks' gestation. Her fourth pregnancy resulted in the birth of a baby boy, now alive and well.

   G: _____   T: _____   P: _____   A: _____   L: _____

G. Nutrition During Pregnancy

1. Brianna Flint is in your medical office for her first prenatal visit. This is her first pregnancy, and she is concerned about adequate nutrition during her pregnancy. Explain why the following nutrients are of particular importance during pregnancy and provide good food sources of each. The pregnancy and childbirth Internet sites listed under "On the Web" at the end of Chapter 8 in your textbook can be used to obtain information to complete this activity.

2. In a classroom situation, select a partner. In a role-playing situation, one student takes the role of the medical assistant, and the other plays the role of the patient. Explain to the patient the importance of these nutrients, and list good food sources of each.

Nutrient	Importance During Pregnancy	Food Sources
Iron		
Calcium		
Protein		
Folic acid		

H. Minor Discomforts of Pregnancy

1. Listed here are the minor discomforts that a prenatal patient may experience during pregnancy. Indicate measures the patient can take to help prevent or relieve each discomfort. The pregnancy and childbirth Internet sites listed under "On the Web" at the end of Chapter 8 in your textbook can be used to obtain information to complete this activity.

2. In a classroom situation, select a partner. In a role-playing situation, one student takes the role of the medical assistant, and the other plays the role of the patient. The patient should indicate that she has a problem with each of these discomforts, and the medical assistant should respond by describing measures the patient can take to help prevent or relieve each problem.

a. Nausea (morning sickness)

_____

_____

b. Heartburn

_____

_____

c. Fatigue

_____

_____

d. Constipation

_____

_____

e. Backache

_____

_____

f. Breathing difficulties

_____

_____

g. Varicose veins

_____

_____

h. Hemorrhoids

_____

_____

i. Leg cramps

_____

_____

j. Swelling of the lower legs and feet

_____

_____

I. Health Promotion During Pregnancy

1. Obtain a prenatal guidebook, and list the guidelines the patient should follow with respect to each of the areas provided. The pregnancy and childbirth Internet sites listed under "On the Web" at the end of Chapter 8 in your textbook can be used to obtain information to complete this activity.

2. In a classroom situation, select a partner. In a role-playing situation, one student takes the role of the medical assistant, and the other plays the role of the patient. The patient should ask for guidance regarding each of these areas, and the medical assistant should respond with appropriate information.

a. Nutrition

_____

_____

b. Employment

_____

_____

c. Exercise

_____

_____

d. Travel

_____

_____

e. Smoking

_____

_____

f. Alcohol

_____

_____

g. Medication

_____

_____

J. Breast-Feeding

1. Lucy Clark asks you for information regarding the advantages and disadvantages of breast-feeding and bottle-feeding. List these in the following chart. The pregnancy and childbirth Internet sites listed under "On the Web" at the end of Chapter 8 in your textbook can be used to obtain information to complete this activity.

2. In a classroom situation, select a partner. In a role-playing situation, one student takes the role of the medical assistant, and the other plays the role of the patient. The patient should ask for information regarding the advantages and disadvantages of both methods, and the medical assistant should respond with appropriate information.

Bottle-feeding	
Advantages	*Disadvantages*

Breast-feeding	
Advantages	*Disadvantages*

K. Prenatal Ultrasound

View obstetric ultrasound scans at the following Internet sites:

www.ob-ultrasound.net/frames.htm

www.layyous.com/ultasound/ultrasound_video.htm

The following scans can be viewed at these sites:

1. Gestational sac

2. Fetus at various gestational ages

3. Fetal measurements

4. Fetal organs

5. Three-dimensional (3D) and four-dimensional (4D) images of the fetus

L. Crossword Puzzle: Gynecology and Obstetrics

Directions: Complete the crossword puzzle using the clues presented below.

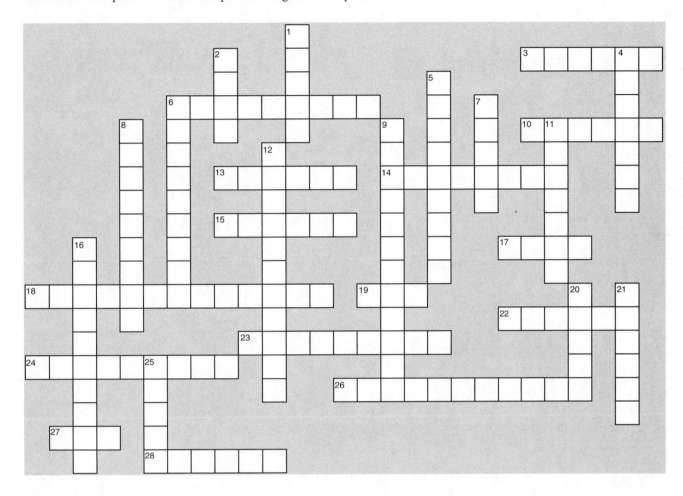

Across

3 STD preventer
6 Breast radiograph
10 Malignant or benign?
13 What most breast lumps are
14 May not occur with STD, especially females
15 Age to begin BSE
17 Definite minor Pap changes
18 Abnormal reported as normal
19 Screening test for GDM
22 Breast exam position
23 Pelvic exam position
24 STD symptom
26 Freezes the cervix
27 Cause of most cervical cancers
28 How cervical cancer develops

Down

1 Birth size of macrosomia baby
2 Warning sign of breast cancer
4 Risk factor for GDM
5 Antibiotics cure this STD
6 Menstrual cycle ceases
7 HPV symptom
8 What all STDs can be
9 Cervical cancer surgery
11 What a GDM mother may need
12 Serious STD complication
16 Examination of the cervix
20 Breast cancer increases (age)
21 A viral STD
25 Slightly abnormal Pap cells

Notes

Name: _____

Directions:
a. Watch the indicated videos.
b. Mark each true statement with a T and each false statement with an F. For each false statement, change the wording of the question so that it becomes a true statement.

Video: Procedure 8-1: Breast Self-Examination Instructions

_____ 1. Breast cancer is one of the most common types of cancer among American women.

_____ 2. Early detection of breast cancer has a high survival rate.

_____ 3. Breast cancer that has spread to the lymph nodes greatly reduces the survival rate.

_____ 4. Most breast lumps are cancerous.

_____ 5. A woman with regular periods should examine her breasts 2 to 3 days after her menstrual period has started.

_____ 6. A woman who does not have menstrual periods as a result of menopause or a hysterectomy does not need to examine her breasts.

_____ 7. A complete breast self-examination should be performed in two ways—in front of a mirror and while lying down.

_____ 8. Using more than one method to examine the breasts makes it more likely that breast changes will be detected.

_____ 9. Puckering and dimpling of the skin of the breast may mean that a tumor is pulling the skin inward.

_____ 10. It is abnormal for one breast to be slightly different in size than the other breast.

_____ 11. When the arms are moved at the same time into the same position, both breasts and nipples should react to the movement in the same way.

_____ 12. Flexing the chest muscles allows breast abnormalities to become more apparent.

_____ 13. The fingertips of the middle three fingers should be used to perform the breast examination.

_____ 14. When examining the breast, small, rotating motions (about the size of a dime) should be used along with continuous, firm pressure.

_____ 15. A circular, vertical strip, or wedge pattern should be used to move around the breast during the exam.

_____ 16. A different pattern should be used each time the patient examines her breasts.

_____ 17. The breast should be palpated for lumps, hard knots, and thickening.

_____ 18. Breast tissue normally feels a little lumpy and uneven.

_____ 19. An enlarged node in the armpit can be a sign of breast cancer even if nothing can be felt in the breast.

_____ 20. Instruct the patient to report lumps and other changes to the physician immediately.

Video: Procedure 8-2: Assisting with a Gynecologic Examination

_____ 1. Gynecology is the branch of medicine that deals with diseases of the reproductive organs of women.

_____ 2. The gynecologic examination is frequently performed in the medical office and includes a breast examination and an abdominal examination.

_____ 3. The expiration date on the ThinPrep Pap test vial must be checked to prevent inaccurate test results.

_____ 4. If the patient's bladder is full, it is easier for the physician to examine the patient, and it is more comfortable for the patient.

_____ 5. The patient must be positioned in the prone position for the breast examination.

_____ 6. The patient is positioned in the lithotomy position for the pelvic examination.

_____ 7. Help the patient to relax during the examination by telling her to breathe deeply, slowly, and evenly through her mouth.

_____ 8. The ectocervical specimen is collected first for the Pap test.

_____ 9. Vigorous swirling of the collection device in the ThinPrep vial removes cervical cells from the spatula and deposits them in the solution.

_____ 10. The physician uses a spatula to collect the endocervical specimen for the Pap test.

_____ 11. Tighten the cap on the ThinPrep vial so the torque line on the cap is opposite the torque line on the vial.

_____ 12. The ectocervical and endocervical specimens can be collected at the same time with the broom.

_____ 13. The SurePath method allows 100% of the collected cells to be used for the Pap test.

_____ 14. After use, a disposable vaginal speculum should be discarded in a regular waste container.

_____ 15. The physician performs a bimanual examination to palpate the size, shape, and position of the uterus and ovaries and to detect tenderness or lumps.

_____ 16. The Hemoccult test is used to test for sexually transmitted diseases.

_____ 17. The patient should be told how and when she will be notified of the Pap test results.

Video: Procedure 8-3: Assisting with a Return Prenatal Examination

_____ 1. Prenatal care is important for promoting the health of the mother and fetus during the pregnancy.

_____ 2. The equipment and supplies needed for the prenatal examination depend on the stage of the pregnancy.

_____ 3. In a normal pregnancy, a vaginal examination is performed approximately 6 to 8 weeks from the due date.

_____ 4. The purpose of the vaginal examination is to confirm the presenting part of the fetus and to determine whether there is any cervical dilation or effacement.

_____ 5. Maternal weight gain or loss assists in assessing fetal development.

_____ 6. The patient's urine specimen is tested for glucose and blood.

_____ 7. The patient is positioned in the supine position for the prenatal examination.

_____ 8. A percussion hammer is used to determine the fundal height measurement.

_____ 9. A stethoscope is used to measure the fetal heart tones.

_____ 10. After the examination, assist the patient off of the examining table to prevent falls.

Notes

Procedure 8-1: Breast Self-Examination. Instruct an individual about the procedure for performing a breast self-examination and record the procedure in the chart provided.

	CHART
Date	

CHART	
Date	

Chapter **8** **The Gynecologic Examination and Prenatal Care**

Procedure 8-2: Gynecologic Examination

1. Complete the cytology request form provided using a female classmate as the patient.
2. Practice the procedure for assisting with a gynecologic examination. Record the vital signs and height and weight in the chart provided.

CHART	
Date	

GYN CYTOLOGY REQUISITION

THOMAS WOODSIDE, MD
501 MAIN ST
ST. LOUIS, MO 63146
(314) 883–0093

PATIENT INFO

| Patient's Name (Last) | (First) | (MI) | Date of Birth MO / DAY / YR | Collection Time : AM PM | Collection Date MO / DAY / YR | Patient's ID # |

Patient's Address   Phone

City   State   ZIP

RESP. PARTY

Name of Responsible Party (if different from patient)

Address of Responsible Party   APT #

City   State   ZIP

INSURANCE

Patient's Relationship to Responsible Party   ☐ 1. Self   ☐ 2. Spouse   ☐ 3. Child   ☐ 4. Other

Insurance Company Name	Plan	Carrier Code
Subscriber/Member #	Location	Group #
Insurance Address		Physician's Provider #
City	State	ZIP
Employer's Name or Number	Insured SSN	

Diagnosis/Signs/Symptoms in ICD-9 Format (Highest Specificity)

REQUIRED

ICD-9 codes are the internationally accepted method of describing the clinical picture of the patient. All diagnoses should be provided by the ordering physician or his or her authorized designee. The following is a partial list of common diagnoses in ICD-9 format. Most third party payers require an ICD-9 code to indicate the medical necessity of the test(s) and/or profile(s) ordered. For a complete list of all ICD-9 codes, please refer to a current ICD-9 manual.

V76.2	Routine Cervical Pap Smear	616.0	Cervicitis	626.8	Abnormal Bleeding
V15.89	High Risk Cervical Screening	616.10	Vaginitis	627.1	Postmenopausal Bleeding
V22.2	Pregnancy	617.0	Endometriosis, Uterus	627.3	Atrophic Vaginitis
079.4	Human Papillomavirus	622.1	Dysplasia, Cervix	795.0	Abnormal Cervical Pap Smear
180.0	Malignant Neoplasm, Cervix	623.0	Dysplasia, Vagina		

COLLECTION METHOD

Liquid-Based Prep
192055 ☐ Thin Prep Pap Test

192039 ☐ Thin Prep Pap Test w/reflex to HPV
Hybrid Capture when ASC-US or SIL

192047 ☐ Thin Prep Pap Test w/reflex to high-risk only
HPV Hybrid Capture when ASC-US

Pap Smear
009100 ☐ 1 Slide   009191 ☐ 2 Slides

Pap Smear and Maturation Index
009209 ☐ 1 Slide   190074 ☐ 2 Slides

SOURCE OF SPECIMEN

☐ Cervical
☐ Endocervical
☐ Vaginal

Date LMP

___/___/___
Mo   Day   Year

COLLECTION TECHNIQUE

☐ Spatula
☐ Brush
☐ Broom
☐ Other
_____

PATIENT HISTORY

☐ Pregnant
☐ Lactating
☐ Oral Contraceptives
☐ Postmenopausal
☐ Hormone Replacement Therapy

☐ PMP Bleeding
☐ Postpartum
☐ IUD
☐ Postcoital Bleeding
☐ DES Exposure
☐ Previous Abnormal Pap Test

☐ Other _____

PREVIOUS TREATMENT   Date/Results

☐ None
☐ Colposcopy and Bx   _____
☐ Cryosurgery   _____
☐ LEEP   _____
☐ Laser Vaporization   _____
☐ Conization   _____
☐ Hysterectomy   _____
☐ Radiation   _____
☐ Chemotherapy   _____

Copyright © 2015, 2012, 2008, 2004, 2000, 1995, 1990 by Saunders, an imprint of Elsevier Inc.
All rights reserved.

Procedure 8-3: Return Prenatal Examination

1. Complete the prenatal health history form provided by using a female classmate as the patient.
2. Prepare the patient and assist with a return prenatal examination. Record the results of procedures you performed on the chart provided.

CHART	
Date	

CHART	
Date	

PRENATAL HEALTH HISTORY

PATIENT INFORMATION

Date: _____ EDD: _____

Name: _____
LAST   FIRST   MIDDLE

Address: _____
CITY   STATE   ZIP

Date of Birth: ___/___/___ Age: ____ Marital Status: _____

Occupation: _____

Education: ☐ High School ☐ College ☐ Post-graduate

Referred By: _____

Phone (home): _____

Phone (work): _____

Emergency Contact: _____

Phone: _____

PAST MEDICAL HISTORY

	O Neg + Pos	DETAIL POSITIVE REMARKS INCLUDE DATE AND TREATMENT		O Neg + Pos	DETAIL POSITIVE REMARKS INCLUDE DATE AND TREATMENT
1. DIABETES			16. D (Rh) SENSITIZED		
2. HYPERTENSION			17. PULMONARY (TB, ASTHMA)		
3. HEART DISEASE			18. RHEUMATIC FEVER		
4. AUTOIMMUNE DISORDER			19. BLEEDING TENDENCY		
5. KIDNEY DISEASE/UTI			20. GYN SURGERY		
6. NEUROLOGIC/EPILEPSY					
7. PSYCHIATRIC			21. OPERATIONS/HOSPITALIZATIONS (YEAR AND REASON)		
8. HEPATITIS/LIVER DISEASE					
9. VARICOSITIES/PHLEBITIS					
10. THYROID DYSFUNCTION			22. ANESTHETIC COMPLICATIONS		
11. TRAUMA/DOMESTIC VIOLENCE			23. HISTORY OF ABNORMAL PAP		
12. BLOOD TRANSFUSION			24. UTERINE ANOMALY/DES		

	AMT/DAY PREPREG.	AMT/DAY PREG.	# YEARS USE			
				25. INFERTILITY		
13. TOBACCO				26. SEXUALLY TRANSMITTED DISEASE		
14. ALCOHOL						
15. STREET DRUGS				27. OTHER		

IMMUNIZATIONS:

Mark an X next to those you have had.

☐ Influenza ☐ Chickenpox

☐ Hepatitis B ☐ Pneumococcal

☐ Hib ☐ Tuberculin Test

☐ Polio ☐ Tetanus Booster

☐ MMR

ALLERGIES:

List all allergies (foods, drugs, environment). ☐ None

_____
_____
_____
_____
_____
_____

MENSTRUAL HISTORY

Menarche: Age of Onset _____

Frequency: Q _____ Days

Duration: _____ Days

Amount of Flow: ☐ Small ☐ Moderate ☐ Large

GYN Disorders (List): _____
_____
_____

On contraceptive at conception? ☐ Yes ☐ No

OBSTETRIC HISTORY

G _____ T _____ P _____ A _____ L _____
(Total Pregnancies)   (Term)   (Preterm)   (Abortions)   (Living Children)

PREVIOUS PREGNANCIES:

DATE MONTH/ YEAR	WEEKS GEST.	LENGTH OF LABOR	BIRTH WEIGHT	SEX M/F	TYPE DELIVERY	ANES.	MATERNAL COMPLICATIONS	INFANT COMPLICATIONS

PRESENT PREGNANCY HISTORY

NAUSEA			ABDOMINAL PAIN		
VOMITING			URINARY COMPLAINTS		
FATIGUE			VAGINAL BLEEDING		
BREAST CHANGES			VAGINAL DISCHARGE		
INDIGESTION			PRURITUS		
CONSTIPATION			ACCIDENTS		
PERSISTENT HEADACHES			SURGERY		
DIZZINESS			X-RAYS		
VISUAL DISTURBANCE			RUBELLA EXPOSURE		
EDEMA (SPECIFY AREA)			OTHER VIRAL INFECTIONS		

LMP _____ / _____ / _____   Amount of Flow: ☐ Small   ☐ Moderate ☐ Large
        Mo   Day   Year

CURRENT MEDICATIONS: (Include prescription, OTC, herbal, and vitamins). ☐ None

Medication _____ **Frequency** _____

_____

_____

INITIAL PHYSICAL EXAMINATION

DATE ____ / ____ / ____

1. HEENT	☐ NORMAL	☐ ABNORMAL	12. VULVA	☐ NORMAL	☐ CONDYLOMA	☐ LESIONS
2. FUNDI	☐ NORMAL	☐ ABNORMAL	13. VAGINA	☐ NORMAL	☐ INFLAMMATION	☐ DISCHARGE
3. TEETH	☐ NORMAL	☐ ABNORMAL	14. CERVIX	☐ NORMAL	☐ INFLAMMATION	☐ LESIONS
4. THYROID	☐ NORMAL	☐ ABNORMAL	15. UTERUS SIZE	_____ WEEKS		☐ FIBROIDS
5. BREASTS	☐ NORMAL	☐ ABNORMAL	16. ADNEXA	☐ NORMAL	☐ MASS	
6. LUNGS	☐ NORMAL	☐ ABNORMAL	17. RECTUM	☐ NORMAL	☐ ABNORMAL	
7. HEART	☐ NORMAL	☐ ABNORMAL	18. DIAGONAL CONJUGATE	☐ REACHED	☐ NO	_____CM
8. ABDOMEN	☐ NORMAL	☐ ABNORMAL	19. SPINES	☐ AVERAGE	☐ PROMINENT	☐ BLUNT
9. EXTREMITIES	☐ NORMAL	☐ ABNORMAL	20. SACRUM	☐ CONCAVE	☐ STRAIGHT	☐ ANTERIOR
10. SKIN	☐ NORMAL	☐ ABNORMAL	21. SUBPUBIC ARCH	☐ NORMAL	☐ WIDE	☐ NARROW
11. LYMPH NODES	☐ NORMAL	☐ ABNORMAL	22. GYNECOID PELVIC TYPE	☐ YES	☐ NO	

COMMENTS (Number and explain abnormals): _____

_____

_____

_____ **EXAM BY** _____

PATIENT'S NAME _____

INTERVAL PRENATAL HISTORY

Date 20___	Weeks Gestation	Height of Fundus (cm)	Weight	B/P	Urine Glucose	Urine Protein	FHT	Vaginal Examination	Presentation	Edema	Discharge	Bleeding	Contractions	Fetal Activity	NST	Next Appt.	Initials

PLANS/EDUCATION (COUNSELED ☑)

☐ ANESTHESIA PLANS _____
☐ TOXOPLASMOSIS PRECAUTIONS (CATS/RAW MEAT) _____
☐ CHILDBIRTH CLASSES _____
☐ PHYSICAL/SEXUAL ACTIVITY _____
☐ LABOR SIGNS _____
☐ NUTRITION COUNSELING _____
☐ BREAST OR BOTTLE FEEDING _____
☐ NEWBORN CAR SEAT _____
☐ POSTPARTUM BIRTH CONTROL _____
☐ ENVIRONMENTAL/WORK HAZARDS _____

☐ TUBAL STERILIZATION _____
☐ VBAC COUNSELING _____
☐ CIRCUMCISION _____
☐ TRAVEL _____
☐ LIFESTYLE, TOBACCO, ALCOHOL _____

REQUESTS _____
_____

TUBAL STERILIZATION
CONSENT SIGNED   DATE ___/___/___   INITIALS _____

LABORATORY			PATIENT'S NAME _____			
INITIAL LABS	DATE		RESULTS		REVIEWED	COMMENTS
BLOOD TYPE	/ /	A	B	AB	O	
Rh FACTOR	/ /	☐ Pos	☐ Neg			
Rh ANTIBODY SCREEN	/ /	☐ Pos	☐ Neg			
HCT/HGB	/ /	_____ % _____ g/dL				
RUBELLA ANTIBODY TITER	/ /	Immune	Nonimmune			
VDRL	/ /	☐ NR	☐ R			
HBsAg (HEPATITIS B)	/ /	☐ Pos	☐ Neg			
HIV	/ /	☐ Pos	☐ Neg ☐ Declined			
URINE CULTURE/SCREEN	/ /					
PAP TEST	/ /	☐ Normal ☐ Abnormal				
CHLAMYDIA (DNA PROBE)	/ /	☐ Pos	☐ Neg			
GONORRHEA (DNA PROBE)	/ /	☐ Pos	☐ Neg			
7–20 WEEK LABS (WHEN INDICATED/ELECTED)	DATE		RESULTS		REVIEWED	COMMENTS
ULTRASOUND #1 (7–13 WEEKS)	/ /	EDD:				
ULTRASOUND #2 (18–20 WEEKS)	/ /	EFW:				
TRIPLE SCREEN (15–20 WEEKS)	/ /					
CVS	/ /					
AMNIOCENTESIS	/ /					
24–28 WEEK LABS (WHEN INDICATED)	DATE		RESULTS		REVIEWED	COMMENTS
HCT/HGB	/ /	_____ % _____ g/dL				
GCT (24–28 WKS)	/ /	1 Hour _____				
GTT (IF SCREEN ABNORMAL)	/ /	_____ FBS _____ 1 Hour _____ 2 Hour _____ 3 Hour				
D (Rh) ANTIBODY SCREEN	/ /					
D IMMUNE GLOBULIN (RhIG) GIVEN (28 WKS)	/ /	SIGNATURE				
32–36 WEEK LABS	DATE		RESULTS		REVIEWED	COMMENTS
HCT/HGB (32 WKS)	/ /	_____ % _____ g/dL				
ULTRASOUND #3 (34 WKS)	/ /	EFW:				
GROUP B STREP (35–37 WKS)	/ /	☐ Pos	☐ Neg			
ADDITIONAL LAB TESTS	DATE		RESULTS		REVIEWED	COMMENTS
	/ /					
	/ /					
	/ /					
	/ /					
	/ /					

Procedure 8-1: Breast Self-Examination Instructions

Name: _____ Date: _____

Evaluated by: _____ Score: _____

Performance Objective

Outcome:	Instruct a patient in the procedure for performing a breast self-examination.
Conditions:	Small pillow.
Standards:	Time: 10 minutes. Student completed procedure in _____ minutes.
	Accuracy: Satisfactory score on the Performance Evaluation Checklist.

Performance Evaluation Checklist

Trial 1	Trial 2	Point Value	Performance Standards
		•	Greeted the patient and introduced yourself.
		•	Identified the patient and explained that you will be instructing the patient in a BSE.
		•	Explained the purpose of the exam, when to perform it, and the three methods of examination.
		▷	Explained why three methods are used to examine the breasts.
			Instructed the patient:
			1. Before a mirror
		•	Remove clothing from the waist up.
		•	Place arms at the sides and inspect the breasts.
		•	Inspect for a change in size or shape; swelling, puckering, or dimpling; change in skin texture; nipple retraction; change in nipple size or position compared with other breast.
		▷	Described what may cause puckering or dimpling of the skin.
		•	Slowly raise arms over the head and inspect the breasts.
		▷	Stated what should normally occur when the arms are moved at the same time.
		•	Rest palms on the hips, press down firmly, and inspect the breasts.
		▷	Stated the purpose of flexing the chest muscles.
		•	Gently squeeze each nipple and look for a discharge.
			2. Lying down
		•	Place a pillow (or folded towel) under the right shoulder.
		•	Place the right hand behind the head.
		▷	Stated the purpose of the pillow and hand placement.
		•	Use the finger pads of the middle three fingers of the left hand.
		▷	Explained why the finger pads should be used.
		•	Use small, rotating motions and continuous firm pressure.

Trial 1	Trial 2	Point Value	Performance Standards
		•	Use one of the following patterns to move around the breast: circular, vertical strip, or wedge.
		▷	Stated why a pattern is used.
			Circular pattern:
		•	Visualize the breast as a clock face.
		•	Start at the outside edge of the breast.
		•	Proceed clockwise until you return to the starting point.
		•	Move in 1 inch, and repeat the circle.
		•	Continue until the nipple is reached.
			Vertical strip:
		•	Divide the breast into strips.
		•	Start at the underarm.
		•	Slowly move fingers down until they are below the breast.
		•	Move fingers 1 inch toward the middle and move back up.
		•	Repeat until the entire breast has been examined.
			Wedge:
		•	Divide the breasts into wedges.
		•	Start at the outer edge of the breast.
		•	Move fingers toward the nipple and back to the edge of the breast.
		•	Repeat until the entire breast has been examined.
			Use the following techniques during the examination:
		•	Press firmly enough to feel the different breast tissues.
		▷	Explained how to perform each pattern.
		•	Palpate for lumps, hard knots, or thickening.
		▷	Explained how normal breast tissue feels.
		•	Examine the entire chest area from your collarbone to the base of a properly fitted bra and from the breastbone to the underarm.
		•	Pay special attention to the area between the breast and underarm, including the underarm itself.
		▷	Explained why the underarm should be examined.
		•	Continue the examination until every part of the right breast has been examined, including the nipple.
		•	Repeat the procedure on the left breast, with a pillow or rolled towel under the left shoulder, the left hand behind the head, and using the right hand to palpate.
			3. In the shower
		•	Gently lather each breast.
		▷	Explained why the breasts should be examined in the shower.
		•	Place the right hand behind the head.
		•	Use the finger pads of the middle three fingers of the left hand.
		•	Use small, rotating motions and continuous, firm pressure.

Trial 1	Trial 2	Point Value	Performance Standards
		•	Use your preferred pattern to examine the right breast and underarm thoroughly for lumps, hard knots, or thickening.
		•	Repeat the procedure on the left breast by using the pads of your right fingers.
		•	Instructed the patient to report any lumps or changes to the physician immediately.
		▷	Explained why it is important to report changes immediately.
		•	Charted the procedure correctly.
		✴	Completed the procedure within 10 minutes.
			Totals
CHART			
Date			

Evaluation of Student Performance

EVALUATION CRITERIA			COMMENTS
Symbol	**Category**	**Point Value**	
✴	Critical Step	16 points	
•	Essential Step	6 points	
▷	Theory Question	2 points	

Score calculation: 100 points

− _____ points missed

_____ Score

Satisfactory score: 85 or above

CAAHEP Competencies Achieved

Psychomotor (Skills)

☑ IV. 5. Instruct patients according to their needs to promote health maintenance and disease prevention.

☑ IV. 9. Document patient education.

Affective (Behavior)

☑ I. 2. Use language/verbal skills that enable patients' understanding.

☑ IV. 3. Use appropriate body language and other nonverbal skills in communicating with patients, family, and staff.

ABHES Competencies Achieved

☑ 8. e. Locate resources and information for patients and employers.

☑ 8. cc. Communicate on the recipient's level of comprehension.

☑ 8. ii. Recognize and respond to verbal and nonverbal communication.

☑ 9. r. Teach patients methods of health promotion and disease prevention.

EVALUATION OF COMPETENCY

Procedure 8-2: Assisting with a Gynecologic Examination

Name: _____   Date: _____

Evaluated by: _____   Score: _____

Performance Objective

Outcome:	Assist with a gynecologic examination.
Conditions:	Using an examining table.
	Given the following: disposable gloves, examining gown and drape, disposable vaginal speculum, lubricant, gauze pads, collection vial, plastic spatula and endocervical brush or cytology broom, Hemoccult slide and developing solution, tissues, biohazard waste container, cytology request form and biohazard specimen transport bag.
Standards:	Time: 15 minutes. Student completed procedure in _____ minutes.
	Accuracy: Satisfactory score on the Performance Evaluation Checklist.

Performance Evaluation Checklist

Trial 1	Trial 2	Point Value	Performance Standards
		•	Sanitized hands.
		•	Assembled the equipment.
		•	Completed as much of the cytology request form as possible.
		•	Checked the expiration date and labeled the collection vial.
		•	Greeted the patient and introduced yourself.
		•	Escorted the patient to the examining room.
		•	Identified the patient.
		•	Asked the patient whether she has any problems or concerns and charted the information.
		•	Completed the cytology request by asking necessary questions.
		•	Measured the vital signs and height and weight and charted the results correctly.
			Prepared the patient for the examination:
		•	Asked the patient whether she needs to empty her bladder.
		▷	Explained why the bladder should be empty for the examination.
		•	Instructed the patient to undress and put on the examining gown with the opening in front.
		•	Informed the patient that physician would be in soon.
		•	Left the room to provide patient privacy.
		•	Made the medical record available for review by the physician (if using a PPR).
		•	Checked to make sure the patient is ready.
		•	Informed the physician that the patient was ready.

367

Trial 1	Trial 2	Point Value	Performance Standards
			Assisted the physician:
		•	Positioned and draped the patient in a supine position for the breast examination.
		•	Positioned and draped the patient in the lithotomy position for the pelvic examination.
		•	Prepared the vaginal speculum and handed it to the physician.
		•	Prepared the light for the physician.
		•	Handed the vaginal speculum to the physician.
		•	Reassured the patient and helped her to relax during the examination.
		▷	Explained why the patient should be relaxed during the examination.
			Assisted with Pap specimen collection:
		•	Applied gloves and removed the cap from the collection vial.
			1a. ThinPrep spatula and brush method
		•	Held the vial to receive the collection device from the physician.
		•	Correctly rinsed each collection device in the liquid preservative.
		▷	Explained why the collection device should be swirled vigorously.
		•	Discarded each collection device in a biohazard waste container.
		•	Tightened the cap on the vial.
			1b. ThinPrep broom method
		•	Held the vial to receive the broom from the physician.
		•	Correctly rinsed the broom in the liquid preservative.
		•	Discarded the broom in a biohazard waste container.
		•	Tightened the cap on the vial.
			2. SurePath spatula and brush method
		•	Held the vial to receive each collection device from the physician.
		•	Broke off or disconnected tip of each collection device.
		•	Discarded each handle in a regular waste container.
		•	Tightened cap on the vial.
			Assisted with the remainder of the examination:
		•	Removed the light source.
		•	Discarded the vaginal speculum in a biohazard waste container.
		•	Provided the physician with lubricant for the bimanual and rectal-vaginal examinations.
		•	Assisted as required with the collection of the fecal occult blood specimen.
		•	Assisted the patient into a sitting position and allowed her to rest.
		▷	Explained why the patient should be allowed to rest.
		•	Offered the patient tissues to remove lubricant from the perineum.
		•	Assisted the patient from the examining table.
		•	Instructed the patient to get dressed.
		•	Informed the patient of the method used by the medical office to relay test results.
		•	Tested the fecal occult blood specimen and charted the results.

368

Trial 1	Trial 2	Point Value	Performance Standards
		•	Prepared the Pap specimen for transport to the laboratory.
		•	Placed the specimen in a biohazard specimen bag and sealed the bag.
		•	Inserted the cytology requisition into the outside pocket of bag.
		•	Placed the bag in appropriate location for pickup by the laboratory.
		•	Charted the transport of the Pap specimen to an outside laboratory.
		•	Cleaned the examining room.
		✱	Completed the procedure within 15 minutes.
			Totals

CHART

Date	

Evaluation of Student Performance

EVALUATION CRITERIA			COMMENTS
Symbol	**Category**	**Point Value**	
✱	Critical Step	16 points	
•	Essential Step	6 points	
▷	Theory Question	2 points	

Score calculation: 100 points

$$- \underline{\qquad} \text{ points missed}$$
$$\underline{\qquad} \text{ Score}$$

Satisfactory score: 85 or above

CAAHEP Competencies Achieved

Psychomotor (Skills)

☑ 1. 10. Assist physician with patient care.

☑ IV. 5. Instruct patients according to their needs to promote health maintenance and disease prevention.

☑ IV. 6. Prepare a patient for procedures and/or treatments.

Affective (Behavior)

☑ III. 3. Show awareness of patients' concerns.

☑ IV. 1. Demonstrate empathy in communicating with patients, family, and staff.

GYN CYTOLOGY REQUISITION

THOMAS WOODSIDE, MD
501 MAIN ST
ST. LOUIS, MO 63146
(314) 883–0093

PATIENT INFO

Patient's Name (Last)	(First)	(MI)	Date of Birth MO	DAY	YR	Collection Time : AM PM	Collection Date MO	DAY	YR	Patient's ID #

Patient's Address   Phone

City   State   ZIP

RESP. PARTY

Name of Responsible Party (if different from patient)

Address of Responsible Party   APT #

City   State   ZIP

INSURANCE

Patient's Relationship to Responsible Party   ☐ 1. Self   ☐ 2. Spouse   ☐ 3. Child   ☐ 4. Other

Insurance Company Name	Plan	Carrier Code
Subscriber/Member #	Location	Group #

Insurance Address   Physician's Provider #

City   State   ZIP

Employer's Name or Number   Insured SSN

Diagnosis/Signs/Symptoms in ICD-9 Format (Highest Specificity)

REQUIRED

ICD-9 codes are the internationally accepted method of describing the clinical picture of the patient. All diagnoses should be provided by the ordering physician or his or her authorized designee. The following is a partial list of common diagnoses in ICD-9 format. Most third party payers require an ICD-9 code to indicate the medical necessity of the test(s) and/or profile(s) ordered. For a complete list of all ICD-9 codes, please refer to a current ICD-9 manual.

V76.2	Routine Cervical Pap Smear	616.0	Cervicitis	626.8	Abnormal Bleeding
V15.89	High Risk Cervical Screening	616.10	Vaginitis	627.1	Postmenopausal Bleeding
V22.2	Pregnancy	617.0	Endometriosis, Uterus	627.3	Atrophic Vaginitis
079.4	Human Papillomavirus	622.1	Dysplasia, Cervix	795.0	Abnormal Cervical Pap Smear
180.0	Malignant Neoplasm, Cervix	623.0	Dysplasia, Vagina		

COLLECTION METHOD

Liquid-Based Prep
192055 ☐ Thin Prep Pap Test

192039 ☐ Thin Prep Pap Test w/reflex to HPV Hybrid Capture when ASC-US or SIL

192047 ☐ Thin Prep Pap Test w/reflex to high-risk only HPV Hybrid Capture when ASC-US

Pap Smear
009100 ☐ 1 Slide   009191 ☐ 2 Slides

Pap Smear and Maturation Index
009209 ☐ 1 Slide   190074 ☐ 2 Slides

SOURCE OF SPECIMEN

☐ Cervical
☐ Endocervical
☐ Vaginal

Date LMP

___ / ___ / ___
Mo   Day   Year

COLLECTION TECHNIQUE

☐ Spatula
☐ Brush
☐ Broom
☐ Other ___

PATIENT HISTORY

☐ Pregnant
☐ Lactating
☐ Oral Contraceptives
☐ Postmenopausal
☐ Hormone Replacement Therapy

☐ PMP Bleeding
☐ Postpartum
☐ IUD
☐ Postcoital Bleeding
☐ DES Exposure
☐ Previous Abnormal Pap Test

☐ Other ___

PREVIOUS TREATMENT   Date/Results

☐ None
☐ Colposcopy and Bx ___
☐ Cryosurgery ___
☐ LEEP ___
☐ Laser Vaporization ___
☐ Conization ___
☐ Hysterectomy ___
☐ Radiation ___
☐ Chemotherapy ___

EVALUATION OF COMPETENCY

Procedure 8-3: Assisting with a Return Prenatal Examination

Name: _____   Date: _____

Evaluated by: _____   Score: _____

Performance Objective

Outcome:	Prepare the patient and assist with a return prenatal examination.
Conditions:	Using an examining table.
	Given the following: centimeter tape measure, Doppler fetal pulse detector, ultrasound coupling agent, paper towel, disposable vaginal speculum, disposable gloves, lubricant, gauze pads, examining gown and drape, and a biohazard waste container.
Standards:	Time: 15 minutes. Student completed procedure in _____ minutes.
	Accuracy: Satisfactory score on the Performance Evaluation Checklist.

Performance Evaluation Checklist

Trial 1	Trial 2	Point Value	Performance Standards
		•	Sanitized hands.
		•	Set up the tray for the prenatal examination.
		•	Greeted the patient and introduced yourself.
		•	Identified the patient and explained the procedure.
		•	Asked the patient to obtain a urine specimen.
		•	Escorted the patient to the examining room and asked her to be seated.
		•	Asked the patient whether she has experienced any problems since her last visit and recorded information in the prenatal record.
		•	Measured the patient's blood pressure and charted the results correctly.
		•	Weighed the patient and charted the results correctly.
		▷	Stated the importance of weighing the patient.
		•	Instructed and prepared the patient for the examination.
		•	Left room to provide the patient with privacy.
		•	Made the medical record available for review by the physician (if using a PPR).
		•	Tested the urine specimen for glucose and protein and charted the results correctly.
		•	Checked to make sure the patient is ready to be seen by physician.
		•	Informed physician that patient is ready.
		▷	Stated how the physician can be informed that the patient is ready.
		•	Assisted the patient into a supine position and properly draped her.
			Assisted physician during the examination:
		•	Handed the physician the tape measure for determination of fundal height.

371

Trial 1	Trial 2	Point Value	Performance Standards
		•	Applied coupling gel to the patient's abdomen and handed the physician the Doppler device.
		•	Removed gel from the patient's abdomen.
		•	Cleaned the probe head of the Doppler device.
		•	Assisted the patient into the lithotomy position if a vaginal specimen is to be obtained or if vaginal examination is to be performed.
			After completion of the examination:
		•	Assisted the patient into a sitting position and allowed her to rest.
		•	Assisted the patient from the examining table.
		•	Provided patient teaching and explanation of the physician's instructions as required.
		•	Escorted the patient to the reception area.
		•	Cleaned the examining room in preparation for the next patient.
		•	Prepared any specimens collected for transport to an outside laboratory.
		✶	Completed the procedure within 15 minutes.
			Totals

CHART

Date	

Evaluation of Student Performance

EVALUATION CRITERIA			COMMENTS
Symbol	**Category**	**Point Value**	
✶	Critical Step	16 points	
•	Essential Step	6 points	
▷	Theory Question	2 points	

Score calculation: 100 points

     − _____ points missed

     ____ Score

Satisfactory score: 85 or above

CAAHEP Competencies Achieved

Psychomotor (Skills)

☑ 1. 10. Assist physician with patient care.

☑ II. 2. Maintain laboratory test results using flow sheets.

☑ IV. 1. Use reflection, restatement, and clarification techniques to obtain a patient history.

☑ IV. 5. Instruct patients according to their needs to promote health maintenance and disease prevention.

☑ IV. 6. Prepare a patient for procedures and/or treatments.

☑ IX. 7. Document accurately in the patient record.

Affective (Behavior)

☑ IV. 2. Apply active listening skills.

☑ IV. 8. Analyze communications in providing appropriate responses or feedback.

ABHES Competencies Achieved

☑ 4. a. Document accurately.

☑ 8. e. Locate resources and information for patients and employers.

☑ 8. ff. Interview effectively.

☑ 9. f. Screen and follow up patient test results.

☑ 9. k. Prepare and maintain examination and treatment area.

☑ 9. l. Prepare patient for examinations and treatments.

☑ 9. m. Assist physician with routine and specialty examinations and treatments.

☑ 9. r. Teach patients methods of health promotion and disease prevention.

PATIENT'S NAME _____

INTERVAL PRENATAL HISTORY

Date 20___	Weeks Gestation	Height of Fundus (cm)	Weight	B/P	Urine Glucose	Urine Protein	FHT	Vaginal Examination	Presentation	Edema	Discharge	Bleeding	Contractions	Fetal Activity	NST	Next Appt.	Initials

Chapter **8** **The Gynecologic Examination and Prenatal Care**

9 The Pediatric Examination

CHAPTER ASSIGNMENTS

√ After Completing	Date Due	Textbook Pages	TEXTBOOK ASSIGNMENTS	Possible Points	Points You Earned
		319–352	Read Chapter 9: The Pediatric Examination		
		320 349	Read Case Study 1 Case Study 1 questions	5	
		334 349	Read Case Study 2 Case Study 2 questions	5	
		342 349–350	Read Case Study 3 Case Study 3 questions	5	
			Total points		
√ After Completing	**Date Due**	**Study Guide Pages**	**STUDY GUIDE ASSIGNMENTS (CTA = Critical Thinking Activity)**	**Possible Points**	**Points You Earned**
		379	Pretest	10	
		380	Term Key Term Assessment	12	
		380–383	Evaluation of Learning questions	30	
		383	CTA A: Pediatric Weight	7	
			Evolve Site: Chapter 9 Pounds and Ounces: Measuring Pediatric Weight (Record points earned)		
		384	CTA B: Pediatric Length	8	
			Evolve Site: Chapter 9 Inch by Inch: Measuring Pediatric Length (Record points earned)		
		384–385	CTA C: Growth Charts	18	
		386–388	CTA D: Motor and Social Development (5 points/each category)	65	
		389	CTA E: Intramuscular Injection	15	

√ After Completing	Date Due	Study Guide Pages	STUDY GUIDE ASSIGNMENTS (CTA = Critical Thinking Activity)	Possible Points	Points You Earned
		389–390	CTA F: Vaccine Information Statement	10	
		390	CTA G: Locating and Interpreting a Vaccine Information Statement	20	
		390–391	CTA H: Immunization Administration Record	40	
		392	CTA I: Crossword Puzzle	30	
		394–400	CTA J: Choose-a-Clue Game (Record points earned)		
			e Evolve Site: Chapter 9 Nutrition Nugget: Nutrition and Breastfeeding	10	
			e Evolve Site: Apply Your Knowledge questions	10	
		401–402	*e* Video Evaluation	31	
		379	?≣ Posttest	10	
			ADDITIONAL ASSIGNMENTS		
			Total points		

√ When Assigned by Your Instructor	Study Guide Pages	Practices Required	LABORATORY ASSIGNMENTS (Procedure Number and Name)	Score*
	403	3	Practice for Competency 9-A: Carrying an Infant Textbook reference: pp. 322–323	
	407–408		Evaluation of Competency 9-A: Carrying an Infant	*
	404	5	Practice for Competency 9-1: Measuring the Weight and Length of an Infant Textbook reference: pp. 325–326	
	409–411		Evaluation of Competency 9-1: Measuring the Weight and Length of an Infant	*
	404	5	Practice for Competency 9-2: Measuring Head and Chest Circumference of an Infant Textbook reference: pp. 326–327	
	413–414		Evaluation of Competency 9-2: Measuring Head and Chest Circumference of an Infant	*
	404	5	Practice for Competency 9-3: Calculating Growth Percentiles Textbook reference: pp. 328–332	
	415–416		Evaluation of Competency 9-3: Calculating Growth Percentiles	*
	405	5	Practice for Competency 9-4: Applying a Pediatric Urine Collector Textbook reference: pp. 335–336	
	417–419		Evaluation of Competency 9-4: Applying a Pediatric Urine Collector	*
	405–406	5	Practice for Competency 9-5: Newborn Screening Test Textbook reference: pp. 347–348	
	421–424		Evaluation of Competency 9-5: Newborn Screening Test	*
			ADDITIONAL ASSIGNMENTS	

Notes

Name: _____ Date: _____

True or False

_____ 1. A pediatrician is a medical doctor who specializes in the diagnosis and treatment of disease in children.

_____ 2. The first well-child visit is usually scheduled 4 weeks after birth of the infant.

_____ 3. Length is measured with the child standing with his or her back to the measuring device.

_____ 4. Blood pressure should be taken for a child starting at 8 years of age.

_____ 5. It is best not to tell a child that an immunization will hurt.

_____ 6. The vastus lateralis muscle site is recommended for administering an injection to an infant.

_____ 7. An MMR injection includes the following immunizations: measles, meningitis, and rubella.

_____ 8. A Vaccine Information Statement explains the benefits and risks of a vaccine in lay terminology.

_____ 9. The hepatitis B vaccine can be given to a newborn.

_____ 10. The blood specimen for a newborn screening test is obtained from the infant's earlobe.

? POSTTEST

True or False

_____ 1. A well-child visit is also referred to as a health maintenance visit.

_____ 2. A reason for weighing a child is to determine proper medication dosage.

_____ 3. Growth charts can be used to identify children with growth abnormalities.

_____ 4. Measuring pediatric blood pressure helps to identify children at risk for type 1 diabetes.

_____ 5. Using a blood pressure cuff that is too large for the child can result in a falsely low reading.

_____ 6. The length of the needle used for a pediatric IM injection depends on the amount of medication being administered.

_____ 7. The resistance of the body to pathogenic microorganisms or their toxins is known as *inflammation*.

_____ 8. The recommended route of administration for an MMR vaccine is subcutaneous.

_____ 9. Before administering a pediatric immunization, the National Childhood Vaccine Injury Act (NCVIA) requires that the parent sign a consent form.

_____ 10. If PKU is left untreated, it can lead to malnutrition.

Directions: Match each medical term (numbers) with its definition (letters).

———— 1. Immunity

———— 2. Immunization

———— 3. Infant

———— 4. Length

———— 5. Pediatrician

———— 6. Pediatrics

———— 7. Preschooler

———— 8. School-aged child

———— 9. Toddler

———— 10. Toxoid

———— 11. Vaccine

———— 12. Vertex

A. A physician who specializes in the care and development of children and the diagnosis and treatment of children's diseases
B. A child between 1 and 3 years old
C. The top of the head
D. The resistance of the body to the effects of a harmful agent such as a pathogenic microorganism or its toxins
E. The branch of medicine that deals with the care and development of children and the diagnosis and treatment of children's diseases
F. A suspension of attenuated or killed microorganisms administered to an individual to prevent an infectious disease
G. The process of becoming immune or of rendering an individual immune through the use of a vaccine or toxoid
H. The measurement from the vertex of the head to the heel of the foot in a supine position
I. A toxin that has been treated by heat or chemicals to destroy its harmful properties administered to an individual to prevent an infectious disease
J. A child from birth to 12 months old
K. A child from 3 to 6 years old
L. A child from 6 to 12 years old

EVALUATION OF LEARNING

Directions: Fill in each blank with the correct answer.

1. What are the components of the well-child visit?

———————————————————————————————————

———————————————————————————————————

2. What is the usual schedule for well-child visits?

———————————————————————————————————

———————————————————————————————————

———————————————————————————————————

3. What is the purpose of the sick-child visit?

———————————————————————————————————

———————————————————————————————————

4. What procedures are often performed by the medical assistant during pediatric office visits?

———————————————————————————————————

———————————————————————————————————

———————————————————————————————————

5. Why is it important for the medical assistant to develop a rapport with the pediatric patient?

_____

_____

_____

6. List the two positions that can be used to carry an infant safely.

_____

7. Why is it important to measure the growth (weight and height or length) of the child during each office visit?

_____

8. What is the difference between height and length?

_____

_____

9. What is the purpose of measuring head circumference?

_____

_____

10. What is the primary use of growth charts?

_____

_____

11. What is the primary cause of childhood obesity?

_____

12. What problems are associated with childhood obesity?

_____

_____

13. List five guidelines for preventing childhood obesity.

_____

_____

_____

14. According to the American Academy of Pediatrics, at what age and how often should blood pressure be measured in children?

_____

_____

15. What is the importance of measuring blood pressure in children?

_____

_____

16. What criteria must be followed to determine the correct cuff size for a child?

_____

_____

17. What occurs if the blood pressure cuff is too small or too large?

_____

_____

18. What three factors must be taken into consideration when determining whether a child has hypertension?

_____

_____

_____

19. List three reasons for collecting a urine specimen from a child.

_____

_____

_____

20. Why should the child's genitalia be cleansed before applying a pediatric urine collector?

_____

_____

21. What gauge and length (range) of needle are recommended for giving an intramuscular injection to a child?

_____

22. Why is the dorsogluteal site not recommended for use as an intramuscular injection site in infants and young children?

_____

_____

_____

23. Why is the vastus lateralis muscle recommended as a good site for giving an intramuscular injection to an infant or young child?

_____

_____

_____

24. What is the difference between a vaccine and a toxoid?

_____

_____

_____

25. According to the American Academy of Pediatrics, what immunizations are recommended for each of the following pediatric patients?

    a. 2-month-old infant _____

    b. 6-month-old infant _____

    c. 12-month-old infant _____

    d. 5-year-old child _____

26. What information must be provided to parents as required by the NCVIA?

_____

_____

27. According to the NCVIA, what information must be recorded in the patient's medical record after a pediatric immunization has been administered?

_____

_____

_____

28. The newborn screening test screens for which metabolic diseases?

_____

_____

29. What are the symptoms of phenylketonuria (PKU) if left untreated?

_____

30. Why can the PKU screening test be performed earlier on infants on formula compared with breast-fed babies?

_____

_____

CRITICAL THINKING ACTIVITIES

A. Pediatric Weight

Locate the following weight values on a pediatric balance scale. Place a check mark next to each one after it has been correctly located.

1. 7 pounds, 9 ounces   _____

2. 8 pounds, 5 ounces   _____

3. 12 pounds, 10 ounces   _____

4. 15 pounds, 11 ounces   _____

5. 19 pounds, 7 ounces   _____

6. 23 pounds, 6 ounces   _____

7. 25 pounds, 3 ounces   _____

B. Pediatric Length

Locate the following length values on your pediatric measuring device. Place a check mark next to each after it has been correctly located.

1. 20 ½ inches _____

2. 22 ½ inches _____

3. 24 inches _____

4. 25 ¾ inches _____

5. 28 ½ inches _____

6. 31 inches _____

7. 33 ¼ inches _____

8. 36 ½ inches _____

C. Growth Charts

Matthew Williams, age 2 years (24 months), has had health maintenance visits at the intervals listed below. His length and weight measurements were taken during each visit and are recorded here. Plot these on the growth chart provided on the following page. You can also print out a growth chart from your computer by going to the following Web site: www.cdc.gov/growthcharts (choose Clinical Growth Charts: Set 1). Calculate the percentile for each and record it in the space provided. (*Note:* His birth weight was 7 pounds, 8 ounces, and his length was 20 inches.)

Well-Child Visit				
Age	**Weight**	**Percentile**	**Length**	**Percentile**
1 month	9 lb, 10 oz		22 in	
2 months	12 lb, 4 oz		23 ½ in	
4 months	16 lb, 5 oz		25 ¼ in	
6 months	18 lb, 8 oz		27 in	
9 months	22 lb, 4 oz		29 ¼ in	
12 months	24 lb, 4 oz		30 ½ in	
15 months	26 lb, 8 oz		31 ½ in	
18 months	27 lb		32 ½ in	
24 months	28 lb		35 ¾ in	

Birth to 36 months: Boys
Length-for-age and Weight-for-age percentiles

NAME _____

RECORD# _____

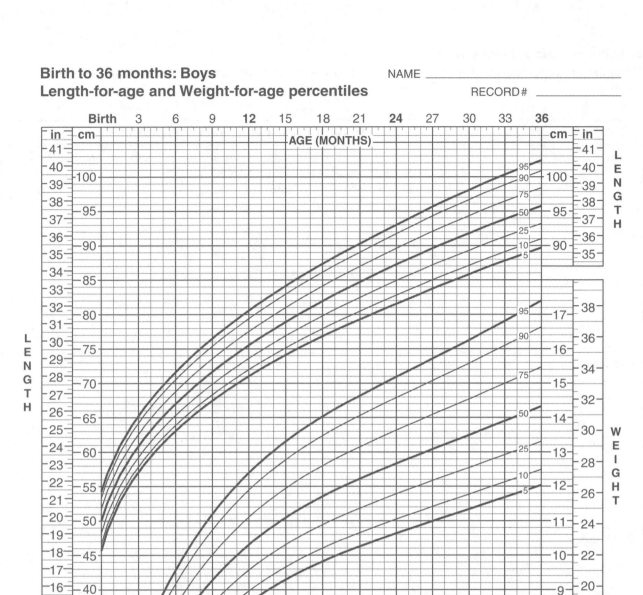

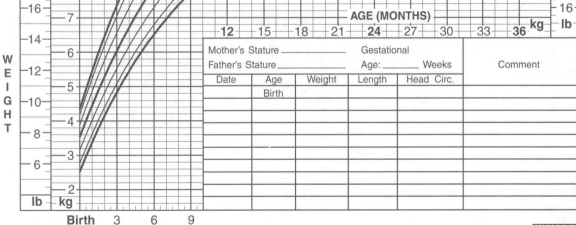

Mother's Stature		Gestational		
Father's Stature		Age: _____ Weeks		Comment
Date	Age	Weight	Length	Head Circ.
	Birth			

Published May 30, 2000 (modified 4/20/01).
SOURCE: Developed by the National Center for Health Statistics in collaboration with
the National Center for Chronic Disease Prevention and Health Promotion (2000).
http://www.cdc.gov/growthcharts

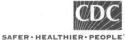

SAFER · HEALTHIER · PEOPLE™

D. Motor and Social Development

Using a reference source, describe the motor and social development of the age groups listed here. The first one is done for you.

AGE	MOTOR AND SOCIAL DEVELOPMENT
Birth to 3 months	Raises head but not stable, can turn head from side to side, activities are limited to reflexes, cries when hungry, responsive social smile, coos, eyes can focus on an object and follow a moving object 180 degrees.
4 to 6 months	
7 to 9 months	
10 to 12 months	

AGE	MOTOR AND SOCIAL DEVELOPMENT
1 year	
2 years	
3 years	
4 years	
5 years	

Chapter **9** **The Pediatric Examination**

AGE	MOTOR AND SOCIAL DEVELOPMENT
6 years	
7 years	
8 to 10 years	
Preadolescent	
Adolescent	

Chapter **9** **The Pediatric Examination**

E. Intramuscular Injection

How would you prepare the following children for an intramuscular injection of penicillin to reduce apprehension and fear? Table 9-2, Techniques for Interacting with Children, on page 322 of your textbook can be used as a reference for this activity.

a. Katie Waugh, age 5

_____

_____

_____

b. Patrick Williams, age 8

_____

_____

_____

c. Julie Anderson, age 15

_____

_____

_____

F. Vaccine Information Statement

Refer to the Diphtheria, Tetanus, and Pertussis Vaccine Information Statement (VIS) in your textbook (pages 343 and 344), and answer the following questions:

1. How does an individual contract tetanus?

_____

_____

2. What are the symptoms of the following diseases?

   a. Diphtheria _____

   b. Tetanus _____

   c. Pertussis _____

3. Why is DTaP now used instead of DTP?

_____

_____

4. What is the immunization schedule for DTaP?

_____

_____

5. Who should not receive a DTaP immunization?

_____

_____

389

6. What does Td protect against, and what is the recommended immunization schedule for Td?

_____

_____

7. What mild problems may occur from a DTaP vaccine?

_____

_____

8. What moderate problems may occur from a DTaP vaccine?

_____

_____

9. What should be done if the patient develops fever and pain after receiving DTaP?

_____

_____

10. What should be done if a moderate or severe reaction occurs after a DTaP immunization?

_____

_____

G. Locating and Interpreting a Vaccine Information Statement

Obtain a VIS for a vaccine that you would like to know more about (other than the DTaP vaccine already included in your textbook). List the information that would be important for a parent to know before this immunization is administered to his or her child. The following Internet sites can be used to obtain a VIS:

www.cdc.gov/vaccines/pubs/vis

www.immunize.org/vis

Name of Immunization: _____

Publication Date: _____

Information to Relay to a Parent:

_____

_____

_____

_____

_____

_____

_____

_____

_____

H. Immunization Administration Record

Complete the following immunization record form for an infant at his 2-month, 4-month, and 6-month visit using Figure 9-11 (immunization schedule) in the textbook to determine which immunizations are administered during these well-child visits. The Web site (www.immunize.org/catg.d/p2022.pdf) provides an example of a completed immunization administration form to assist you in completing this form.

IMMUNIZATION ADMINISTRATION RECORD

Name _____
    (first)   (MI)   (last)

DOB _____

Physician _____

Address _____

_____

SITE ABBREVIATIONS:

RVL: **Right vastus lateralis**
LVL: **Left vastus lateralis**
RD: **Right deltoid**
LD: **Left deltoid**
PO: **By mouth**
IN: **Intranasal**

Vaccine	Type of Vaccine[1] (generic abbreviation)	Date Given (mo/day/yr)	Dose	Site	Vaccine Lot #	Vaccine Mfr.	Vaccine Information Statement Date on VIS	Vaccine Information Statement Date Given	Signature and Title of Vaccinator
Hepatitis B[2] (e.g., HepB, Hib-HepB, DTaP-HepB-IPV) Give IM.									
Diphtheria, Tetanus, Pertussis[2] (e.g., DTaP, DTaP-Hib, DTaP-HepB-IPV, DT, DTaP-HiB-IPV, Tdap, DTaP-IPV, Td) Give IM.									
Haemophilus influenzae **type b**[2] (e.g., Hib, Hib-HepB, DTaP-HiB-IPV, DTaP-Hib) Give IM.									
Polio[2] (e.g., IPV, DTaP-HepB-IPV, DTaP-HiB-IPV, DTaP-IPV) Give IPV SC or IM. Give all others IM.									
Pneumococcal (e.g., PCV, conjugate; PPV, polysaccharide) Give PCV IM. Give PPV SC or IM.									
Rotovirus Give oral.									
Measles, Mumps, Rubella (e.g., MMR, MMRV) Give SC.									
Varicella (e.g., Var, MMRV) Give SC.									
Hepatitis A (HepA) Give IM									
Meningococcal (e.g., MCV4, MPSV4) Give MCV4 IM and MPSV4 SC.									
Human papillomavirus (e.g., HPV) Give IM									
Influenza (e.g., TIV, inactivated; LAIV, live attenuated) Give TIV IM. Give LAIV IN.									
Other									

1. Record the generic abbreviation for the type of vaccine given (e.g., DTaP-Hib, PCV), *not* the trade name.
2. For combination vaccines, fill in a row for each separate antigen in the combination.

I. Crossword Puzzle: Pediatrics

Directions: Complete the crossword puzzle using the clues presented below.

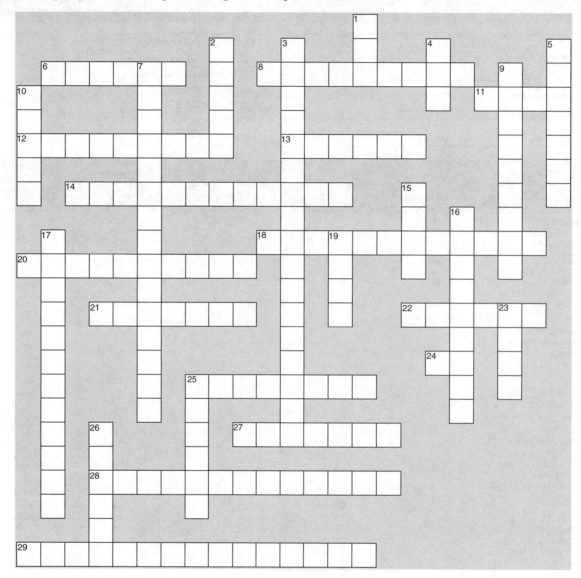

Across

6 Vertex to heel
8 Whooping cough
11 Not a kid reward
12 Not caused by chickens
13 Hold-me position
14 Helps identify nutrition abnormalities
18 MMR administration route
20 Can give at birth vaccine
21 German measles
22 Stand up straight
24 Begin at 3 years
25 Resistance to MOs
27 Much easier to prevent
28 Required for school entrance
29 Injection site for babies

Down

1 No phenylalanine enzyme
2 Kid's vaccine act
3 Screens for macroencephaly
4 Immunization explainer
5 From 1 to 3
7 Childhood obesity can cause this
9 First breast milk
10 Common immunization side effect
15 3-in-1 vaccine
16 Do not weigh infant in this
17 Baby doctor
19 Right size for kid's BP?
23 Newborn screening puncture site
25 Title expires at 1 year
26 Used to determine drug dosage

Notes

J. Choose-a-Clue Game

Object: The object of the game is to become familiar with childhood diseases.

Directions:

1. Cut out the game cards on the following pages.
2. List three clues for each condition specified on the reverse of the card. Your clues should include information on symptoms, prevention, and treatment. Do *not* write the name of the disease on this side of the card.
3. Use the game cards as flash cards to study the diseases.
4. Get into a group of three students.
5. Place your game cards on the table in front of you with the clues facing up.
6. One of the players should name the first disease on the list provided.
7. Each player places the appropriate game card on the table with the clues facing upward.
8. When all players have placed a card on the table, turn the cards over.
9. Award yourself 5 points if you have correctly determined the disease.
10. Review the information each player listed on his or her game card.
11. Keep track of your points on the score card provided.
12. Continue playing until all the diseases have been identified.

Internet sources can help you find clues:

www.kidshealth.org

www.merck.org/mmpe

Childhood diseases

1. Conjunctivitis
2. Fifth disease
3. Head lice
4. Impetigo
5. Influenza
6. Meningococcal meningitis
7. Methicillin-resistant *Staphylococcus aureus* (MRSA)
8. Otitis media
9. Pertussis
10. Pinworms
11. Roseola
12. Respiratory syncytial virus (RSV)
13. Scarlet fever
14. Strep throat
15. Urinary tract infection
16. Varicella (chickenpox)

CHOOSE-A-CLUE
SCORE CARD

Name: _____

Recording Points:
Cross off a number each time you properly identify a disease (starting with 5 and continuing in sequence). Your total points will be equal to the last number you crossed off. Record this number in the space provided, and place a check mark next to the level you achieved.

Points:	
5	75
10	80
15	85
20	90
25	95
30	100
35	105
40	110
45	115
50	120
55	125
60	130
65	135
70	140

Total points: _____

LEVEL: _____

☐ 75 points and above: **Free from Infection**

☐ 65 to 70 points: **Putting Up a Good Fight**

☐ 55 to 60 points: **Susceptible**

☐ 50 points and under: **Infected**

Notes

Conjunctivitis	**Fifth disease**
Head lice	**Impetigo**
Influenza	**Meningococcal meningitis**
Otitis media	**Pertussis**

Sym:

_____

_____

Prev:

_____

_____

Tx:

_____

_____

Sym:

_____

_____

Prev:

_____

_____

Tx:

_____

_____

Sym:

_____

_____

Prev:

_____

_____

Tx:

_____

_____

Sym:

_____

_____

Prev:

_____

_____

Tx:

_____

_____

Sym:

_____

_____

Prev:

_____

_____

Tx:

_____

_____

Sym:

_____

_____

Prev:

_____

_____

Tx:

_____

_____

Sym:

_____

_____

Prev:

_____

_____

Tx:

_____

_____

Sym:

_____

_____

Prev:

_____

_____

Tx:

_____

_____

Pinworms

MRSA

Roseola

Respiratory syncytial virus (RSV)

Scarlet fever

Strep throat

Urinary tract infection

Varicella (chickenpox)

Sym:

_____

_____

Prev:

_____

_____

Tx:

_____

_____

Sym:

_____

_____

Prev:

_____

_____

Tx:

_____

_____

Sym:

_____

_____

Prev:

_____

_____

Tx:

_____

_____

Sym:

_____

_____

Prev:

_____

_____

Tx:

_____

_____

Sym:

_____

_____

Prev:

_____

_____

Tx:

_____

_____

Sym:

_____

_____

Prev:

_____

_____

Tx:

_____

_____

Sym:

_____

_____

Prev:

_____

_____

Tx:

_____

_____

Sym:

_____

_____

Prev:

_____

_____

Tx:

_____

_____

Name _____

Directions:

a. Watch the indicated videos.

b. Mark each true statement with a T and each false statement with an F. For each false statement, change the wording of the question so that it becomes a true statement.

Video: Procedure 9-1: Measuring the Weight and Length of an Infant

_____ 1. Pediatrics deals with the care and development of children and the diagnosis and treatment of diseases in children.

_____ 2. The height of a child is used to determine nutritional needs and the proper dosage of medication to give the child.

_____ 3. Length is the measurement of the child in a standing position.

_____ 4. Weighing an infant with a wet diaper may increase the weight of the infant considerably.

_____ 5. Placing a paper protector on the scale prevents cross-contamination among patients.

_____ 6. The scale should be balanced without the paper protector in place.

_____ 7. If the scale is properly balanced, the indicator point rests in the center of the balance area.

_____ 8. When measuring an infant's weight, the lower weight must be seated firmly in its groove to ensure an accurate reading.

_____ 9. To measure the infant's weight, slowly slide the upper weight along its calibration bar by tapping it gently until the indicator point comes to a rest at the center of the balance area.

_____ 10. The infant's weight is read in pounds and ounces.

_____ 11. When measuring the infant's length, the knees should be straightened.

_____ 12. The infant's length should be read in inches, to the nearest inch.

Video: Procedure 9-2: Measuring Head and Chest Circumference of an Infant

_____ 1. The head circumference of children younger than 6 years old is routinely measured at each office visit to screen for microencephaly and macroencephaly.

_____ 2. The chest circumference is usually measured only when a heart or lung abnormality is suspected.

_____ 3. Between 6 months and 2 years of age, the chest and head circumference measurements are about the same.

_____ 4. To measure head circumference, the measuring device is positioned around the infant's head at the greatest circumference.

_____ 5. To measure chest circumference, the measuring device is positioned around the infant's chest at the nipple line.

Video: Procedure 9-3: Calculating Growth Percentiles

_____ 1. Growth percentiles are used to monitor the individual growth pattern of a child.

_____ 2. Growth charts for weight are calibrated in pounds and kilograms.

_____ 3. Growth charts for length are calibrated only in centimeters.

Video: Procedure 9-4: Applying a Pediatric Urine Collector

_____ 1. A pediatric urine collector is used with an infant or young child who cannot urinate voluntarily.

_____ 2. The child's genitalia must be cleansed to prevent contaminants from entering the urine specimen.

_____ 3. A back-to-front motion should be used to cleanse the genitalia.

_____ 4. After cleansing the genitalia, allow the area to dry completely so that the bag will adhere to the skin.

_____ 5. When applying the urine collector bag, make sure there is no puckering, to prevent leakage of urine.

_____ 6. Check the urine collector bag every 5 minutes until a urine specimen is obtained.

_____ 7. If you wait too long to check the collector bag, moisture from the urine may loosen the adhesive surface, and the bag may leak.

_____ 8. The collector bag should be removed slowly to prevent discomfort and irritation of the infant's skin.

_____ 9. After removing the collector bag, clean the genital area with an alcohol wipe.

_____ 10. Transfer the urine into a specimen container and tightly apply the lid.

_____ 11. Dispose of the collector bag in a biohazard waste container.

Procedure 9-A: Carrying an Infant

Practice the procedure for carrying an infant, using a pediatric training mannequin in the following positions: cradle and upright.

CARRYING POSITION	NUMBER OF PRACTICES

Procedures 9-1 and 9-3: Weight, Length, and Growth Charts

1. **Weight and Length.** Measure the weight of an infant using a pediatric training mannequin. Record the results in the chart provided.
2. **Growth Charts.** Calculate growth percentiles on a growth chart using the values presented below. Assume these values were taken from the same (female) child over the course of her first year of life.

Age	Weight	Length
2 months	9 pounds	21 inches
4 months	11 pounds, 8 ounces	23 ½ inches
6 months	14 pounds, 8 ounces	25 ¼ inches
9 months	18 pounds, 8 ounces	27 ¼ inches
12 months	21 pounds, 6 ounces	28 ¾ inches

Procedure 9-2: Head and Chest Circumference. Measure the head and chest circumference of an infant using a pediatric training mannequin. Record the results in the chart provided.

CHART	
Date	

Procedure 9-4: Pediatric Urine Collector. Practice the procedure for applying a pediatric urine collector, using a pediatric training mannequin. Record the procedure in the chart provided.

Procedure 9-5: Newborn Screening Test

1. Complete the information section of the Newborn Screening Test Card provided for you.
2. Practice the procedure for specimen collection for the newborn screening test using a pediatric training mannequin. Record the procedure in the chart provided.

Date	CHART

Newborn Screening Test

USE BALL POINT PEN-PRESS HARD

ALL INFORMATION MUST BE PRINTED

Birth date: ____ / ____ / ____

Baby's name: (last, first)

Hospital provider number:

Hospital of birth or transfer:

Mom's name: (last, first, initial)

Mom's address:

Mom's city: ____ Ohio ____ Zip: ____

Mom's race:

Mom's age:

Mom's SSN: ____ - ____ - ____

Mom's phone: (____) ____ - ____

Mom's county:

Mom's ID:

Baby's ID:

Specimen date ____ / ____ / ____

Baby's physician: (last name first)

Physician address:

City: ____ Ohio ____ Zip ____

Physician phone: (____) ____ - ____

Physician provider number:

Time ____ : ____ (Use 24 hour time only)

Time ____ : ____ (Use 24 hour time only)

1. SPECIMEN: ☐ FIRST ☐ SECOND
   ☐ other

2. BIRTH NUMBER/ SEX:
   ☐ SINGLE ☐ MULTIPLE A, B, C, etc.
   ☐ FEMALE ☐ MALE

3. BIRTH WEIGHT: ____ GRAMS

4. PREMATURE: ☐ YES ☐ NO

5. ANTIBIOTICS: ☐ YES ☐ NO

6. TRANSFUSION: ☐ YES ☐ NO

7. FEEDING: ☐ YES ☐ NO
   Type 1. Breast 2. Milk-base
   NO. 3. Soy 4. TPN 5. IV-only

8. SUBMITTER:
   ☐ HOSPITAL/BIRTH CENTER
   ☐ HEALTH DEPARTMENT
   ☐ PHYSICIAN
   ☐ HOME HEALTH CARE AGENCY
   ☐ CLINICAL LAB
   ☐ OTHER

   ☐ SPECIMEN REJECTED

EVALUATION OF COMPETENCY

Procedure 9-A: Carrying an Infant

Name: _____   Date: _____

Evaluated by: _____   Score: _____

Performance Objective

Outcome:	Carry an infant in the following positions: cradle and upright.
Conditions:	Given a pediatric training mannequin.
Standards:	Time: 5 minutes. Student completed procedure in _____ minutes.
	Accuracy: Satisfactory score on the Performance Evaluation Checklist.

Performance Evaluation Checklist

Trial 1	Trial 2	Point Value	Performance Standards
			Cradle position:
		•	Slid the left hand and arm under the infant's back.
		•	Grasped the infant's upper arm from behind.
		•	Encircled the infant's upper arm with the thumb and fingers.
		•	Supported the infant's head, shoulders, and back on your arm.
		•	Slipped the right arm up and under the infant's buttocks.
		•	Cradled the infant in your arms with the infant's body resting against your chest.
			Upright position:
		•	Slipped the right hand under the infant's head and shoulders.
		•	Spread the fingers apart to support the infant's head and neck.
		•	Slipped the left forearm under the infant's buttocks.
		•	Allowed the infant to rest against your chest.
		✱	Completed the procedure within 5 minutes.
			Totals
CHART			
Date			

Evaluation of Student Performance

EVALUATION CRITERIA			COMMENTS
Symbol	**Category**	**Point Value**	
✳	Critical Step	16 points	
•	Essential Step	6 points	
▷	Theory Question	2 points	

Score calculation: 100 points

− _____ points missed

_____ Score

Satisfactory score: 85 or above

CAAHEP Competencies Achieved

Psychomotor (Skills)

☑ IV. 6. Prepare a patient for procedures and/or treatments.

Affective (Behavior)

☑ IV. 1. Demonstrate empathy in communicating with patients, family, and staff.

ABHES Competencies Achieved

☑ 9. 1. Prepare patient for examinations and treatments.

Procedure 9-1: Measuring the Weight and Length of an Infant

Name: _____   Date: _____

Evaluated by: _____   Score: _____

Performance Objective

Outcome:	Measure the weight and length of an infant.
Conditions:	Using a pediatric training mannequin and a pediatric balance scale (table model).
	Given a paper protector.
Standards:	Time: 5 minutes. Student completed procedure in _____ minutes.
	Accuracy: Satisfactory score on the Performance Evaluation Checklist.

Performance Evaluation Checklist

Trial 1	Trial 2	Point Value	Performance Standards
			Weight:
		•	Sanitized hands.
		•	Greeted the infant's parent and introduced yourself.
		•	Identified the infant.
		•	Explained the procedure to the child's parent.
		•	Based on the medical office policy asked parent to: (a) remove the infant's clothing and put on a dry diaper; and (b) remove the infant's clothing including the diaper.
		▷	Stated why the infant should not be weighed with a wet diaper.
		•	Unlocked the pediatric scale and placed a clean paper protector on it.
		▷	Stated the purpose of the paper protector.
		•	Checked the balance scale for accuracy.
		▷	Stated the purpose for balancing the scale.
		•	Gently placed the infant on his or her back on the scale.
		•	Placed one hand slightly above the infant.
		•	Balanced the scale.
		•	Read the results while the infant was lying still.
		•	Jotted down the value or made a mental note of it.
		✶	The reading was identical to the evaluator's reading.
		•	Returned the balance to its resting position and locked the scale.

Trial 1	Trial 2	Point Value	Performance Standards
			Length:
		•	Placed the vertex of the infant's head against the headboard at the zero mark.
		•	Asked the parent to hold the infant's head in position.
		•	Straightened the infant's knees and placed the soles of the infant's feet firmly against the upright footboard.
		•	Read the infant's length in inches from the measure.
		•	Jotted down the value or made a mental note of it.
		✳	The reading was identical to the evaluator's reading.
		•	Removed the infant from the scale and handed him or her to the parent.
		•	Returned the headboard and footboard to their resting positions.
		•	Sanitized hands.
		•	Charted the results correctly.
		✳	Completed the procedure within 5 minutes.
			Totals
CHART			
Date			

Evaluation of Student Performance

EVALUATION CRITERIA			COMMENTS
Symbol	**Category**	**Point Value**	
✳	Critical Step	16 points	
•	Essential Step	6 points	
▷	Theory Question	2 points	

Score calculation: 100 points

− _____ points missed

_____ Score

Satisfactory score: 85 or above

<table>
<tr><td colspan="2">CAAHEP Competencies Achieved</td></tr>
<tr><td colspan="2">Psychomotor (Skills)</td></tr>
<tr><td colspan="2">☑ IV. 6. Prepare a patient for procedures and/or treatments.</td></tr>
<tr><td colspan="2">Affective (Behavior)</td></tr>
<tr><td colspan="2">☑ I. 2. Use language/verbal skills that enable patients' understanding.</td></tr>
<tr><td colspan="2">☑ IV. 7. Demonstrate recognition of the patient's level of understanding in communications.</td></tr>
</table>

<table>
<tr><td>ABHES Competencies Achieved</td></tr>
<tr><td>☑ 5. f. Identify and discuss developmental stages of life.</td></tr>
<tr><td>☑ 8. cc. Communicate on the recipient's level of comprehension.</td></tr>
<tr><td>☑ 9. l. Prepare patient for examinations and treatments.</td></tr>
</table>

Notes

EVALUATION OF COMPETENCY

Procedure 9-2: Measuring Head and Chest Circumference of an Infant

Name: _____   Date: _____

Evaluated by: _____   Score: _____

Performance Objective

Outcome:	Measure the head and chest circumference of an infant.
Conditions:	Given a flexible, nonstretch tape measure (in centimeters).
Standards:	Time: 5 minutes. Student completed procedure in _____ minutes.
	Accuracy: Satisfactory score on the Performance Evaluation Checklist.

Performance Evaluation Checklist

Trial 1	Trial 2	Point Value	Performance Standards
			Measurement of head circumference:
		•	Sanitized hands.
		•	Assembled the equipment.
		•	Positioned the infant.
		▷	Stated what positions can be used to measure head circumference.
		•	Positioned the measuring device around the infant's head.
		•	The tape measure was placed slightly above the eyebrows and pinna of the ears and around the occipital prominence at the back of the skull.
		•	Read the results in centimeters (or inches).
		•	Jotted down the value or made a mental note of it.
		✶	The reading was identical to the evaluator's reading.
		•	Sanitized hands.
		•	Charted the results correctly.
			Measurement of chest circumference:
		•	Positioned the infant on his or her back on the examining table.
		•	Encircled the measuring device around the infant's chest at the nipple line.
		•	Ensured that the measuring device was snug but not too tight.
		•	Read the results in centimeters (or inches).
		•	Jotted down this value or made a mental note of it.
		✶	The reading was identical to the evaluator's reading.

Trial 1	Trial 2	Point Value	Performance Standards
		•	Charted the results correctly.
		✱	Completed the procedure within 5 minutes.
			Totals

CHART

Date	

Evaluation of Student Performance

EVALUATION CRITERIA			COMMENTS
Symbol	**Category**	**Point Value**	
✱	Critical Step	16 points	
•	Essential Step	6 points	
▷	Theory Question	2 points	

Score calculation: 100 points

     −   _____ points missed

         ____ Score

Satisfactory score: 85 or above

CAAHEP Competencies Achieved

Psychomotor (Skills)

☑ IV. 6. Prepare a patient for procedures and/or treatments.

Affective (Behavior)

☑ I. 1. Apply critical thinking skills in performing patient assessment and care.

ABHES Competencies Achieved

☑ 9. 1. Prepare patient for examinations and treatments.

Procedure 9-3: Calculating Growth Percentiles

Name: _____   Date: _____

Evaluated by: _____   Score: _____

Performance Objective

Outcome:	Plot a pediatric growth value on a growth chart.
Conditions:	Given a pediatric growth chart.
Standards:	Time: 5 minutes. Student completed procedure in _____ minutes.
	Accuracy: Satisfactory score on the Performance Evaluation Checklist.

Performance Evaluation Checklist

Trial 1	Trial 2	Point Value	Performance Standards
		•	Selected the proper growth chart.
		•	Located the child's age in the horizontal column at the bottom of the chart.
		•	Located the growth value in the vertical column under the appropriate category.
		•	Drew a (imaginary) vertical line from the child's age mark and an imaginary horizontal line from the growth mark.
		•	Found the site at which the two lines intersected on the graph.
		•	Placed a dot on this site.
		•	Determined the percentile by following the curved percentile line upward.
		•	Read the value located on the right side of the chart.
		•	Estimated the results if the value did not fall exactly on a percentile line.
		•	Charted the results correctly.
		✻	The value was within ±2 percentage points of the evaluator's determination.
		✻	Completed the procedure within 5 minutes.
			Totals
CHART			
Date			

Evaluation of Student Performance

EVALUATION CRITERIA			COMMENTS
Symbol	**Category**	**Point Value**	
✱	Critical Step	16 points	
•	Essential Step	6 points	
▷	Theory Question	2 points	

Score calculation: 100 points

      − _____ points missed

          _____ Score

Satisfactory score: 85 or above

CAAHEP Competencies Achieved

Psychomotor (Skills)

☑ II. 3. Maintain growth charts.

Affective (Behavior)

☑ II. 2. Distinguish between normal and abnormal test results.

ABHES Competencies Achieved

☑ 8. hh. Receive, organize, prioritize, and transmit information expediently.

☑ 5. f. Identify and discuss developmental stages of life.

Procedure 9-4: Applying a Pediatric Urine Collector

Name: _____   Date: _____

Evaluated by: _____   Score: _____

Performance Objective

Outcome:	Apply a pediatric urine collector.
Conditions:	Using a pediatric training mannequin.
	Given the following: disposable gloves, personal antiseptic wipes, pediatric urine collector bag, urine specimen container and label, and a waste container.
Standards:	Time: 10 minutes. Student completed procedure in _____ minutes.
	Accuracy: Satisfactory score on the Performance Evaluation Checklist.

Performance Evaluation Checklist

Trial 1	Trial 2	Point Value	Performance Standards
		•	Sanitized hands.
		•	Assembled the equipment.
		•	Greeted the child's parent and introduced yourself.
		•	Identified the child and explained the procedure to the parent.
		•	Applied gloves.
		•	Positioned the child on his or her back with legs spread apart.
			Cleanse the area and apply the bag:
			Females
		•	Cleansed each side of the meatus with a separate wipe using a front-to-back motion.
		•	Cleansed directly down the middle with a third wipe.
		•	Discarded each wipe after cleansing.
		▷	Stated the reason for cleansing the urinary meatus.
		•	Allowed the area to dry completely.
		▷	Explained why the area should be allowed to dry.
		•	Removed the paper backing from the urine collector bag.
		•	Placed the bottom of the adhesive ring on the perineum and worked upward.
		•	Firmly pressed the adhesive surface firmly to the skin surrounding the external genitalia.
		•	Made sure there was no puckering.

Trial 1	Trial 2	Point Value	Performance Standards
		•	The opening of the bag was placed directly over the urinary meatus.
		•	Excess length of the bag was positioned toward the feet.
			Males
		•	Retracted the foreskin of the penis if the child is not circumcised.
		•	Cleansed each side of the urethral orifice with a separate wipe.
		•	Cleansed directly over the urethral orifice.
		•	Cleansed the scrotum.
		•	Discarded each wipe after cleansing.
		•	Allowed the area to dry completely.
		•	Removed the paper backing from urine collector bag.
		•	Positioned the bag so that child's penis and scrotum are projected through the opening of the bag.
		•	Firmly pressed the adhesive surface firmly to the skin.
		•	Excess length of the bag was positioned toward the feet.
			Completed the procedure:
		•	Loosely diapered the child.
		•	Checked the bag every 15 minutes until the urine specimen was obtained.
		•	Gently removed the collector bag from top to bottom.
		•	Cleansed the genital area with a personal antiseptic wipe and rediapered the child.
		•	Transferred the urine specimen into the specimen container and tightly applied the lid.
		•	Applied a label to the container.
		•	Disposed of the collector bag in a regular waste container.
		•	Tested the specimen or prepared it for transfer to an outside laboratory.
		▷	Explained why the urine specimen should not be allowed to stand at room temperature.
		•	Removed gloves and sanitized hands.
		•	Charted the procedure correctly.
		✷	Completed the procedure within 10 minutes.
			Totals

CHART	
Date	

Evaluation of Student Performance

EVALUATION CRITERIA			COMMENTS
Symbol	**Category**	**Point Value**	
✴	Critical Step	16 points	
•	Essential Step	6 points	
▷	Theory Question	2 points	

Score calculation: 100 points

− _____ points missed

_____ Score

Satisfactory score: 85 or above

CAAHEP Competencies Achieved

Psychomotor (Skills)

☑ IV. 6. Prepare a patient for procedures and/or treatments.

Affective (Behavior)

☑ III. 2. Explain the rationale for performance of a procedure to the patient.

ABHES Competencies Achieved

☑ 10. d. Collect, label, and process specimens.

Notes

![icon] **EVALUATION OF COMPETENCY**

Procedure 9-5: Newborn Screening Test

Name: _____   Date: _____

Evaluated by: _____   Score: _____

Performance Objective

Outcome:	Collect a capillary blood specimen for a newborn screening test.
Conditions:	Using a pediatric training mannequin.
	Given the following: disposable gloves, sterile lancet, heel warmer or warm compress, antiseptic wipe, newborn testing card, mailing envelope, sterile gauze pad, adhesive bandages, and a biohazard sharps container.
Standards:	Time: 10 minutes. Student completed procedure in _____ minutes.
	Accuracy: Satisfactory score on the Performance Evaluation Checklist.

Performance Evaluation Checklist

Trial 1	Trial 2	Point Value	Performance Standards
		•	Sanitized hands.
		•	Assembled the equipment.
		•	Greeted the infant's parent and introduced yourself.
		•	Identified the infant and explained the procedure to the parent.
		•	Completed the information section of the newborn screening card.
		•	Selected an appropriate puncture site.
		•	Identified the sites that can be used for the heel puncture.
		▷	Explained what could occur if a different site is used.
		•	Warmed the puncture site.
		▷	Stated the purpose of warming the site.
		•	Cleaned the puncture site with an antiseptic wipe and allowed it to air-dry.
		•	Applied gloves and grasped infant's foot around the puncture site.
		•	Punctured the heel using a sterile lancet, and disposed of the lancet.
		•	Wiped away the first drop of blood with a gauze pad.
		▷	Explained why the first drop of blood should be wiped away.
		•	Encouraged a large drop of blood to form by exerting gentle pressure on the heel.
		•	Did not excessively squeeze the heel.
		▷	Explained why the excessive squeezing should be avoided.
		•	Touched the drop of blood to the center of the first circle on the test card.

Trial 1	Trial 2	Point Value	Performance Standards
		•	Completely filled the circle on the test card with blood.
		•	Continued until all the circles are completely filled with blood.
		▷	Explained why each circle must be completely filled with blood.
		•	Did not touch the blood specimen with your gloved hand.
		▷	Stated why the specimen should not be touched.
		•	Held a gauze pad over the puncture site and applied pressure.
		•	Remained with the infant until bleeding stopped. Applied an adhesive bandage if needed.
		•	Removed gloves and sanitized hands.
		•	Allowed the test card to air-dry horizontally for 3 hours at room temperature.
		•	Did not allow the blood specimen to come in contact with any other surface.
		•	Did not place the specimen in a plastic bag.
		▷	Explained what occurs if the specimen is placed in a plastic bag.
		•	Placed the test card in its protective envelope.
		•	Mailed the card to the laboratory within 48 hours.
		▷	Stated why the specimen must be mailed within 48 hours.
		•	Charted the procedure correctly.
		✶	Completed the procedure within 10 minutes.
			Totals
		CHART	
Date			

Evaluation of Student Performance

EVALUATION CRITERIA			COMMENTS
Symbol	Category	Point Value	
✶	Critical Step	16 points	
•	Essential Step	6 points	
▷	Theory Question	2 points	

Score calculation: 100 points

      − _____ points missed

         _____ Score

Satisfactory score: 85 or above

CAAHEP Competencies Achieved
Psychomotor (Skills)
☑ I. 3. Perform capillary puncture.
Affective (Behavior)
☑ III. 2. Explain the rationale for performance of a procedure to the patient.

ABHES Competencies Achieved
☑ 10. d. Collect, label, and process specimens. (2) Perform capillary puncture.

Newborn Screening Test

USE BALL POINT PEN—PRESS HARD

ALL INFORMATION MUST BE PRINTED

Birth date: ___ / ___ / ___

Time ___ : ___ (Use 24 hour time only)

Baby's name: (last, first)

Hospital provider number:

Hospital of birth or transfer:

Mom's name: (last, first, initial)

Mom's address:

Mom's city: Ohio **Zip:** ___ - ___

Mom's race:

Mom's age:

Mom's SSN: ___ - ___ - ___

Mom's phone: (___) ___ - ___

Mom's county:

Mom's ID:

Baby's ID:

Specimen date ___ / ___ / ___

Time ___ : ___ (Use 24 hour time only)

Baby's physician: (last name first)

Physician address:

City: Ohio **Zip** ___ - ___

Physician provider number:

Physician phone: (___) ___ - ___

1. SPECIMEN: ☐ FIRST ☐ SECOND ☐ other

2. BIRTH NUMBER/ SEX: ☐ SINGLE ☐ MULTIPLE A, B, C, etc. ☐ FEMALE ☐ MALE

3. BIRTH WEIGHT: ___ GRAMS

4. PREMATURE: ☐ YES ☐ NO

5. ANTIBIOTICS: ☐ YES ☐ NO

6. TRANSFUSION: ☐ YES ☐ NO

7. FEEDING: ☐ YES ☐ NO
Type 1. Breast 2. Milk-base No. 3. Soy 4. TPN 5. IV-only

8. SUBMITTER:
☐ HOSPITAL/BIRTH CENTER
☐ HEALTH DEPARTMENT
☐ PHYSICIAN
☐ HOME HEALTH CARE AGENCY
☐ CLINICAL LAB
☐ OTHER

☐ SPECIMEN REJECTED

10 Minor Office Surgery

CHAPTER ASSIGNMENTS

√ After Completing	Date Due	Textbook Pages	TEXTBOOK ASSIGNMENTS	Possible Points	Points You Earned
		353–413	Read Chapter 10: Minor Office Surgery		
		376 409	Read Case Study 1 Case Study 1 questions	5	
		387 409	Read Case Study 2 Case Study 2 questions	5	
		401 409	Read Case Study 3 Case Study 3 questions	5	
			Total points		
√ After Completing	**Date Due**	**Study Guide Pages**	**STUDY GUIDE ASSIGNMENTS (CTA = Critical Thinking Activity)**	**Possible Points**	**Points You Earned**
		429	Pretest	10	
		430 431	Key Term Assessment A. Definitions B. Word Parts (Add 1 point for each medical term)	26 9	
		431–436	Evaluation of Learning questions	50	
		436–437	CTA A: Medical and Surgical Asepsis	10	
		437–438	CTA B: Violation of Surgical Asepsis	10	
		439–441	CTA C: Surgical Instruments (2 points each)	26	
			Evolve Site: Chapter 10 It's Instrumental: Identify Instruments (Record points earned)		
			Evolve Site: Chapter 10 Keep It Sterile: Set Up a Sterile Tray (Record points earned)		

√ After Completing	Date Due	Study Guide Pages	STUDY GUIDE ASSIGNMENTS (CTA = Critical Thinking Activity)	Possible Points	Points You Earned
		441	CTA D: Pioneers in Surgical Asepsis (5 points each)	15	
		442	CTA E: Crossword Puzzle	24	
		443–445	CTA F: Patient Instruction Sheet	20	
			e Evolve Site: Chapter 10 Animations (2 points each)	10	
			e Evolve Site: Chapter 10 Nutrition Nugget: Nutrition and Weight Loss Surgery	10	
			e Evolve Site: Apply Your Knowledge questions	10	
		447–450	*e* Video Evaluation	70	
		429	?▤ Posttest	10	
			ADDITIONAL ASSIGNMENTS		
			Total points		

√ When Assigned by Your Instructor	Study Guide Pages	Practices Required	LABORATORY ASSIGNMENTS (Procedure Number and Name)	Score*
	451	5	*e* Practice for Competency 10-1: Applying and Removing Sterile Gloves Textbook reference: pp. 363–365	
	453–454		Evaluation of Competency 10-1: Applying and Removing Sterile Gloves	*
	451	5	*e* Practice for Competency 10-2: Opening a Sterile Package Textbook reference: pp. 365–367	
	455–456		Evaluation of Competency 10-2: Opening a Sterile Package	*
	451	5	Practice for Competency Using Commercially Prepared Sterile Packages Textbook reference: p. 362	
	457–458		Evaluation of Competency Using Commercially Prepared Sterile Packages	*
	451	3	*e* Practice for Competency 10-3: Pouring a Sterile Solution Textbook reference: p. 367	
	459–460		Evaluation of Competency 10-3: Pouring a Sterile Solution	*
	451	5	*e* Practice for Competency 10-4: Changing a Sterile Dressing Textbook reference: pp. 370–372	
	461–463		Evaluation of Competency 10-4: Changing a Sterile Dressing	*
	451	Sutures: 3 Staples: 3	*e* Practice for Competency 10-5: Removing Sutures and Staples Textbook reference: pp. 377–379	
	465–467		Evaluation of Competency 10-5: Removing Sutures and Staples	*
	451	3	*e* Practice for Competency 10-6: Applying and Removing Adhesive Skin Closures Textbook reference: pp. 380–384	

√ When Assigned by Your Instructor	Study Guide Pages	Practices Required	LABORATORY ASSIGNMENTS (Procedure Number and Name)	Score*
	469–471		Evaluation of Competency 10-6: Applying and Removing Adhesive Skin Closures	*
	451	5	*e* Practice for Competency 10-7: Assisting with Minor Office Surgery Textbook reference: pp. 388–392	
	473–476		Evaluation of Competency 10-7: Assisting with Minor Office Surgery	*
	451	Each bandage turn: 3	*e* Practice for Competency 10-A: Bandage Turns Textbook reference: pp. 404–405	
	477–478		Evaluation of Competency 10-A: Bandage Turns	*
	452	3	Practice for Competency 10-8: Applying a Tubular Gauze Bandage Textbook reference: pp. 407–408	
	479–480		Evaluation of Competency 10-8: Applying a Tubular Gauze Bandage	*
			ADDITIONAL ASSIGNMENTS	

Name: _____ Date: _____

True or False

_____ 1. Surgical asepsis refers to practices that keep objects and areas free from all microorganisms.

_____ 2. Something that is sterile is contaminated if it comes in contact with a pathogen.

_____ 3. Reaching over a sterile field is a violation of sterile technique.

_____ 4. An incision is a jagged tearing of the tissues.

_____ 5. The skin is the first line of defense of the body.

_____ 6. One of the local signs of inflammation is fever.

_____ 7. Sutures approximate the edges of a wound until proper healing occurs.

_____ 8. A biopsy is usually performed to determine whether an infection is present.

_____ 9. An ingrown toenail can be caused by shoes that are too tight.

_____ 10. One of the functions of a bandage is to hold a dressing in place.

? POSTTEST

True or False

_____ 1. Measuring a patient's temperature requires the use of surgical asepsis.

_____ 2. Hemostatic forceps are used to clamp off blood vessels.

_____ 3. An instrument with a ratchet should be kept in a closed position when not in use.

_____ 4. The physician would most likely order a tetanus booster for an abrasion.

_____ 5. Inflammation is the protective response of the body to trauma and the entrance of foreign substances.

_____ 6. A serous exudate is red in color.

_____ 7. Size 4-0 sutures have a smaller diameter than size 3 sutures.

_____ 8. Sebaceous cysts are commonly found on the palm of the hand.

_____ 9. Colposcopy is frequently used to evaluate lesions of the cervix.

_____ 10. Cryosurgery is used in the treatment of cervical cancer.

A. Definitions

Directions: Match each medical term (numbers) with its definition (letters).

_____	1. Abrasion		A. A protective response of the body to trauma and the entrance of foreign matter
_____	2. Abscess		B. To cause a sterile object or surface to become unsterile
_____	3. Absorbable suture		C. A wound made by a sharp pointed object piercing the skin
_____	4. Approximation		D. The condition in which the body is invaded by a pathogen
_____	5. Bandage		E. A collection of pus in a cavity surrounded by inflamed tissue
_____	6. Biopsy		F. The arrest of bleeding by natural or artificial means
_____	7. Capillary action		G. Free of all living microorganisms and bacterial spores
_____	8. Colposcope		H. A wound in which the tissues are torn apart, leaving ragged and irregular edges
_____	9. Colposcopy		I. A lighted instrument with a binocular magnifying lens used to examine the vagina and cervix
_____	10. Contaminate		J. A localized staphylococcal infection that originates deep within a hair follicle; also known as a boil
_____	11. Contusion		K. An injury to the tissues under the skin that causes blood vessels to rupture, allowing blood to seep into the tissues
_____	12. Cryosurgery		L. The surgical removal and examination of tissue from the living body
_____	13. Fibroblast		M. A wound in which the outer layers of the skin are damaged
_____	14. Forceps		N. The action that causes liquid to rise along a wick, a tube, or a gauze dressing
_____	15. Furuncle		O. A two-pronged instrument for grasping and squeezing
_____	16. Hemostasis		P. Practices that keep objects and areas sterile or free from microorganisms
_____	17. Incision		Q. A break in the continuity of an external or internal surface caused by physical means
_____	18. Infection		R. The therapeutic use of freezing temperatures to destroy abnormal tissue
_____	19. Inflammation		S. The visual examination of the vagina and cervix using a lighted instrument with a magnifying lens
_____	20. Laceration		T. Suture material that is gradually digested and absorbed by the body
_____	21. Nonabsorbable suture		U. The process of bringing two parts, such as tissue, together through the use of sutures or other means
_____	22. Puncture		V. A strip of woven material used to wrap or cover a part of the body
_____	23. Sterile		W. A clean cut caused by a cutting instrument
_____	24. Surgery		X. Suture material that is not absorbed by the body
_____	25. Surgical asepsis		Y. An immature cell from which connective tissue can develop
_____	26. Wound		Z. The branch of medicine that deals with operative and manual procedures for correction of deformities and defects, repair of injuries, and diagnosis and treatment of certain diseases

B. Word Parts

Directions: Indicate the meaning of each word part in the space provided. List as many medical terms as possible that incorporate the word part in the space provided.

Word Part	Meaning of Word Part	Medical Terms That Incorporate Word Part
1. bi/o		
2. -opsy		
3. colp/o		
4. -scope		
5. -scopy		
6. cry/o		
7. fibr/o		
8. hem/o		
9. stasis		

EVALUATION OF LEARNING

Directions: Fill in each blank with the correct answer.

1. List the characteristics of a minor surgical procedure.

_____

_____

_____

_____

2. List the responsibilities of the medical assistant during a minor surgical operation.

_____

_____

_____

_____

3. What is the purpose of serrations found on some instruments?

_____

_____

4. What is the difference in function between mosquito hemostatic forceps and standard hemostatic forceps?

_____

_____

_____

5. What is the function of a speculum?

   _____

   _____

6. List five guidelines that should be followed in caring for instruments.

   _____

   _____

   _____

   _____

   _____

7. What is the difference between a closed and an open wound?

   _____

   _____

8. Why does a puncture wound encourage the growth of tetanus bacteria?

   _____

   _____

9. What is the purpose of inflammation?

   _____

   _____

10. List the four local signs that occur during inflammation.

   _____

11. What occurs during the inflammatory phase of wound healing?

   _____

   _____

12. What occurs during the granulation phase of wound healing?

   _____

   _____

13. What occurs during the maturation phase of wound healing?

   _____

14. What is an exudate?

   _____

   _____

15. Describe the appearance of the following types of exudates:

   a. Serous _____

   b. Sanguineous _____

   c. Purulent _____

    d. Serosanguineous _____

    e. Purosanguineous _____

16. List two functions of a sterile dressing.

    _____

    _____

17. The names and sizes of sutures are listed. In each set, circle the suture that has the smaller diameter:
    a. 4-0 silk
       2-0 silk
    b. 0 chromic surgical gut
       3-0 chromic surgical gut
    c. 2-0 polypropylene
       2 polypropylene

18. List five examples of materials used for nonabsorbable sutures.

    _____

    _____

19. What is a swaged needle? List advantages of using a swaged needle.

    _____

    _____

20. Why are sutures inserted in the head and neck generally removed sooner than other sutures?

    _____

    _____

21. List two advantages of using surgical skin staples to approximate a wound.

    _____

    _____

22. List three advantages of adhesive skin closures.

    _____

    _____

    _____

23. What is the purpose of preparing the patient's skin before minor office surgery?

    _____

24. What is the purpose of a fenestrated drape?

    _____

    _____

25. What is the name of the local anesthetic most frequently used in the medical office during minor office surgery?

    _____

26. Explain how an instrument should be handed to the physician during minor office surgery.

_____

27. What is a sebaceous cyst, and what causes it to form?

_____

_____

28. What is the purpose of using gauze packing or a rubber Penrose drain after incising a localized infection?

_____

_____

29. What is the difference between congenital nevi and acquired nevi?

_____

_____

30. What are skin tags? Where are they most frequently found on the body?

_____

_____

_____

31. Describe the appearance of dysplastic nevi. What concern exists with dysplastic nevi?

_____

_____

_____

32. List the characteristics of melanoma.

_____

_____

_____

33. What are the most common methods used to remove moles?

_____

_____

34. What is the purpose of a biopsy?

_____

_____

35. What is an ingrown toenail?

_____

_____

434

Chapter **10 Minor Office Surgery**

36. List three causes of an ingrown toenail.

_____

_____

_____

37. List two reasons for performing a colposcopy.

_____

_____

38. What is the purpose of performing a cervical punch biopsy?

_____

_____

39. List the postoperative instructions that must be relayed to the patient after a cervical punch biopsy.

_____

_____

_____

40. List two uses of cryosurgery.

_____

_____

41. List the postoperative instructions that must be relayed to the patient after cervical cryosurgery.

_____

_____

_____

42. List three functions of a bandage.

_____

_____

_____

43. List four guidelines to follow when applying a bandage.

_____

_____

_____

_____

44. List four signs that may indicate a bandage is too tight.

_____

_____

45. Why should the medical assistant be careful when applying an elastic bandage?

_____

_____

46. What is the purpose of reversing the spiral during a spiral-reverse turn?

_____

_____

47. List two uses of the figure-eight bandage turn.

_____

_____

48. What type of bandage turn is used to anchor a bandage?

_____

49. List four examples of body parts to which a tubular bandage can be applied.

_____

_____

_____

_____

50. List two advantages for using a tubular bandage (compared with a roller bandage).

_____

_____

CRITICAL THINKING ACTIVITIES

A. Medical and Surgical Asepsis

Refer to Chapter 2, and describe the difference between medical asepsis and surgical asepsis.

_____

_____

_____

Which technique (medical asepsis or surgical asepsis) would be employed during the following procedures? For procedures requiring surgical asepsis, indicate which of the following reasons necessitate the use of surgical asepsis: caring for broken skin, penetrating a skin surface, or entering a body cavity that is normally sterile.

1. Administering oral medication

_____

_____

2. Inserting sutures

_____

_____

3. Measuring oral temperature

_____

_____

4. Applying a bandage to the forearm

_____

_____

5. Performing a needle biopsy

_____

_____

6. Removing a sebaceous cyst

_____

_____

7. Obtaining a Pap specimen

_____

_____

8. Inserting a urinary catheter

_____

_____

9. Incision and drainage of an abscess

_____

_____

10. Applying a dressing to an open wound

_____

_____

B. Violation of Surgical Asepsis

In the situations that follow, the principles of surgical asepsis have been violated. In the space provided, explain why the techniques should not be performed in this manner.

1. Placing a sterile 4 × 4 gauze pad within the 1-inch border around the sterile field

_____

_____

2. Wearing rings during the application of sterile gloves

_____

_____

3. Talking over a sterile field

_____

_____

4. Reaching over a sterile field

_____

_____

5. Holding sterile gauze below waist level

_____

_____

6. Not palming the label when pouring an antiseptic solution

_____

_____

7. Spilling an antiseptic solution on the sterile field

_____

_____

8. Passing a soiled dressing over the sterile field

_____

_____

9. Placing a vial of Xylocaine on the sterile field

_____

_____

10. Using bare hands to arrange articles on the sterile field

_____

_____

C. Surgical Instruments

In the space provided, state the name and use of each of the following types of surgical instruments. Identify any of the following parts present on each instrument by labeling the instrument: box lock, spring handle, ratchets, serrations, cutting edge, and teeth.

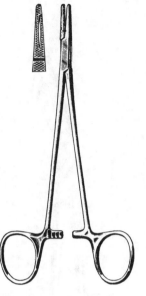

1. Name: _____

   Use: _____

   _____

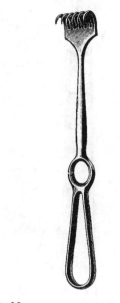

2. Name: _____

   Use: _____

   _____

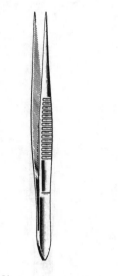

3. Name: _____

   Use: _____

   _____

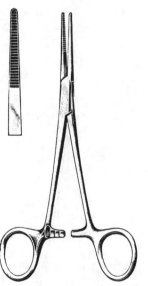

4. Name: _____

   Use: _____

   _____

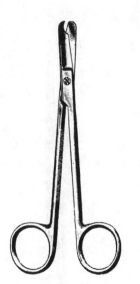

5. Name: _____

   Use: _____

   _____

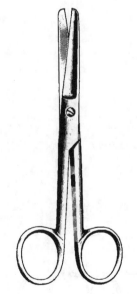

6. Name: _____

   Use: _____

   _____

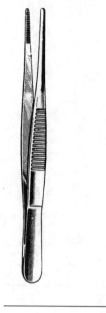

7. Name: _____

    Use: _____

    _____

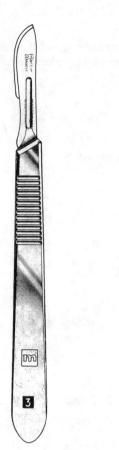

8. Name: _____

    Use: _____

    _____

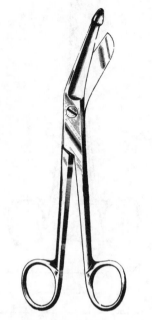

9. Name: _____

    Use: _____

    _____

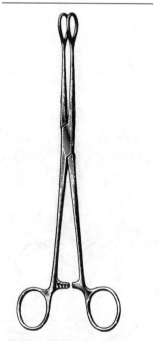

10. Name: _____

     Use: _____

     _____

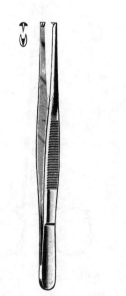

11. Name: _____

     Use: _____

     _____

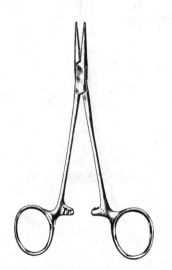

12. Name: _____

     Use: _____

     _____

440

Chapter **10 Minor Office Surgery**

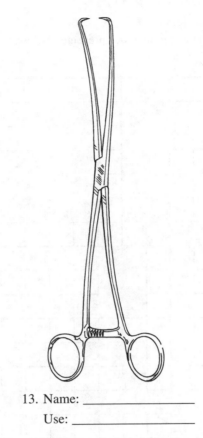

13. Name: _____

Use: _____

_____

(Courtesy of Elmed Incorporated, Addison, IL.)

D. Pioneers in Surgical Asepsis

Using a reference source, describe the contributions the following men made to medicine, especially regarding surgical asepsis:

1. Ignaz Semmelweis

_____

_____

_____

2. Louis Pasteur

_____

_____

_____

3. Joseph Lister

_____

_____

_____

E. Crossword Puzzle: Minor Office Surgery

Directions: Complete the crossword puzzle using the clues presented below.

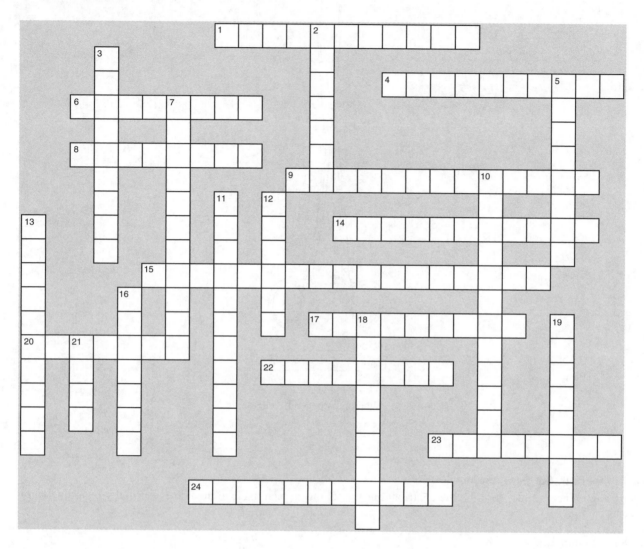

Across

1 Drape with a hole
4 Produces collagen
6 Clean, smooth cut
8 Boil
9 Sac containing oil secretions
14 Pus formation
15 Clamps off blood vessels
17 Local anesthetic brand name
20 Pus in a cavity
22 Tetanus may grow here
23 A local sign of inflammation
24 Bring together

Down

2 Free of all MOs and spores
3 Bruise
5 Scrape
7 Exudate containing blood
10 Suture/needle combination
11 Tx for chronic cervicitis
12 Father of modern surgery
13 Ragged and irregular wound
16 Discovered penicillin
18 Position for colposcopy
19 Antiseptic brand name
21 Nonabsorbable suture material

F. Patient Instruction Sheet

1. You are working for a surgeon, and she would like you to develop a patient instruction sheet for minor surgery. Select one of the minor operations provided. Using the following instruction sheet, develop a sheet that would be informative and visually appealing to a patient. Be as creative as possible in designing your sheet.

2. Select a partner. Have your partner play the role of a patient who is going to have the minor surgery performed, and explain the information on the sheet. Ask the patient to sign the sheet, and witness the patient's signature.

Minor office operations
 a. Sebaceous cyst removal
 b. Mole removal
 c. Needle biopsy
 d. Ingrown toenail removal
 e. Colposcopy and biopsy
 f. Cervical cryosurgery

Notes

PATIENT INSTRUCTION SHEET

NAME OF THE PROCEDURE:

DESCRIPTION OF PROCEDURE:

PURPOSE OF THE PROCEDURE:

HOW TO PREPARE FOR THE PROCEDURE:

WHAT TO DO FOLLOWING THE PROCEDURE:

I have received and understand the above instructions:

Patient's Signature _____

Witness: _____ Date: _____

Notes

VIDEO EVALUATION FOR CHAPTER 10: MINOR OFFICE SURGERY

Name: _____

Directions:

a. Watch the indicated videos.
b. Mark each true statement with a T and each false statement with an F. For each false statement, change the wording of the question so that it becomes a true statement.

Video: Procedure 10-1: Applying and Removing Sterile Gloves

_____ 1. Sterile gloves must be worn when changing a sterile dressing.

_____ 2. Rings do not need to be removed before applying sterile gloves.

_____ 3. Before applying sterile gloves, the hands must be rinsed with Betadine.

_____ 4. If your gloves are too small, they may rip as you apply them or become uncomfortable to wear.

_____ 5. The inside of the glove wrapper is considered contaminated.

_____ 6. The first glove should be picked up by the folded-back cuff with the fingers of the opposite hand.

_____ 7. The hands should be kept below waist level while gloving.

_____ 8. When removing gloves, the bare hands should not be allowed to come in contact with the outside of the gloves.

_____ 9. Gloves that are visibly contaminated with blood or other potentially infectious materials should be discarded in a biohazard waste container.

_____ 10. After gloves are removed, OSHA requires that the hands be sanitized to remove any microorganisms that may have come in contact with the hands.

Video: Procedures 10-2 and 10-3: Sterile Technique

_____ 1. The items included in a sterile pack depend on the type of procedure to be performed.

_____ 2. The inside of a sterile package can be used as a sterile field.

_____ 3. A sterile pack that is wet, torn, or opened is contaminated and cannot be used.

_____ 4. Autoclave tape that has changed color indicates that the contents of the pack are sterile.

_____ 5. An outdated antiseptic solution should not be used because it may produce an undesirable effect.

_____ 6. Talking, laughing, coughing, or sneezing over a sterile field contaminates it.

_____ 7. Reaching over the contents of a sterile field contaminates it.

_____ 8. A 4-inch border around the sterile field is considered contaminated because this area may become contaminated while setting up the sterile field.

_____ 9. A 4 × 4 gauze pad should be gently ejected onto the center of the sterile field.

_____ 10. The label of the antiseptic solution should be palmed while pouring the solution.

_____ 11. After removing the cap from the antiseptic solution, it should be placed on the sterile field with the open end facing up.

_____ 12. Holding the solution bottle too high while pouring it may cause the antiseptic to splash onto the sterile field and contaminate it.

Video: Procedure 10-4: Changing a Sterile Dressing

_____ 1. Surgical asepsis must be maintained when caring for an open wound and applying a sterile dressing.

_____ 2. The size, type, and amount of dressing material used depend on the size and location of the wound and the amount of drainage from the wound.

_____ 3. The function of a sterile dressing is to protect an open wound from contamination and trauma.

_____ 4. A soiled dressing should be removed by gently dragging it horizontally across the wound.

_____ 5. The inside of the dressing should not be touched to prevent transferring an infected discharge to your gloves.

_____ 6. The wound should be inspected for the amount of healing and the presence of drainage.

_____ 7. The antiseptic should be applied from the top to the bottom of the wound, by working from the outside to the center of the wound.

_____ 8. The sterile dressing should be placed over the wound by lightly dropping it in place.

_____ 9. The patient should be instructed to keep the wound clean and moist.

_____ 10. Signs indicating that the wound is infected include swelling, discharge, and pain.

_____ 11. The original signed copy of the wound care instructions protects the physician legally in the event the patient does not follow the wound care instructions and causes harm to the wound.

_____ 12. The bag of contaminated items should be discarded in a biohazard waste container.

Video: Procedure 10-5: Removing Sutures and Staples

_____ 1. Sutures approximate the edges of a wound and hold them in place until healing occurs.

_____ 2. Sutures and staples minimize the amount of scar formation.

_____ 3. The sutures should not be removed if the incision line is not approximated or if redness, swelling, or discharge is present.

_____ 4. Removing dried exudates from the suture line makes it more difficult to remove the sutures.

_____ 5. Do not allow any portion of the suture that was previously outside to be pulled through the tissue lying beneath the incision line.

_____ 6. The number of sutures should be counted as they are removed.

_____ 7. Suturing is the fastest method of closure of long skin incisions.

_____ 8. The patient should be told that a pulling sensation may be felt as each staple is removed.

_____ 9. When staples are removed, the bottom jaws of the staple remover are placed under the staple to be removed.

_____ 10. The staple remover should be lifted at an angle to remove the staple from the incision line.

Video: Procedure 10-6: Applying Adhesive Skin Closures

_____ 1. Adhesive skin closures consist of sterile strips of tape available in different lengths.

_____ 2. A local anesthetic must be used when applying adhesive skin closures.

_____ 3. Sutures have a lower incidence of wound infection than adhesive skin closures.

_____ 4. An antiseptic must be applied to the site before applying adhesive skin closures.

_____ 5. Applying Betadine helps the adhesive strips adhere to the patient's skin.

_____ 6. The first adhesive strip should be positioned over the center of the wound.

_____ 7. The adhesive strips should be applied at 1-inch intervals until the edges of the wound are approximated.

_____ 8. The skin closures will loosen and fall off on their own approximately 5 to 10 days after they have been applied.

Video: Procedure 10-7: Assisting with Minor Office Surgery

_____ 1. Nonsterile articles needed for the minor office surgery are set up on a side table or counter.

_____ 2. The sterile tray can be set up using a prepackaged setup or by transferring articles to a sterile field.

_____ 3. A fenestrated drape exposes only the operative site and maintains a sterile field around the site.

_____ 4. The patient should be asked to sign a consent to treatment form after the surgery is completed.

_____ 5. The patient should be asked whether he or she needs to void before the minor office surgery.

_____ 6. If the patient sneezes on the sterile field, microorganisms from the mouth, nose, and lungs can be transferred to the sterile field.

_____ 7. Clean gloves must be worn when handing the physician a sterile instrument during the minor office surgery.

_____ 8. A biopsy request form must accompany the tissue specimen to the laboratory.

_____ 9. Blood and body secretions should be rinsed off the instruments immediately to prevent them from drying and hardening on the instruments.

Video: Procedure 10-A: Bandage Turns

_____ 1. Bandages are used for support, immobilization, and holding a dressing in place.

_____ 2. The bandage turn that is used depends on the patient's age and physical condition.

_____ 3. The _circular turn_ is applied to a part of uniform width, such as toes, fingers, or the head.

_____ 4. The circular turn is used to anchor a bandage.

_____ 5. The _spiral turn_ is applied to a part of uniform circumference, such as the fingers, arms, legs, chest, or abdomen.

_____ 6. Each spiral turn is carried upward at a slight angle and should overlap the previous turn by one half to two thirds of the width of the bandage.

_____ 7. The _spiral-reverse turn_ is used to bandage a part that varies in width, such as the forearm or lower leg.

———— 8. Reversing each spiral turn allows for a smoother fit and prevents gaping caused by the variation in the contour of the limb.

———— 9. The *figure-eight turn* is used to hold a dressing in place or to support and immobilize an injured joint, such as the ankle, knee, elbow, or wrist.

PRACTICE FOR COMPETENCY

Sterile Technique

Procedure 10-1: Applying and Removing Sterile Gloves. Apply and remove sterile gloves.

Procedure 10-2: Sterile Package. Open a sterile package. Add a sterile article to a sterile field using a commercially prepared peel-apart package. Practice each of the methods used to transfer articles to a sterile field as shown in Figure 10-4 of your textbook.

Procedure 10-3: Sterile Solution. Pour a sterile solution into a container on a sterile field.

Minor Surgical Procedures

Procedure 10-4: Sterile Dressing. Change a sterile dressing and record the procedure in the chart provided.

Procedure 10-5: Suture and Staple Removal. Practice the procedure for removing sutures and staples, and record the procedure in the chart provided.

Procedure 10-6: Adhesive Skin Closures. Practice the procedure for applying and removing adhesive skin closures, and record the procedure in the chart provided.

Procedure 10-7: Assisting with Minor Office Surgery. Obtain eight index cards. For each of the following minor office surgical procedures, indicate (on one side of the card) the equipment and supplies required for the side table. On the other side of the card, indicate the equipment and supplies required for the sterile tray setup. Set up a surgical tray for the procedures listed using your index cards. In the chart provided, record the instructions relayed to the patient following the surgery.

a. Suture insertion
b. Sebaceous cyst removal
c. Incision and drainage of a localized infection
d. Mole removal
e. Needle biopsy
f. Ingrown toenail removal
g. Colposcopy
h. Cervical punch biopsy
i. Cervical cryosurgery

Procedure 10-A: Bandage Turns. Practice the following bandage turns:

a. Circular turn
b. Spiral turn
c. Spiral-reverse turn
d. Figure-eight turn
e. Recurrent turn

Procedure 10-8: Tubular Gauze Bandage. Practice the procedure for applying a tubular gauze bandage, and record the procedure in the chart provided.

	CHART
Date	

Procedure 10-1: Applying and Removing Sterile Gloves

Name: _____   Date: _____

Evaluated by: _____   Score: _____

Performance Objective

Outcome:	Apply and remove sterile gloves.
Conditions:	Given the appropriate-sized sterile gloves.
	Using a clean flat surface.
Standards:	Time: 5 minutes. Student completed procedure in _____ minutes.
	Accuracy: Satisfactory score on the Performance Evaluation Checklist.

Performance Evaluation Checklist

Trial 1	Trial 2	Point Value	Performance Standards
			Application of gloves:
		•	Removed rings and washed hands with an antimicrobial soap.
		▷	Explained why the hands should be washed.
		•	Selected the appropriate-sized gloves.
		▷	Explained what may occur if the gloves are too small or too large.
		•	Placed the glove package on a clean flat surface.
		•	Opened the sterile glove package without touching the inside of the wrapper.
		•	Picked up the first glove on the inside of the cuff without contaminating.
		•	Did not touch the outside of the glove with the bare hand.
		•	Stepped back and pulled on the glove and allowed the cuff to remain turned back on itself.
		•	Picked up the second glove by slipping sterile gloved fingers under its cuff and grasping the opposite side with the thumb.
		•	Pulled the glove on and turned back the cuff.
		•	Turned back the cuff of the first glove without contaminating.
		•	Adjusted the gloves to a comfortable position.
		•	Inspected the gloves for tears.
		▷	Explained what should be done if a glove is torn.
			Removal of gloves:
		•	Grasped the outside of the right glove 1 to 2 inches from the top with the gloved left hand.
		•	Slowly pulled right glove off the hand.
		•	Pulled the right glove free and scrunched it into a ball with the gloved left hand.
		•	Placed the index and middle fingers of the right hand on the inside of left glove.

Trial 1	Trial 2	Point Value	Performance Standards
		•	Did not allow the clean hand to touch the outside of the glove.
		•	Pulled the glove off the left hand, thus enclosing the balled-up right glove.
		•	Discarded both gloves in an appropriate waste container.
		▷	Stated how to discard gloves if they are visibly contaminated with blood.
		•	Sanitized hands.
		✱	Completed the procedure within 5 minutes.
			Totals

Evaluation of Student Performance

EVALUATION CRITERIA			COMMENTS
Symbol	**Category**	**Point Value**	
✱	Critical Step	16 points	
•	Essential Step	6 points	
▷	Theory Question	2 points	

Score calculation: 100 points

− _____ points missed

_____ Score

Satisfactory score: 85 or above

CAAHEP Competencies Achieved

Psychomotor (Skills)

☑ III. 3. Select appropriate barrier/personal protective equipment (PPE) for potentially infectious situations.

ABHES Competencies Achieved

☑ 9. b. Apply principles of aseptic techniques and infection control.

☑ 9. i. Use standard precautions.

Procedure 10-2: Opening a Sterile Package

Name: _____   Date: _____

Evaluated by: _____   Score: _____

Performance Objective

Outcome:	Open a sterile package.
Conditions:	Given a sterile package.
	Using a clean flat surface.
Standards:	Time: 5 minutes. Student completed procedure in _____ minutes.
	Accuracy: Satisfactory score on the Performance Evaluation Checklist.

Performance Evaluation Checklist

Trial 1	Trial 2	Point Value	Performance Standards
		•	Sanitized hands.
		•	Assembled the equipment.
		•	Checked the pack to make sure it is not wet, torn, or opened.
		•	Checked the autoclave tape on the pack.
		▷	Stated the purpose of the autoclave tape.
		•	Positioned the pack on the table so that the top flap of wrapper will open away from the body.
		•	Removed the fastener on the wrapped package and discarded it.
		•	Opened the first flap away from the body.
		•	Opened the left and right flaps without contaminating contents.
		•	Opened the flap closest to the body.
		•	In all cases, touched only the outside of the wrapper.
		•	In all cases, did not reach over the sterile contents of the package.
		▷	Stated why the medical assistant should not reach over the contents of the package.
		•	Adjusted the sterile wrapper by the corners as needed.
		•	Checked the sterilization indicator on the inside of the pack.
		▷	Stated the reason for checking the sterilization indicator.
		✶	Completed the procedure within 5 minutes.
			Totals

Evaluation of Student Performance

EVALUATION CRITERIA			COMMENTS
Symbol	**Category**	**Point Value**	
✷	Critical Step	16 points	
•	Essential Step	6 points	
▷	Theory Question	2 points	

Score calculation: 100 points

– _____ points missed

_____ Score

Satisfactory score: 85 or above

CAAHEP Competencies Achieved

Psychomotor (Skills)

☑ I. 10. Assist physician with patient care.

ABHES Competencies Achieved

☑ 9. n. Assist physician with minor office surgical procedures.

456

Chapter **10 Minor Office Surgery**

Using Commercially Prepared Sterile Packages

Name: _____   Date: _____

Evaluated by: _____   Score: _____

Performance Objective

Outcome:	Add a sterile article to a sterile field from a peel-apart package by ejecting its contents onto the field.
Conditions:	Given the following: peel-apart package and a sterile field.
Standards:	Time: 3 minutes. Student completed procedure in _____ minutes.
	Accuracy: Satisfactory score on the Performance Evaluation Checklist.

Performance Evaluation Checklist

Trial 1	Trial 2	Point Value	Performance Standards
		•	Sanitized hands.
		•	Grasped the two unsterile flaps of the peel-pack between the thumbs.
		•	Pulled the package apart using a rolling-outward motion.
		▷	Stated what parts of the peel-pack must remain sterile.
		•	Stepped back slightly from the sterile field.
		▷	Explained the reason for stepping back.
		•	Gently ejected the contents of the peel-pack onto the center of the sterile field.
		✱	Completed the procedure within 3 minutes.
			Totals

Evaluation of Student Performance

EVALUATION CRITERIA			COMMENTS
Symbol	**Category**	**Point Value**	
✱	Critical Step	16 points	
•	Essential Step	6 points	
▷	Theory Question	2 points	

Score calculation: 100 points

−   _____ points missed

_____ Score

Satisfactory score: 85 or above

CAAHEP Competencies Achieved

Psychomotor (Skills)

☑ I. 10. Assist physician with patient care.

ABHES Competencies Achieved

☑ 9. n. Assist physician with minor office surgical procedures.

EVALUATION OF COMPETENCY

Procedure 10-3: Pouring a Sterile Solution

Name: _____   Date: _____

Evaluated by: _____   Score: _____

Performance Objective

Outcome:	Pour a sterile solution.
Conditions:	Given the following: sterile solution, sterile container, and a sterile towel.
Standards:	Time: 5 minutes. Student completed procedure in _____ minutes.
	Accuracy: Satisfactory score on the Performance Evaluation Checklist.

Performance Evaluation Checklist

Trial 1	Trial 2	Point Value	Performance Standards
		•	Checked the label of the solution.
		•	Checked the expiration date on the solution.
			Explained why an outdated solution should not be used.
		•	Checked the solution label a second time.
		•	Palmed the label of the bottle.
		▷	Explained why the label should be palmed.
		•	Removed the cap and placed it on a flat surface with the open end up.
		▷	Stated why the cap should be placed with the open end up.
		•	Rinsed the lip of the bottle.
		▷	Explained why the lip of the bottle should be rinsed.
		•	Poured the proper amount of solution into a sterile container at a height of 6 inches.
		•	Did not allow the neck of the bottle to come in contact with container.
		•	Did not allow any of the solution to splash onto the sterile field.
		▷	Explained why the sterile solution should not be allowed to splash onto the sterile field.
		•	Replaced the cap on the container without contaminating.
		•	Checked the label a third time.
		✶	Completed the procedure within 5 minutes.
			Totals

EVALUATION CRITERIA			COMMENTS
Symbol	**Category**	**Point Value**	
✷	Critical Step	16 points	
•	Essential Step	6 points	
▷	Theory Question	2 points	

Score calculation: 100 points

− _____ points missed

_____ Score

Satisfactory score: 85 or above

CAAHEP Competencies Achieved

Psychomotor (Skills)

☑ I. 10. Assist physician with patient care.

ABHES Competencies Achieved

☑ 9. n. Assist physician with minor office surgical procedures.

EVALUATION OF COMPETENCY

Procedure 10-4: Changing a Sterile Dressing

Name: _____   Date: _____

Evaluated by: _____   Score: _____

Performance Objective

Outcome:	Change a sterile dressing.
Conditions:	Given the following: Mayo stand, biohazard waste container, clean and disposable gloves, antiseptic swabs, sterile gloves, plastic waste bag, adhesive tape and scissors, sterile dressing, and thumb forceps.
Standards:	Time: 10 minutes. Student completed procedure in _____ minutes.
	Accuracy: Satisfactory score on the Performance Evaluation Checklist.

Performance Evaluation Checklist

Trial 1	Trial 2	Point Value	Performance Standards
		•	Washed hands with an antimicrobial soap.
		•	Assembled the equipment.
		•	Set up nonsterile items on a side table or counter.
		•	Positioned the plastic waste bag in a convenient location.
		•	Greeted the patient and introduced yourself.
		•	Identified the patient and explained the procedure.
		•	Instructed the patient not to move during procedure.
		•	Adjusted the light.
		•	Applied clean gloves.
		•	Loosened the tape and carefully removed the soiled dressing by pulling it upward.
		•	Did not touch the inside of the dressing next to the wound.
		▷	Explained why the inside of the dressing should not be touched.
		▷	Described what should be done if the dressing is stuck to the wound.
		•	Placed the soiled dressing in the waste bag without touching the outside of the bag.
		•	Inspected the wound.
		▷	Stated what type of inspection should be performed.
		•	Opened the antiseptic swabs, and placed the pouch in a convenient location or held the pouch in your hand.
		•	Applied the antiseptic to the wound.
		•	Used a new swab for each motion.
		•	Discarded each contaminated swab in the waste bag after use.
		•	Removed gloves and discarded them without contaminating.
		•	Sanitized hands and prepared the sterile field.

Trial 1	Trial 2	Point Value	Performance Standards
		•	Instructed the patient not to talk, laugh, sneeze, or cough over the sterile field.
		•	Opened a sterile glove package and applied sterile gloves.
		•	Picked up a sterile dressing from the tray using sterile gloves or sterile forceps.
		•	Placed the sterile dressing over the wound by lightly dropping it in place.
		•	Did not move the dressing after dropping it in place.
		▷	Explained why the dressing should be dropped onto the wound and then not moved.
		•	Discarded the gloves (and forceps) in the waste bag.
		•	Applied hypoallergenic tape to hold the sterile dressing in place.
		•	Provided the patient with written wound care instructions.
		•	Instructed the patient in wound care.
		▷	Described the wound care that should be relayed to the patient.
		•	Asked the patient to sign the instruction sheet.
		•	Witnessed the patient's signature.
		•	Gave a signed copy to the patient.
		•	Filed the original in the patient's medical record.
		▷	Stated the purpose of filing the original in the patient's chart.
		•	Returned the equipment.
		•	Disposed of the plastic bag in a biohazard waste container.
		•	Sanitized hands.
		•	Charted the procedure correctly.
		✷	Completed the procedure within 10 minutes.
			Totals
			CHART
Date			

Evaluation of Student Performance

EVALUATION CRITERIA			COMMENTS
Symbol	**Category**	**Point Value**	
✱	Critical Step	16 points	
•	Essential Step	6 points	
▷	Theory Question	2 points	

Score calculation: 100 points

$-$ _____ points missed

_____ Score

Satisfactory score: 85 or above

CAAHEP Competencies Achieved

Psychomotor (Skills)

☑ IV. 5. Instruct patients according to their needs to promote health maintenance and disease prevention.

☑ IV. 6. Prepare a patient for procedures and/or treatments.

☑ IV. 8. Document patient care.

☑ IV. 9. Document patient education.

Affective (Behavior)

☑ III. 2. Explain the rationale for performance of a procedure to the patient.

☑ III. 3. Show awareness of patients' concerns regarding their perceptions related to the procedure being performed.

ABHES Competencies Achieved

☑ 4. a. Document accurately.

☑ 8. cc. Communicate on the recipient's level of comprehension.

☑ 9. l. Prepare patient for examinations and treatments.

☑ 9. r. Teach patients methods of health promotion and disease prevention.

Notes

EVALUATION OF COMPETENCY

Procedure 10-5: Removing Sutures and Staples

Name: _____   Date: _____

Evaluated by: _____   Score: _____

Performance Objective

Outcome:	Remove sutures and staples.
Conditions:	Given the following: Mayo stand, antiseptic swabs, clean and disposable gloves, sterile 4 × 4 gauze, surgical tape, biohazard waste container, suture removal kit, and staple removal kit.
Standards:	Time: 10 minutes. Student completed procedure in _____ minutes.
	Accuracy: Satisfactory score on the Performance Evaluation Checklist.

Performance Evaluation Checklist

Trial 1	Trial 2	Point Value	Performance Standards
		•	Washed hands with an antimicrobial soap.
		•	Assembled the equipment.
		•	Greeted the patient and introduced yourself.
		•	Identified the patient and explained the procedure.
		•	Positioned the patient as required.
		•	Adjusted the light.
		•	Checked to make sure the sutures (or staples) were intact.
		•	Checked to make sure the incision line was approximated and free from infection.
		▷	Explained what to do if the incision line is not approximated.
		•	Opened the suture or staple removal kit.
		•	Applied clean gloves.
		•	Cleaned the incision line with antiseptic swabs by using a new swab for each motion.
		•	Allowed the skin to dry.
		•	Informed the patient that he or she would feel a pulling sensation as each suture (or staple) is removed.
			Removed sutures as follows:
		•	Picked up the knot of suture with thumb forceps.
		•	Placed the curved tip of suture scissors under the suture.
		•	Cut the suture below the knot on the side of the suture closest to the skin.
		•	Gently pulled the suture out of the skin by using a smooth, continuous motion.
		•	Did not allow any portion of suture previously on the outside to be pulled through the tissue lying beneath the incision line.
		•	Placed the suture on the gauze.
		•	Repeated this sequence until all sutures were removed.

Trial 1	Trial 2	Point Value	Performance Standards
			Removed staples as follows:
		•	Gently placed the jaws of the staple remover under the staple.
		•	Squeezed the staple handles until they were fully closed.
		•	Lifted the staple remover upward to remove the staple.
		•	Placed the staple on gauze.
		•	Continued until all the staples were removed.
		•	Counted the number of sutures or staples and checked the number with the chart.
		•	Cleansed the site with an antiseptic swab.
		•	Applied adhesive skin closures if directed by the physician.
		•	Applied DSD, if directed to do so by the physician.
		•	Disposed of the sutures or staples and gauze in a biohazard waste container.
		•	Removed gloves and sanitized hands.
		•	Charted the procedure correctly.
		✶	Completed the procedure within 10 minutes.
			Totals
CHART				
Date			

Evaluation of Student Performance

EVALUATION CRITERIA			COMMENTS
Symbol	**Category**	**Point Value**	
✶	Critical Step	16 points	
•	Essential Step	6 points	
▷	Theory Question	2 points	

Score calculation: 100 points

− _____ points missed

_____ Score

Satisfactory score: 85 or above

CAAHEP Competencies Achieved

Psychomotor (Skills)

☑ IV. 5. Instruct patients according to their needs to promote health maintenance and disease prevention.

☑ IV. 6. Prepare a patient for procedures and/or treatments.

☑ IV. 8. Document patient care.

Affective (Behavior)

☑ III. 3. Show awareness of patients' concerns regarding their perceptions related to the procedure being performed.

☑ IV. 1. Demonstrate empathy in communicating with patients, family, and staff.

ABHES Competencies Achieved

☑ 4. a. Document accurately.

☑ 8. bb. Are impartial and show empathy when dealing with patients.

☑ 8. cc. Communicate on the recipient's level of comprehension.

☑ 9. l. Prepare patient for examinations and treatments.

☑ 9. r. Teach patients methods of health promotion and disease prevention.

Notes

Procedure 10-6: Applying and Removing Adhesive Skin Closures

Name: _____ Date: _____

Evaluated by: _____ Score: _____

Performance Objective

Outcome:	Apply and remove adhesive skin closures.
Conditions:	Given the following: clean and disposable gloves, sterile gloves, antiseptic solution, surgical scrub brush, antiseptic swabs, tincture of benzoin, sterile cotton-tipped applicator, adhesive skin closure strips, sterile 4 × 4 gauze pads, surgical tape, and a biohazard waste container.
Standards:	Time: 10 minutes. Student completed procedure in _____ minutes.
	Accuracy: Satisfactory score on the Performance Evaluation Checklist.

Performance Evaluation Checklist

Trial 1	Trial 2	Point Value	Performance Standards
			Application of adhesive skin closures:
		•	Washed hands with an antimicrobial soap.
		•	Assembled the equipment.
		•	Checked the expiration date on the adhesive skin closures.
		•	Greeted the patient and introduced yourself.
		•	Identified the patient and explained the procedure.
		•	Positioned the patient as required.
		•	Adjusted the light.
		•	Applied clean gloves.
		•	Inspected the wound for redness, swelling, and drainage.
		•	Scrubbed the wound with an antiseptic solution.
		•	Allowed the skin to dry or patted dry with gauze pads.
		•	Applied antiseptic by using a new swab for each motion.
		•	Allowed the skin to dry.
		▷	Explained why the skin must be completely dry.
		•	Applied tincture of benzoin without letting it touch the wound.
		▷	Stated the purpose of tincture of benzoin.
		•	Allowed the skin to dry.
		•	Removed gloves and washed hands.
		•	Opened the package of adhesive strips and laid them on a flat surface.
		•	Applied sterile gloves and tore the tab off the card of strips.
		•	Peeled a strip of tape off the card.

Trial 1	Trial 2	Point Value	Performance Standards
		•	Checked to make sure the skin surface was dry.
		•	Positioned the first strip over the center of the wound.
		•	Secured one end of the strip to the skin by pressing down firmly on the tape.
		•	Stretched the strip across the incision until the edges of the wound were approximated.
		•	Secured the strip to the skin on the other side of the wound.
		•	Applied the second strip on one side of center strip at a ⅛-inch interval.
		•	Applied a third strip at a ⅛-inch interval on the other side of the center strip.
		•	Continued applying the strips at ⅛-inch intervals until the edges of the wound were approximated.
		▷	Explained why the strips should be spaced at ⅛-inch intervals.
		•	Applied two closures approximately ½-inch from the ends of the strips.
			Stated the purpose of applying a strip along each edge.
		•	Applied a sterile dressing over the strips if indicated by the physician.
		•	Removed gloves and sanitized hands.
		•	Provided the patient with written wound care instructions.
		•	Explained the wound care instructions to the patient.
		•	Asked the patient to sign instruction sheet and witnessed the patient's signature.
		•	Gave a signed copy to the patient and filed original in the patient's medical record.
		•	Charted the procedure correctly.
			Removal of adhesive skin closures:
		•	Sanitized hands.
		•	Greeted the patient and introduced yourself.
		•	Identified the patient and explained the procedure.
		•	Positioned the patient as required.
		•	Adjusted the light.
		•	Checked to make sure the incision line was approximated and free from infection.
		•	Positioned a 4 × 4 gauze pad in a convenient location.
		•	Applied clean gloves.
		•	Peeled off each half of the strip from the outside toward the wound margin.
		•	Stabilized the skin with one finger.
		•	Gently lifted the strip up and away from the wound and placed it on the gauze.
		•	Continued until all closures were removed.
		•	Cleansed the site with an antiseptic swab.
		•	Applied a sterile dressing if indicated by the physician.
		•	Disposed of the strips and gauze in a biohazard waste container.
		•	Removed gloves and sanitized hands.
		•	Charted the procedure correctly.
		✱	Completed the procedure within 10 minutes.
			Totals

<table>
<tr><th colspan="2">CHART</th></tr>
<tr><td>Date</td><td></td></tr>
<tr><td></td><td></td></tr>
<tr><td></td><td></td></tr>
<tr><td></td><td></td></tr>
<tr><td></td><td></td></tr>
</table>

Evaluation of Student Performance

EVALUATION CRITERIA			COMMENTS
Symbol	**Category**	**Point Value**	
✶	Critical Step	16 points	
•	Essential Step	6 points	
▷	Theory Question	2 points	

Score calculation: 100 points

$$- \underline{\hspace{3cm}} \text{ points missed}$$

$$\underline{\hspace{2cm}} \text{ Score}$$

Satisfactory score: 85 or above

CAAHEP Competencies Achieved

Psychomotor (Skills)

☑ IV. 5. Instruct patients according to their needs to promote health maintenance and disease prevention.

☑ IV. 6. Prepare a patient for procedures and/or treatments.

☑ IV. 8. Document patient care.

Affective (Behavior)

☑ III. 2. Explain the rationale for performance of a procedure to the patient.

☑ III. 3. Show awareness of patients' concerns regarding their perceptions about the procedure being performed.

ABHES Competencies Achieved

☑ 4. a. Document accurately.

☑ 8. bb. Are impartial and show empathy when dealing with patients.

☑ 8. cc. Communicate on the recipient's level of comprehension.

☑ 9. l. Prepare patient for examinations and treatments.

☑ 9. r. Teach patients methods of health promotion and disease prevention.

Notes

Procedure 10-7: Assisting with Minor Office Surgery

Name: _____   Date: _____

Evaluated by: _____   Score: _____

Performance Objective

Outcome:	Set up the surgical tray and assist with minor office surgery.
Conditions:	Given a Mayo stand, biohazard waste container, and the instruments and supplies required for a specific minor office surgery as designed by the instructor.
Standards:	Time: 15 minutes. Student completed procedure in _____ minutes.
	Accuracy: Satisfactory score on the Performance Evaluation Checklist.

Performance Evaluation Checklist

Trial 1	Trial 2	Point Value	Performance Standards
		•	Determined the type of minor office surgery to be performed.
		•	Prepared examining room.
		•	Sanitized hands.
		•	Set up the articles required that are not sterile on a side table or counter.
		•	Labeled the specimen container (if included in the setup).
		•	Washed hands with an antimicrobial soap.
		•	Set up the minor office surgery tray on a clean, dry, flat surface, by using the principles of surgical asepsis.
			Prepackaged sterile setup:
		•	Selected the appropriate package from supply shelf, and placed it on a flat surface.
		•	Opened the setup using the inside of wrapper as the sterile field.
		•	Checked the sterilization indicator on the inside of the pack.
		•	Added any additional articles required for the surgery, and covered the tray setup with a sterile towel.
			Transferring articles to a sterile field:
		•	Placed a sterile towel on a flat surface by two corner ends, making sure not to contaminate it.
		•	Transferred sterile articles to the field from wrapped or peel-apart packages.
		•	Applied a sterile glove.
		•	Arranged articles neatly on the sterile field with a sterile glove.
		•	Checked to make sure all articles were available on the sterile field.
		•	Covered the tray setup with a sterile towel without allowing the arms to pass over the sterile field.

Trial 1	Trial 2	Point Value	Performance Standards
			Prepared the patient:
		•	Greeted the patient and introduced yourself.
		•	Identified the patient, explained the procedure, and reassured the patient.
		•	Asked the patient whether he or she needs to void before the surgery.
		•	Instructed the patient on clothing removal.
		•	Instructed the patient not to move during the procedure or to talk, laugh, sneeze, or cough over the sterile field.
		•	Positioned the patient as required for the type of surgery to be performed.
		•	Adjusted the light so that it was focused on the operative site.
			Prepared the patient's skin:
		•	Applied clean disposable gloves.
		•	Shaved the skin (if required).
		•	Cleansed the skin with an antiseptic solution.
		•	Rinsed and dried the area.
		•	Applied antiseptic using antiseptic swabs.
		•	Allowed the skin to dry.
		•	Removed gloves and sanitized hands.
		•	Checked to make sure that everything was ready and informed the physician.
			Assisted the physician:
		•	Uncovered the tray setup.
		•	Opened the outer glove wrapper for the physician.
		•	Held the vial while the physician withdrew the local anesthetic.
		•	Adjusted the light as required.
		•	Restrained the patient (e.g., child).
		•	Relaxed and reassured the patient.
		•	Handed instruments and supplies to the physician. Sterile gloves are required.
		•	Kept the sterile field neat and orderly. Sterile gloves are required.
		•	Held a basin for the physician to deposit soiled instruments and supplies. Clean gloves are required.
		•	Retracted the tissue. Sterile gloves are required.
		•	Sponged blood from the operative site. Sterile gloves are required.
		•	Added instruments and supplies as necessary to the sterile field.
		•	Held the specimen container to accept the specimen. Clean gloves are required.
		•	Cut the ends of suture material after insertion by the physician. Sterile gloves are required.
			After surgery:
		•	Applied a sterile dressing to the surgical wound if ordered by the physician.
		•	Stayed with the patient as a safety precaution.
		•	Assisted and instructed the patient as required.

Trial 1	Trial 2	Point Value	Performance Standards
		•	Verified that the patient understood the postoperative instructions.
		•	Provided the patient with verbal and written wound care instructions.
		▷	Stated the patient instructions that should be relayed for wound and suture care.
		•	Asked the patient to sign instruction sheet and witnessed the patient's signature.
		•	Gave a signed copy to the patient and filed original in the patient's medical record.
		•	Relayed information regarding the return visit.
		•	Assisted the patient off the table.
		•	Instructed the patient to get dressed.
		•	Prepared any specimens collected for transfer to the laboratory with a completed biopsy request.
		•	Charted correctly.
		•	Cleaned the examining room.
		•	Discarded disposable contaminated articles in a biohazard waste container.
		•	Sanitized and sterilized the instruments.
		✶	Completed the procedure within 15 minutes.
			Totals

CHART

Date	

Evaluation of Student Performance

EVALUATION CRITERIA			COMMENTS
Symbol	**Category**	**Point Value**	
✶	Critical Step	16 points	
•	Essential Step	6 points	
▷	Theory Question	2 points	

Score calculation: 100 points

− _____ points missed

_____ Score

Satisfactory score: 85 or above

CAAHEP Competencies Achieved

Psychomotor (Skills)

☑ I. 10. Assist physician with patient care.

☑ IV. 5. Instruct patients according to their needs to promote health maintenance and disease prevention.

☑ IV. 6. Prepare a patient for procedures and/or treatments.

☑ IV. 8. Document patient care.

☑ IX. 1. Respond to issues of confidentiality.

Affective (Behavior)

☑ III. 2. Explain the rationale for performance of a procedure to the patient.

☑ III. 3. Show awareness of patients' concerns regarding their perceptions related to the procedure being performed.

☑ IV. 6. Demonstrate awareness of how an individual's personal appearance affects anticipated responses.

☑ IX. 3. Recognize the importance of local, state, and federal legislation and regulations in the practice setting.

ABHES Competencies Achieved

☑ 4. a. Document accurately.

☑ 4. f. Comply with federal, state, and local health laws and regulations.

☑ 8. bb. Are impartial and show empathy when dealing with patients.

☑ 8. cc. Communicate on the recipient's level of comprehension.

☑ 9. e. Recognize emergencies and treatments and minor office surgical procedures.

☑ 9. l. Prepare patient for examinations and treatments.

☑ 9. n. Assist physician with minor office surgical procedures.

☑ 9. r. Teach patients methods of health promotion and disease prevention.

EVALUATION OF COMPETENCY

Procedure 10-A: Bandage Turns

Name: _____   Date: _____

Evaluated by: _____   Score: _____

Performance Objective

Outcome:	Apply the following bandage turns: circular, spiral, spiral-reverse, figure-eight, and recurrent.
Conditions:	Given the following: a roller bandage and an elastic bandage.
Standards:	Time: 15 minutes. Student completed procedure in _____ minutes.
	Accuracy: Satisfactory score on the Performance Evaluation Checklist.

Performance Evaluation Checklist

Trial 1	Trial 2	Point Value	Performance Standards
			Circular turn:
		•	Placed the end of a bandage on a slant.
		•	Encircled the body part while allowing the corner of the bandage to extend.
		•	Turned down the corner of the bandage.
		•	Made another circular turn around the body part.
		▷	Stated a use of the circular turn.
			Spiral turn:
		•	Anchored the bandage using a circular turn.
		•	Encircled the body part while keeping the bandage at a slant.
		•	Carried each spiral turn upward at a slight angle.
		•	Overlapped each previous turn by one half to two thirds of the width of the bandage.
		▷	Stated a use of the spiral turn.
			Spiral-reverse turn:
		•	Anchored the bandage by using a circular turn.
		•	Encircled the body part while keeping bandage at a slant.
		•	Reversed the spiral turn by using the thumb or index finger.
		•	Directed the bandage downward and folded it on itself.
		•	Kept the bandage parallel to the lower edge of the previous turn.
		•	Overlapped each previous turn by two thirds the width of the bandage.
		▷	Stated a use of the spiral-reverse turn.
			Figure-eight turn:
		•	Anchored the bandage using a circular turn.
		•	Slanted bandage turns to ascend and descend alternately around the body part.

477

Trial 1	Trial 2	Point Value	Performance Standards
		•	Crossed the turns over one another in the middle to resemble a figure eight.
		•	Overlapped each previous turn by two thirds of the width of the bandage.
		▷	Stated a use of the figure-eight turn.
			Recurrent turn:
		•	Anchored the bandage by using two circular turns.
		•	Passed the bandage back and forth over the tip of the body part being bandaged.
		•	Overlapped each previous turn by two thirds of the width of the bandage.
		▷	Stated a use of the recurrent turn.
		✳	Completed the procedure within 15 minutes.
			Totals

	CHART
Date	

Evaluation of Student Performance

EVALUATION CRITERIA			COMMENTS
Symbol	**Category**	**Point Value**	
✳	Critical Step	16 points	
•	Essential Step	6 points	
▷	Theory Question	2 points	

Score calculation: 100 points

−_____ points missed

_____ Score

Satisfactory score: 85 or above

CAAHEP Competencies Achieved

Psychomotor (Skills)

☑ IV. 5. Instruct patients according to their needs to promote health maintenance and disease prevention.

☑ IV. 6. Prepare a patient for procedures and/or treatments.

Affective (Behavior)

☑ I. 1. Apply critical thinking skills in performing patient assessment and care.

ABHES Competencies Achieved

☑ 9. l. Prepare patient for examinations and treatments.

☑ 9. r. Teach patients methods of health promotion and disease prevention.

Procedure 10-8: Applying a Tubular Gauze Bandage

Name: _____   Date: _____

Evaluated by: _____   Score: _____

Performance Objective

Outcome:	Apply a tubular gauze bandage.
Conditions:	Given the following: applicator, tubular gauze, adhesive tape and bandage scissors.
Standards:	Time: 5 minutes. Student completed procedure in _____ minutes.
	Accuracy: Satisfactory score on the Performance Evaluation Checklist.

Performance Evaluation Checklist

Trial 1	Trial 2	Point Value	Performance Standards
		•	Sanitized hands.
		•	Greeted the patient and introduced yourself.
		•	Identified the patient and explained the procedure.
		•	Assembled the equipment.
		•	Selected the proper applicator.
		•	Pulled a sufficient length of gauze from the dispensing box roll.
		•	Spread apart the open end of the gauze.
		•	Slid the gauze over one end of the applicator.
		•	Continued loading the applicator by gathering enough gauze on it to complete the bandage.
		•	Cut the roll of gauze near the opening of box.
		•	Placed the applicator over the proximal end of the patient's finger.
		•	Moved the applicator from the proximal to the distal end of the patient's finger.
		•	Held the bandage in place with the fingers.
		▷	Explained why the bandage should be held in place.
		•	Pulled the applicator 1 to 2 inches past the end of the patient's finger.
		•	Rotated the applicator one full turn to anchor the bandage.
		•	Moved the applicator forward toward the proximal end of the patient's finger.
		•	Moved the applicator forward approximately 1 inch past the original starting point of the bandage.
		•	Rotated the applicator one full turn.
		▷	Stated the reason for rotating the applicator.
		•	Repeated the procedure for the number of layers desired.
		•	Finished the last layer at the proximal end.

Trial 1	Trial 2	Point Value	Performance Standards
		•	Cut the gauze from the applicator.
		•	Removed the applicator.
		•	Applied adhesive tape at the base of the patient's finger.
		•	Sanitized hands.
		•	Charted the procedure correctly.
		✴	Completed the procedure within 5 minutes.
			Totals

CHART	
Date	

Evaluation of Student Performance

EVALUATION CRITERIA			COMMENTS
Symbol	**Category**	**Point Value**	
✴	Critical Step	16 points	
•	Essential Step	6 points	
▷	Theory Question	2 points	

Score calculation: 100 points

− _____ points missed

_____ Score

Satisfactory score: 85 or above

CAAHEP Competencies Achieved

Psychomotor (Skills)

☑ IV. 5. Instruct patients according to their needs to promote health maintenance and disease prevention.

☑ IV. 6. Prepare a patient for procedures and/or treatments.

Affective (Behavior)

☑ I. 1. Apply critical thinking skills in performing patient assessment and care.

ABHES Competencies Achieved

☑ 9. l. Prepare patient for examinations and treatments.

☑ 9. r. Teach patients methods of health promotion and disease prevention.

11 Administration of Medication and Intravenous Therapy

CHAPTER ASSIGNMENTS

√ After Completing	Date Due	Textbook Pages	TEXTBOOK ASSIGNMENTS	Possible Points	Points You Earned
		414–490	Read Chapter 11: Administration of Medication and Intravenous Therapy		
		420 486	Read Case Study 1 — Case Study 1 questions	5	
		443 486	Read Case Study 2 — Case Study 2 questions	5	
		457 486	Read Case Study 3 — Case Study 3 questions	5	
			Total points		

√ After Completing	Date Due	Study Guide Pages	STUDY GUIDE ASSIGNMENTS (CTA = Critical Thinking Activity)	Possible Points	Points You Earned
		489	Pretest	10	
		490 491	Key Term Assessment A. Definitions B. Word Parts (Add 1 point for each medical term)	26 13	
		491–497	Evaluation of Learning questions	65	
		498–500	CTA A: Using the PDR	34	
		501–502	CTA B: Locating Information in a Drug Insert	12	
		502	CTA C: Drug Classifications (3 points each)	30	
			Evolve Site: Chapter 11 Road to Recovery Game: Abbreviations		
			Evolve Site: Chapter 11 Road to Recovery Game: Drug Classifications		
		503	CTA D: Medication Record	20	
		504	CTA E: Seven Rights of Medication Administration	35	

481

Copyright © 2015, 2012, 2008, 2004, 2000, 1995, 1990 by Saunders, an imprint of Elsevier Inc. All rights reserved.

Chapter 11 Administration of Medication and Intravenous Therapy

√ After Completing	Date Due	Study Guide Pages	STUDY GUIDE ASSIGNMENTS (CTA = Critical Thinking Activity)	Possible Points	Points You Earned
			e Evolve Site: Chapter 11 Script It!: Label Parts of a Prescription (Record points earned)		
		505	CTA F: Liquid Measurement	11	
		505	CTA G: Parts of a Needle and Syringe	11	
			e Evolve Site: Chapter 11 Take the Plunge: Label the Parts of a Needle and Syringe (Record points earned)		
		505–506	CTA H: Hypodermic Syringe Calibrations	10	
			e Evolve Site: Chapter 11 Which Needle?: Administration of Medication (Record points earned)		
		506	CTA I: Insulin Syringe Calibrations	20	
		506–507	CTA J: Tuberculin Syringe Calibrations	14	
			e Evolve Site: Chapter 11 Draw It Up!: Drawing up Medication (Record points earned)		
			e Evolve Site: Chapter 11 Math Review (Record points earned)		
		507	CTA K: Syringe and Needle Labels (3 points each)	12	
		507	CTA L: Angle of Insertion for Injections	3	
		508–509	CTA M: Preparing and Administering Parenteral Medication	18	
		509	CTA N: Measuring Mantoux Test Reactions	5	
		510	CTA O: Interpreting Mantoux Test Reactions	11	
		510–511	CTA P: Anaphylactic Reaction	20	
		512–522	CTA Q: Researching Drugs (5 points per drug researched)	325	
		523	CTA R: Crossword Puzzle	37	

√ After Completing	Date Due	Study Guide Pages	STUDY GUIDE ASSIGNMENTS (CTA = Critical Thinking Activity)	Possible Points	Points You Earned
			e Evolve Site: Chapter 11 Animations (2 points each)	10	
			e Evolve Site: Chapter 11 Nutrition Nugget: Food Allergy	10	
			e Evolve Site: Apply Your Knowledge questions	10	
		525–527	*e* Video Evaluation	60	
		489	Posttest	10	
			ADDITIONAL ASSIGNMENTS		
			Total points		

Notes

√ After Completing	Date Due	Study Guide Pages	STUDY GUIDE ASSIGNMENTS Drug Dosage Calculation: Supplemental Education for Chapter 11	Possible Points	Points You Earned
		557	Unit 1: The Metric System A. Units of Measurement	10	
		557	Unit 1: The Metric System B. Metric Abbreviations	7	
		558	Unit 1: The Metric System C. Metric Notation	20	
		558–559	Unit 2: The Apothecary System A. Units of Measurement	14	
		559	Unit 2: The Apothecary System B. Apothecary Abbreviations	10	
		559–560	Unit 2: The Apothecary System C. Apothecary Notation	20	
		560	Unit 3: The Household System Practice Problems for Units of Measurement	4	
		560–561	Unit 4: Medication Orders A. Medical Abbreviations	20	
		561–562	Unit 4: Medication Orders B. Interpreting Medication Orders (3 points each)	30	
		562–563	Unit 5: Converting Units of Measurement A. Using Conversion Tables (2 points each)	50	
		563–565	Unit 5: Converting Units of Measurement B. Converting Units within the Metric System (2 points each)	40	
		565–568	Unit 5: Converting Units of Measurement C. Converting Units within the Apothecary System (2 points each)	50	
		568–570	Unit 5: Converting Units of Measurement D. Converting Units within the Household System (2 points each)	20	
		570–572	Unit 6: Ratio and Proportion A. Ratio and Proportion Guidelines (6 points each)	48	

485

√ After Completing	Date Due	Study Guide Pages	STUDY GUIDE ASSIGNMENTS Drug Dosage Calculation: Supplemental Education for Chapter 11	Possible Points	Points You Earned
		572–573	Unit 6: Ratio and Proportion B. Converting Units Using Ratio (2 points each)	40	
		574–580	Unit 7: Determining Drug Dosage A. Oral Administration (2 points each)	30	
		580–585	Unit 7: Determining Drug Dosage B. Parenteral Administration (2 points each)	20	
			ADDITIONAL ASSIGNMENTS		
			Total points		

√ When Assigned by Your Instructor	Study Guide Pages	Practices Required	LABORATORY ASSIGNMENTS (Procedure Number and Name)	Score*
	529–530	5	Practice for Competency 11-1: Administering Oral Medication Textbook reference: pp. 447–449	
	533–535		Evaluation of Competency 11-1: Administering Oral Medication	*
	529–530	Vial: 5 Ampule: 5	Practice for Competency 11-2: Preparing an Injection Textbook reference: pp. 458–461	
	537–539		Evaluation of Competency 11-2: Preparing an Injection	*
	529–530	3	Practice for Competency 11-3: Reconstituting Powdered Drugs Textbook reference: pp. 461–462	
	541–542		Evaluation of Competency 11-3: Reconstituting Powdered Drugs	*
	529–530	5	Practice for Competency 11-4: Administering a Subcutaneous Injection Textbook reference: pp. 462–464	
	543–545		Evaluation of Competency 11-4: Administering a Subcutaneous Injection	*
	530	5	Practice for Competency 11-5: Administering an Intramuscular Injection Textbook reference: pp. 464–466	
	547–549		Evaluation of Competency 11-5: Administering an Intramuscular Injection	*
	530	5	Practice for Competency 11-6: Z-Track Intramuscular Injection Technique Textbook reference: p. 467	
	551–552		Evaluation of Competency 11-6: Z-Track Intramuscular Injection Technique	*
	530–531	5	Practice for Competency 11-7: Administering an Intradermal Injection Textbook reference: pp. 480–483	

√ When Assigned by Your Instructor	Study Guide Pages	Practices Required	LABORATORY ASSIGNMENTS (Procedure Number and Name)	Score*
	553–555		Evaluation of Competency 11-7: Administering an Intradermal Injection	*
			ADDITIONAL ASSIGNMENTS	

Name: _____ Date: _____

True or False

_____ 1. A drug is a chemical that is used for treatment, prevention, or diagnosis of disease.

_____ 2. The generic name of a drug is assigned by the pharmaceutical manufacturer that develops the drug.

_____ 3. The Rx symbol comes from the Latin word *recipe* and means "take."

_____ 4. An anaphylactic reaction can be life-threatening.

_____ 5. The dorsogluteal site is the most common site for administering injections in infants.

_____ 6. A subcutaneous injection is given into muscle tissue.

_____ 7. The purpose of aspirating when administering an injection is to make sure the needle is not in a blood vessel.

_____ 8. The Mantoux tuberculin skin test is administered through a subcutaneous injection.

_____ 9. The peripheral veins of the arm and hand are used most often for administering IV therapy.

_____ 10. Chemotherapy is the use of chemicals to treat disease.

?▤ **POSTTEST**

True or False

_____ 1. OSHA is responsible for determining whether drugs are safe before release for human use.

_____ 2. An enteric-coated tablet does not dissolve until it reaches the intestines.

_____ 3. The apothecary system is most often used to administer medication in the medical office.

_____ 4. The parenteral route of administering medications is used when the patient is allergic to the oral form of the drug.

_____ 5. Hypodermic syringes are calibrated in milliliters.

_____ 6. The maximum amount of medication that can be administered through the subcutaneous route is 2 mL.

_____ 7. A patient with latent tuberculosis infection has a negative reaction to a TB test.

_____ 8. A tuberculin skin test result should be read 15 to 20 minutes after administering.

_____ 9. The administration of fluids, medication, or nutrients through the IV route is known as an infusion.

_____ 10. The administration of blood through the IV route is known as an IV push.

A. Definitions

Directions: Match each medical term (numbers) with its definition (letters).

_____ 1. Adverse reaction

_____ 2. Allergen

_____ 3. Allergy

_____ 4. Ampule

_____ 5. Anaphylactic reaction

_____ 6. Chemotherapy

_____ 7. Controlled drug

_____ 8. Dose

_____ 9. Drug

_____ 10. Gauge

_____ 11. Induration

_____ 12. Infusion

_____ 13. Inhalation administration

_____ 14. Intradermal injection

_____ 15. Intramuscular injection

_____ 16. Intravenous therapy

_____ 17. Oral administration

_____ 18. Parenteral

_____ 19. Pharmacology

_____ 20. Prescription

_____ 21. Subcutaneous injection

_____ 22. Sublingual administration

_____ 23. Topical administration

_____ 24. Transfusion

_____ 25. Vial

_____ 26. Wheal

A. Application of a drug to a particular spot, usually for a local action
B. Introduction of medication into the dermal layer of the skin
C. A small, sealed glass container that holds a single dose of medication
D. A physician's order authorizing the dispensing of a drug by a pharmacist
E. An unintended and undesirable effect produced by a drug
F. An abnormal hypersensitivity of the body to substances that are ordinarily harmless
G. The administration of a liquid agent directly into a patient's vein, where it is distributed throughout the body by way of the circulatory system
H. A tense, pale raised area of the skin
I. Introduction of medication beneath the skin, into the subcutaneous or fatty layer of the body
J. An abnormally raised hardened area of the skin with clearly defined margins
K. A closed glass container with a rubber stopper that holds medication
L. The administration of medication by way of air or other vapor being drawn into the lungs
M. A serious allergic reaction that requires immediate treatment
N. Administration of medication by mouth
O. A drug that has restrictions placed on it by the federal government because of its potential for abuse
P. Introduction of medication into the muscular layer of the body
Q. Administration of medication by placing it under the tongue
R. The quantity of a drug to be administered at one time
S. A substance that is capable of causing an allergic reaction
T. A chemical used for the treatment, prevention, or diagnosis of disease
U. The diameter of the lumen of a needle used to administer medication
V. Administration of medication by injection
W. The study of drugs
X. The use of chemicals to treat disease; most often refers to the treatment of cancer using antineoplastic medications
Y. The administration of fluids, medications, or nutrients into a vein
Z. The administration of whole blood or blood products through the intravenous route

B. Word Parts

Directions: Indicate the meaning of each word part in the space provided. List as many medical terms as possible that incorporate the word part in the space provided.

Word Part	Meaning of Word Part	Medical Terms That Incorporate Word Part
1. chem/o		
2. -therapy		
3. intra-		
4. derm/o		
5. muscul/o		
6. -ar		
7. ven/o		
8. -ous		
9. pharmac/o		
10. sub-		
11. cutane/o		
12. lingu/o		
13. trans-		

EVALUATION OF LEARNING

Directions: Fill in each blank with the correct answer.

Administration of Medication

1. What are the differences among administering, prescribing, and dispensing medication at the medical office?

_____

_____

_____

_____

2. What is the difference between the generic name and the brand name of a drug?

_____

_____

_____

_____

3. What is a liniment?

_____

_____

4. What is a spray?

_____

_____

5. What is a syrup?

_____

_____

6. What is a tablet?

_____

7. What is the purpose of scoring a tablet?

_____

8. List two drugs that come in the form of chewable tablets.

_____

9. List two reasons for enterically coating a tablet.

_____

_____

10. What is a capsule?

_____

11. Why must a suppository have a cylindrical or conical shape?

_____

_____

12. What is a transdermal patch?

_____

_____

13. Why is the metric system used most often to administer medication?

_____

_____

14. Define the term *volume*.

_____

15. Describe the use of the household system of measurement.

_____

_____

16. When is conversion required?

_____

_____

17. What is a controlled drug?

_____

18. In what forms can a prescription be authorized?

_____

_____

_____

19. What requirements must be followed when writing a prescription for a schedule II drug?

_____

_____

_____

20. List five brand names of schedule II analgesics.

_____

_____

21. What requirements must be followed when writing a prescription for a schedule III drug?

_____

_____

_____

22. What is a schedule IV drug?

_____

_____

23. List three brand names of schedule IV analgesics.

_____

_____

24. List four brand names of schedule IV antianxiety agents.

_____

_____

25. What is included in each of the following parts of a prescription?

    a. Superscription _____

    b. Inscription _____

    c. Subscription _____

    d. Signatura _____

26. Why is it important for the patient's age to be indicated on a prescription?

_____

_____

27. What functions can be performed by an EMR prescription program?

_____

_____

_____

28. What types of medications should be recorded on a medication record form?

_____

29. List and describe three factors that affect the action of drugs in the body.

_____

_____

_____

30. What are the symptoms and treatment of an anaphylactic reaction?

_____

_____

31. What are the advantages and disadvantages of using the parenteral route of administration?

_____

_____

_____

_____

32. How do safety-engineered syringes reduce the risk of a needlestick injury?

_____

33. What is the purpose of using a filter needle when withdrawing medication from an ampule?

_____

34. What sites are used most frequently to administer a subcutaneous injection?

_____

_____

35. List three medications commonly administered through a subcutaneous injection.

_____

_____

_____

36. Why is medication absorbed faster through the intramuscular route than through the subcutaneous route?

_____

_____

37. List the four intramuscular (IM) injection sites, and explain why these sites must be used to administer an IM injection.

_____

_____

_____

_____

38. What types of medication are given using the Z-track technique?

_____

_____

39. What sites are used most frequently to administer an intradermal injection?

_____

40. What is the most frequent use of an intradermal injection?

_____

41. What are the symptoms of active pulmonary tuberculosis?

_____

42. What is latent tuberculosis infection?

_____

43. What are examples of categories of individuals who should have a tuberculin test?

_____

_____

_____

44. Why might a person who was recently infected with tuberculosis have a negative tuberculin skin test result?

_____

_____

45. What is induration, and what causes it?

_____

_____

46. What procedures are performed if a patient has a positive reaction to a tuberculin skin test?

_____

_____

495

47. Who should have a two-step tuberculin skin test?

_____

_____

48. What does it mean if the first test of a two-step tuberculin skin test is negative and the second test is positive? What does it mean if both tests are negative?

_____

_____

_____

49. What is the name of the blood test for tuberculosis?

_____

50. What are 10 examples of common allergens?

_____

_____

_____

_____

51. What is the general treatment for allergies?

_____

52. What is the purpose of patch testing?

_____

_____

53. How long does it take for a reaction to occur with a skin-prick test?

_____

54. Explain what is meant by each of the following intradermal skin test reactions.

    a. ±1 _____

    b. +2 _____

    c. +3 _____

55. What are the advantages of in vitro blood testing over direct skin testing?

_____

_____

_____

Intravenous Therapy

1. What is intravenous therapy?

   _____

2. Which veins are most often used for IV therapy?

   _____

3. What types of liquid agents are administered through IV therapy?

   _____

4. List examples of outpatient sites in which IV therapy may be administered.

   _____

   _____

5. List five reasons for administering IV therapy in an outpatient setting.

   _____

   _____

   _____

6. What are the advantages of outpatient IV therapy?

   _____

   _____

7. What requirements must be met before an entry-level medical assistant can perform IV therapy at a medical office?

   _____

   _____

8. What must be determined by the physician before prescribing IV therapy?

   _____

   _____

9. What are the responsibilities of the physician in prescribing IV therapy?

   _____

   _____

10. What instructions should the medical assistant relay to a patient scheduled for outpatient IV therapy?

   _____

   _____

CRITICAL THINKING ACTIVITIES

A. Using the PDR

This activity assists you in learning how to use the *Physicians' Desk Reference* (PDR). Refer to Figure 11-1 in your textbook to answer the following questions.

Manufacturer's Index

1. What information is included in the Manufacturer's Index?

_____

_____

2. What company manufactures the drugs listed in the Manufacturer's Index?

_____

3. What number would you call if you had an emergency on the weekend regarding one of these drugs?

_____

4. What page would you turn to in the PDR for product information on Nitrostat tablets?

_____

5. Is a photograph included in the PDR for Dilantin-125 Oral Suspension?

_____

6. What page would you turn to in the PDR to find a color photograph of Nardil tablets?

_____

Brand and Generic Name Index

1. To what page in the current PDR edition would you turn to find product information on Lipitor tablets manufactured by Parke-Davis?

_____

2. What is the generic name of Prinivil tablets?

_____

3. What company manufactures Prinivil tablets?

_____

4. What page would you turn to in the PDR to find product information on Prinivil tablets?

_____

5. What page would you turn to in the PDR to find product identification information on Prinivil tablets?

_____

6. Who manufactures Lisinopril tablets?

_____

7. Does the PDR contain full product information on Lisinopril tablets?

_____

Product Category Index

1. What information is included in the Product Category Index?

2. Who manufactures Soma tablets?

3. What page would you turn to in the current PDR edition to find product information on Skelaxin tablets?

4. Who manufactures Valium tablets?

Product Identification Guide

1. What is included in the Product Identification Guide?

2. How can this section assist the user?

Product Information

Under which heading would you look in this section to find information on the following subjects?

1. Conditions the drug is approved by the FDA to treat

2. Information to relay to the patient to ensure safe and effective use of the drug

3. Route of administration

4. Symptoms associated with an overdose of the drug

5. Situations that require special consideration when the drug is used

6. Generic name of the drug

7. How the drug functions in the body to produce its therapeutic effect

_____

_____

8. Situations in which the drug should not be used

_____

_____

9. Recommended adult dosage and duration of treatment

_____

10. How to pronounce the brand name of the drug

_____

11. Handling and storage conditions

_____

_____

_____

12. Serious adverse reactions that may occur with the drug

_____

_____

_____

13. Symptoms associated with an overdose of the drug

_____

_____

_____

14. Unintended and undesirable effects that may occur with the use of the drug

_____

_____

_____

15. Modification of dosage needed for children

_____

B. Locating Information in a Drug Insert

Obtain a drug insert for a prescription drug, and answer the following questions.

1. What is the brand name of the drug?

_____

2. What is the generic name of the drug?

_____

3. What is the drug category of this medication?

_____

4. What are the dosage forms for this drug?

_____

5. What is the route of administration of this medication?

_____

6. What are the indications and usage for this medication?

_____

_____

_____

7. What are the contraindications for this medication?

_____

_____

_____

8. List the warnings for this drug.

_____

_____

_____

9. What are the general precautions for this medication?

_____

_____

_____

10. What information should be relayed to patients regarding this medication?

_____

_____

_____

11. What are the adverse reactions for this medication?

_____

_____

_____

12. What is the dosage and administration for this medication?

_____

_____

C. Drug Classifications

Inspect the package labels of 10 drugs (or use other means) to assess the classification of each drug based on preparation and action. List the name of each drug along with its appropriate category in the spaces provided. Compare results. Example: drug: Tylenol elixir; classification based on preparation: elixir; classification based on action: analgesic, antipyretic.

Classification Based On

Drug	Preparation	Action
1. _____	_____	_____
2. _____	_____	_____
3. _____	_____	_____
4. _____	_____	_____
5. _____	_____	_____
6. _____	_____	_____
7. _____	_____	_____
8. _____	_____	_____
9. _____	_____	_____
10. _____	_____	_____

D. Medication Record

Complete the following medication record form using yourself as the patient. Make sure to include all prescription medications and OTC medications, including vitamin supplements and herbal products. Use Figure 11-5 in your textbook as a guide in completing this form.

MEDICATION RECORD							
Patient _____					ALLERGY		
Birth date _____							
DATE	MEDICATION AND DOSAGE	FREQUENCY	RX	OTC	REFILLS		STOP

E. Seven Rights of Medication Administration

You are the office manager at a large clinic. Six new medical assistants were just hired. Your physician asks you to design an illustrated poster portraying the seven rights of medication administration to remind the new employees of the importance of following these guidelines. Use the diagram below to design your poster.

Follow the Seven Rights	
Right Drug	Right Dose
Right Time	Right Patient
Right Route	Right Technique
Right Documentation	

F. Liquid Measurement

Obtain a medicine cup that is graduated into the metric (milliliters), apothecary (drams and ounces), and household (teaspoons and tablespoons) systems. Complete the following:

1. What is its capacity?
   _____ ounces

   _____ milliliters

   _____ tablespoons

   _____ drams

2. Practice pouring oral liquid medication by pouring the following amounts of water into the medicine cup. Place a check mark by each amount after it has been properly poured.

   20 mL   _____

   4 drams   _____

   1 ounce   _____

   10 mL   _____

   ½ ounce   _____

   1 tablespoon _____

   2 drams   _____

G. Parts of a Needle and Syringe

Obtain a needle and syringe. Locate the following parts of each and explain their function.

Needle   **Function**

1. Hub _____

2. Shaft _____

3. Lumen _____

4. Point _____

5. Bevel _____

6. What is the gauge of the needle? _____

7. What is the length of the needle? _____

Syringe   **Function**

8. Barrel _____

9. Flange _____

10. Plunger _____

11. What is the capacity of the syringe? _____

H. Hypodermic Syringe Calibrations

1. Obtain a 3-mL syringe that is divided into tenths of a milliliter. Locate the following calibrations on the syringe. Place a check mark in the blank next to each calibration after it has been correctly located.

   0.5 mL _____

   1.0 mL _____

   1.2 mL _____

   2.5 mL _____

   2.7 mL _____

2. Locate each calibration (listed in the previous question) on the illustration of the hypodermic syringe by placing an arrow on the correct calibration line and labeling it with the calibration.

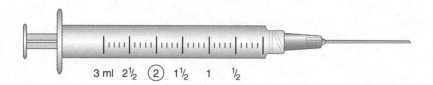

3 ml 2½ ② 1½ 1 ½

I. Insulin Syringe Calibrations

1. Obtain a U-100 insulin syringe. Locate the following calibrations (units) on the syringe, and place a check mark in the blank next to each calibration after it has been correctly located.

10 _____

16 _____

20 _____

44 _____

60 _____

68 _____

70 _____

86 _____

90 _____

100 _____

2. Locate each calibration (listed in the previous question) on the illustration of the insulin syringe by placing an arrow on the correct calibration line and labeling it with the calibration.

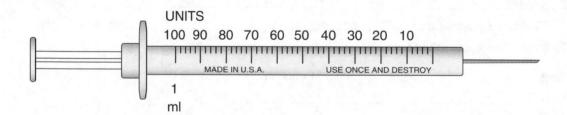

UNITS
100 90 80 70 60 50 40 30 20 10
MADE IN U.S.A. USE ONCE AND DESTROY
1
ml

J. Tuberculin Syringe Calibrations

1. Obtain a 1-mL tuberculin syringe that is divided into tenths and hundredths of a milliliter. Locate the following calibrations on the syringe. Place a check mark in the blank next to each calibration after it has been correctly located.

0.05 mL _____

0.10 mL _____

0.15 mL _____

0.34 mL _____

0.52 mL _____

0.75 mL _____

0.92 mL _____

2. Locate each calibration (listed in the previous question) on the illustration of the tuberculin syringe by placing an arrow on the correct calibration line and labeling it with the calibration.

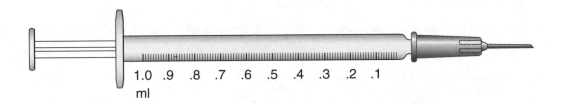

1.0 .9 .8 .7 .6 .5 .4 .3 .2 .1
ml

K. Syringe and Needle Labels

Refer to Figure 11-8 in your textbook, and indicate the following information for each syringe and needle: the syringe capacity and the gauge and length of the needle.

_____

_____

_____

_____

_____

L. Angle of Insertion for Injections

In the diagram that follows, draw three lines indicating the angle of insertion into the correct body tissue for an intradermal, a subcutaneous, and an intramuscular injection. Label the lines.

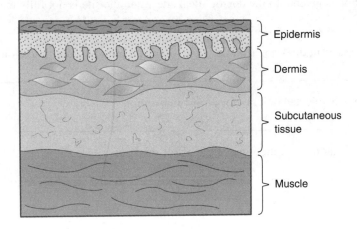

Epidermis

Dermis

Subcutaneous tissue

Muscle

M. Preparing and Administering Parenteral Medication

For each of the following situations involving the preparation and administration of medication, write **C** if the technique is correct and **I** if it is incorrect. If the technique is correct, state the principle underlying the technique. If the technique is incorrect, explain what might happen if it were performed.

_____ 1. The expiration date of the medication is checked before administering the medication.

_____ 2. The medical assistant is unfamiliar with the drug to be administered, so he or she looks it up in a drug reference.

_____ 3. The medical assistant compares the medication label with the physician's instructions three times: as it is taken from the shelf, before preparing the medication, and after preparing the medication.

_____ 4. The rubber stopper of the multidose vial is cleansed with an antiseptic wipe before withdrawing the medication.

_____ 5. Air is not injected into the multidose vial before withdrawing the medication.

_____ 6. Air bubbles are present in the medication in the syringe that has been withdrawn from an ampule.

_____ 7. The injection sites are not rotated when repeated injections are given.

_____ 8. The antiseptic is not allowed to dry before administering an injection.

_____ 9. The skin is stretched taut before an intramuscular injection is given.

_____ 10. The needle is inserted slowly and steadily for an IM injection.

_____ 11. An IM injection is given in the deltoid site to a patient who has a tight sleeve.

_____ 12. An IM injection is given into the dorsogluteal site when the site is not fully exposed.

_____ 13. The medical assistant does not aspirate when giving an intramuscular injection.

_____ 14. The medication is injected quickly for an IM injection.

_____ 15. The needle is withdrawn at the same angle as for insertion.

_____ 16. The intradermal needle is inserted with the bevel facing downward.

_____

_____ 17. The medical assistant does not aspirate when giving an intradermal injection.

_____

_____ 18. Pressure is applied to the injection site after an intradermal injection is given.

_____

N. Measuring Mantoux Test Reactions

Measure the diameter of the following circles, which represent induration from a Mantoux tuberculin skin test. A millimeter ruler is provided below. Cut it out and use it to measure the tuberculin reactions. Record results in the chart provided.

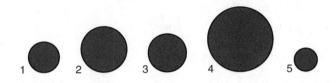

TB Skin Testing
(mm ruler)
0   10   20

CHART	
Date	

O. Interpreting Mantoux Test Reactions

Tuberculin skin test reactions are listed for various individuals. Using Table 11-7 in your textbook as a reference, determine if the individual's test results are positive or negative, and indicate your answer in the space provided.

_____ a. 2 mm of induration; an individual who is caring for a parent with active TB

_____ b. 7 mm of induration; a student attending college

_____ c. 12 mm of induration; an individual who is 12% below ideal body weight

_____ d. 8 mm of induration; an HIV-infected individual

_____ e. Erythema that is 6 mm wide (no induration); an individual with rheumatoid arthritis on Enbrel

_____ f. 16 mm of induration; a dietitian working in a nursing home

_____ g. 12 mm of induration; an individual who recently traveled to Canada

_____ h. 5 mm of induration; a child living with a parent who has active TB

_____ i. 6 mm of induration; an individual with diabetes mellitus

_____ j. 11 mm of induration; a recent immigrant from Africa

_____ k. 9 mm of induration; an individual working in a home and garden center

P. Anaphylactic Reaction

Following these guidelines, create a profile of an individual who is experiencing an anaphylactic reaction:

1. Using colored pencils, crayons, or markers, draw a figure of an individual exhibiting the symptoms of an anaphylactic reaction. Be as creative as possible.

2. Do not use any text on your drawing other than to label items you have drawn in your picture. (A picture is worth a thousand words!)

3. Try to include as many of the symptoms of an anaphylactic reaction as possible.

4. In the classroom, find a partner, and show your drawings. Identify the symptoms in your partner's drawing. With your partner, discuss what causes an anaphylactic reaction and how to prevent it. Also discuss the method of treatment for an anaphylactic reaction.

ANAPHYLACTIC REACTION

Q. Researching Drugs

Obtain a drug reference book, and look up the following information for each of the drugs listed on the Pharmacology Drug Sheets: generic name and drug classification, indications, and patient teaching. Record this information in the appropriate space on the Pharmacology Drug Sheets.

Pharmacology Drug Sheet

Name: _____

Generic Name and Drug Classification	Indications	Patient Teaching
Abilify		
Accupril		
Adderall		
Adrenalin		
Advair Diskus		

Pharmacology Drug Sheet

Name: _____

Ambien		
Amoxil		
Aricept		
Ativan		
Bentyl		
Cardizem		

Chapter **11 Administration of Medication and Intravenous Therapy**

Name: _____

Catapres		
Celebrex		
Cipro		
Coumadin		
Cozaar		
Crestor		

Pharmacology Drug Sheet

Name: _____

Cymbalta		
Depo-Medrol		
Depo-Provera		
Detrol		
Diflucan		
Dilantin		

Chapter **11** **Administration of Medication and Intravenous Therapy**

Pharmacology Drug Sheet

Name: _____

Flagyl		
Flexeril		
Flonase		
Fosamax		
Glucotrol XL		
Humulin		

Pharmacology Drug Sheet

Name: _____

Imitrex		
INFeD		
Keflex		
Lamisil		
Lanoxin		
Lasix		

Chapter **11** **Administration of Medication and Intravenous Therapy**

Pharmacology Drug Sheet

Name: _____

Lipitor		
Loestrin Fe		
Lomotil		
Lyrica		
Macrobid		
Mexate		

Pharmacology Drug Sheet

Name: _____

Nitro-Bid		
Norvasc		
Percocet		
Phenergan		
Plavix		
Premarin		

Chapter **11** **Administration of Medication and Intravenous Therapy**

Pharmacology Drug Sheet

Name: _____

Prevacid		
Prinivil		
Prozac		
Requip		
Rocephin		
Singulair		

Chapter **11** **Administration of Medication and Intravenous Therapy**

Pharmacology Drug Sheet

Name: _____

Synthroid		
Tessalon		
Toprol XL		
Valium		
Valtrex		
Viagra		

Pharmacology Drug Sheet

Name: _____

Vicodin		
Xanax		
Zithromax		
Zyban		
Zyloprim		
Zyrtec		

R. Crossword Puzzle: Administration of Medication

Directions: Complete the crossword puzzle using the clues provided.

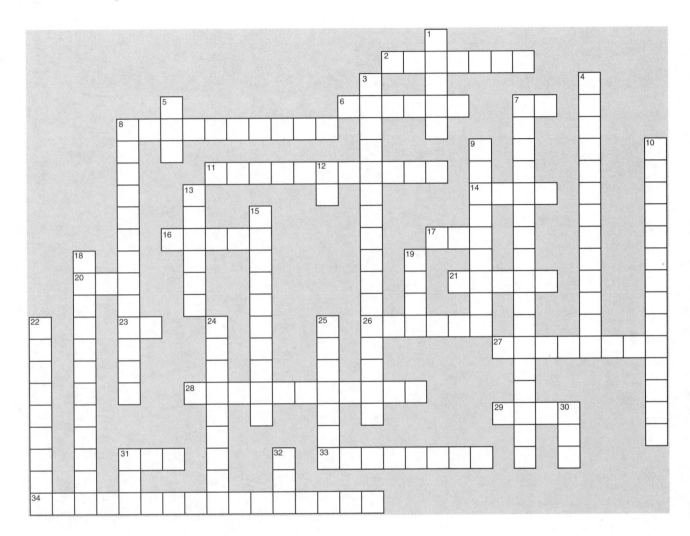

Across
- **2** Discovered penicillin
- **6** Most aggressive Hymenoptera
- **7** 1 mL = 1 _____
- **8** Present with a + Mantoux
- **11** Used to treat anaphylactic reaction
- **14** Metric weight unit
- **16** Ranges between 18 and 27
- **17** Aspirin
- **20** Available w/o a Rx
- **21** Needle opening
- **23** Before meals
- **26** Sym: wheezing and dyspnea
- **27** Allergy to molds and pollen
- **28** Conditions a drug is approved to treat
- **29** Immediately!
- **31** Tuberculin is made of this
- **33** Causes house dust allergy
- **34** Runny and inflamed allergic nose

Down
- **1** Slant of the needle
- **3** Do not use this drug!
- **4** Drug to d/c before allergy testing
- **5** Approves drugs
- **7** Poison ivy causes this
- **8** Abnormal or peculiar reaction
- **9** Medication label info
- **10** Calibrated in units
- **12** By mouth
- **13** Prevents syringe from rolling
- **15** This drug may cause an allergic reaction
- **18** Do not use this IM site for children
- **19** Blood test for allergies
- **22** Hives
- **24** Rx requirement for controlled drug
- **25** Max of 1 mL at this site
- **30** Three times per day
- **31** Drug reference (ex)
- **32** As needed

Notes

Name: _____

Directions:

a. Watch the indicated videos.
b. Mark each true statement with a T and each false statement with an F. For each false statement, change the wording of the question so that it becomes a true statement.

Video: Procedure 11-2: Preparing an Injection

_____ 1. Parenteral refers to the administration of medication by mouth.

_____ 2. The medical assistant must administer medication only under the direction of the physician.

_____ 3. A vial is a closed glass container with a rubber stopper.

_____ 4. When preparing medication, the drug label must be checked just one time to make sure it is the correct medication.

_____ 5. An outdated medication should not be used because it could produce undesirable effects.

_____ 6. The rubber stopper of the vial must be cleansed to remove any dust or bacteria present on the stopper.

_____ 7. Air must be injected into the vial to prevent the formation of a vacuum, which would make it difficult to withdraw medication.

_____ 8. Air bubbles must be removed from the syringe because they take up space the medication should occupy.

_____ 9. An ampule is a small, sealed glass container that holds several doses of medication.

_____ 10. The stem of an ampule is broken off by snapping it quickly and firmly toward the body.

_____ 11. A filter needle should be used to remove medication from an ampule.

_____ 12. When withdrawing fluid from an ampule, the needle opening must be kept below the fluid level to avoid drawing air into the syringe.

Video: Procedure 11-3: Reconstituting a Powdered Drug

_____ 1. Medications that are not stable in a liquid form must be prepared and stored in a powder form in a vial.

_____ 2. The liquid used to reconstitute a powdered drug is known as the solute.

_____ 3. The vial must be shaken vigorously to mix the powdered drug and liquid.

_____ 4. If the vial is for multiple-dose administration, it must be labeled with the date of preparation and your initials.

Video: Procedure 11-4: Administration of a Subcutaneous Injection

_____ 1. The subcutaneous layer consists of collagen and is located just under the skin.

_____ 2. The sites most commonly used for a subcutaneous injection include the upper arm, thigh, back, and abdomen.

_____ 3. Allergy injections should always be administered in the same arm.

_____ 4. After cleansing the skin, the antiseptic must be allowed to dry before administering the injection to prevent patient irritation and discomfort.

_____ 5. When administering an SC injection to an obese patient, the skin should be grasped and held in a cushion fashion.

_____ 6. The skin should be held taut when administering an SC injection to a normal-sized adult.

_____ 7. The needle should be positioned at a 45-degree angle to the arm if you are using a ⅝-inch needle to administer an SC injection.

_____ 8. After inserting the needle, remove your hand from the skin to prevent injecting the medication into compressed tissue, which can result in an allergic reaction.

_____ 9. Rapid injection of the medication can destroy tissue and lead to patient discomfort.

_____ 10. The needle should be removed at the same angle as was used for insertion to minimize patient discomfort.

_____ 11. After removing the needle, vigorously rub the area so that the medication is completely absorbed.

_____ 12. After an allergy injection is administered, the patient must wait for 5 minutes to make sure that an allergic reaction does not occur.

Video: Procedure 11-5: Administering an Intramuscular Injection

_____ 1. Intramuscular injections are administered into the muscular layer that lies beneath the skin and subcutaneous layers.

_____ 2. Numerous nerve fibers located in muscle tissue make absorption of medication more rapid through this route.

_____ 3. The length of the needle used for an IM injection depends on the size of the patient.

_____ 4. Thick and oily medications require a needle with a bigger lumen.

_____ 5. Intramuscular injections must be administered at specific sites to avoid puncturing large nerves or blood vessels.

_____ 6. In an adult, the gluteal muscles are well developed and can absorb a large amount of medication.

_____ 7. The deltoid site is small and cannot accommodate more than 5 mL of medication.

_____ 8. The dorsogluteal site is used to administer medication to infants and young children.

_____ 9. An IM injection should be inserted with the needle held at a 90-degree angle to the patient's skin.

_____ 10. The IM needle should be inserted to the hub.

_____ 11. If a medication intended for intramuscular administration is injected into a blood vessel, the result is faster absorption of the medication, which may produce undesirable results.

_____ 12. After withdrawing the IM needle, apply gentle pressure to the injection site with the gauze pad so that the medication is completely absorbed by the muscle tissue.

Video: Procedure 11-6: Administering an Injection Using the Z-Track Method

_____ 1. Medications that are irritating to subcutaneous tissue or medications that discolor the skin must be given using the Z-track method.

_____ 2. The Z-track method seals off the needle path and prevents the medication from reaching the subcutaneous layers or skin surface.

_____ 3. The dorsogluteal site is located in the upper outer quadrant of the buttocks about 2 to 3 inches below the iliac crest.

_____ 4. The injection site should be cleansed with an antiseptic wipe using a circular motion, starting at the injection site and moving outward.

_____ 5. The skin should be pulled away laterally from the injection site approximately 1 to 1½ inches.

_____ 6. After injecting the medication, wait 60 seconds before withdrawing the needle to allow for initial absorption of the medication.

_____ 7. Releasing the traction on the skin seals off the needle track and prevents the medication from reaching the subcutaneous tissue and skin surface.

_____ 8. Pressure should be applied to the injection site to prevent the medication from seeping out.

Video: Procedure 11-7: Administering an Intradermal Injection

_____ 1. An intradermal injection is administered into the dermal layer of the skin at an angle almost parallel to the skin.

_____ 2. The most frequent use of intradermal injections is to administer skin tests.

_____ 3. The needle used for an intradermal injection ranges from ⅜ inch to ⅝ inch, and the gauge ranges between 25 and 27.

_____ 4. If the antiseptic has not dried when the skin is punctured, it may cause a reaction that could be mistaken for a positive test result.

_____ 5. The needle should be inserted at a 10- to 15-degree angle with the bevel downward.

_____ 6. If a wheal does not form, complete the injection, and chart this information in the patient's medical record.

_____ 7. Applying pressure to the injection site may cause leakage of the testing solution through the needle puncture site, thus resulting in inaccurate test results.

_____ 8. Instruct the patient to cover the test site with a Band-Aid and to rub the arm dry after washing it.

_____ 9. The TB test results must be read within 48 to 72 hours after the test has been administered.

_____ 10. The TB test result should be read horizontally to the long axis of the forearm, meaning _across_ the forearm.

_____ 11. If erythema is present without induration, the results are interpreted as negative.

_____ 12. The TB test results should be recorded in millimeters.

Notes

PRACTICE FOR COMPETENCY

Prerequisite. Complete the Drug Dosage Calculation: Supplemental Education for Chapter 11 (pages 557–585 in this manual).
Procedure 11-1: Oral Medication. Administer oral solid and liquid medication, and record the procedure in the chart provided.
Procedure 11-2: Preparing the Injection. Prepare an injection from an ampule and a vial.
Procedure 11-3: Reconstituting Powdered Drugs. Reconstitute a powdered drug for parenteral administration.
Procedure 11-4: Subcutaneous Injection. Administer an allergy injection, and record the procedure in the allergy injection form provided.

ALLERGY INJECTION (IMMUNOTHERAPY) RECORD

Name _____

Date of Birth _____

ADMINISTRATION GUIDELINES:

Allergy injections are administered weekly. The allergy extract should be increased by 0.05 mL per week until symptomatic improvement is achieved or until a maximum dosage of 0.5 mL is reached.

The patient should remain in the office for 20 minutes following the injection and the reaction should be noted. If no reaction occurs, the abbreviation NR should be recorded. If a reaction occurs, it should be recorded in mm.

Do not administer the allergy injection in the following situations:
    a. The patient is ill with a temperature that is greater than 101° F
    b. The patient is having an acute asthma attack
    c. The patient is experiencing shortness of breath

Vial Number: **Vial Expiration Date:** _____
    _____ 1
    _____ 2
    _____ 3
    _____ 4

DATE	DOSAGE (mL)	Left Arm	Right Arm	REACTION (mm)	ADMINISTERED BY:

Procedure 11-5: Intramuscular Injection. Administer an intramuscular injection, and record the procedure in the chart provided.

Procedure 11-6: Z-Track Method. Administer an intramuscular injection using the Z-track method. Record the procedure in the chart provided.

Procedure 11-7: Intradermal Injection. Administer an intradermal injection, and record the procedure in the chart provided. Read and interpret the test results, and record them in the chart. Complete three TB test record cards located on the following page.

CHART	
Date	

TUBERCULOSIS TEST RECORD

Name	Date Admin: / /
	Date Read: / /
MANTOUX TEST	**RESULT**

____ mm

Logan Family Practice
401 St. George St.
St. Augustine, FL 32084
(904) 555-3933

Performed by _____

TUBERCULOSIS TEST RECORD

Name	Date Admin: / /
	Date Read: / /
MANTOUX TEST	**RESULT**

____ mm

Logan Family Practice
401 St. George St.
St. Augustine, FL 32084
(904) 555-3933

Performed by _____

TUBERCULOSIS TEST RECORD

Name	Date Admin: / /
	Date Read: / /
MANTOUX TEST	**RESULT**

____ mm

Logan Family Practice
401 St. George St.
St. Augustine, FL 32084
(904) 555-3933

Performed by _____

Notes

Chapter **11** **Administration of Medication and Intravenous Therapy**

EVALUATION OF COMPETENCY

Procedure 11-1: Administering Oral Medication

Name: _____   Date: _____

Evaluated by: _____   Score: _____

Performance Objective

Outcome:	Administer oral solid and liquid medication.
Conditions:	Given the following: appropriate medication, medicine cup, and a medication tray.
Standards:	Time: 5 minutes. Student completed procedure in _____ minutes.
	Accuracy: Satisfactory score on the Performance Evaluation Checklist.

Performance Evaluation Checklist

Trial 1	Trial 2	Point Value	Performance Standards
		•	Sanitized hands.
		•	Assembled equipment.
		•	Worked in a quiet, well-lit atmosphere.
		•	Selected the correct medication from the shelf.
		•	Compared the medication with the physician's instructions.
		•	Checked the drug label.
		•	Checked the expiration date.
		•	Calculated the correct dose to be given, if needed.
		•	Removed the bottle cap.
		•	Checked the drug label and poured the medication.
			Solid medication
		✱	Poured the correct number of capsules or tablets into the bottle cap.
		▷	Explained why the medication is poured into the bottle cap.
		•	Transferred the medication to a medicine cup.
			Liquid medication
		•	Placed lid of bottle on a flat surface with the open end facing up.
		•	Palmed the surface of the drug label.
		▷	Explained why the surface of the drug label should be palmed.
		•	Placed thumbnail at the proper calibration on medicine cup.
		•	Held the medicine cup at eye level.
		✱	Poured the correct amount of medication and read the dose at the lowest level of the meniscus.
		•	Replaced the bottle cap.
		•	Checked the drug label and returned the medication to its storage location.

533

Trial 1	Trial 2	Point Value	Performance Standards
		•	Greeted the patient and introduced yourself.
		•	Identified the patient and explained the procedure.
		•	Handed the medicine cup to the patient.
		•	Offered water to the patient.
		▷	Stated one instance when water should not be offered.
		•	Remained with the patient until the medication was swallowed.
		•	Sanitized hands.
		•	Charted the procedure correctly.
		✷	Completed the procedure within 10 minutes.
			Totals

CHART	
Date	

Evaluation of Student Performance

EVALUATION CRITERIA			COMMENTS
Symbol	**Category**	**Point Value**	
✷	Critical Step	16 points	
•	Essential Step	6 points	
▷	Theory Question	2 points	

Score calculation: 100 points

− _____ points missed

_____ Score

Satisfactory score: 85 or above

CAAHEP Competencies Achieved

Psychomotor (Skills)

☑ I. 8. Administer oral medications.

☑ II. 1. Prepare proper dosages of medication for administration.

☑ IX. 7. Document accurately in the patient record.

Affective (Behavior)

☑ II. 1. Verify ordered doses or dosages before administration.

☑ IX. 2. Demonstrate awareness of the consequences of not working within the legal scope of practice.

ABHES Competencies Achieved

☑ 4. a. Document accurately.

☑ 9. j. Prepare and administer oral and parenteral medications as directed by physician.

535

Notes

Procedure 11-2: Preparing an Injection

Name: _____   Date: _____

Evaluated by: _____   Score: _____

Performance Objective

Outcome:	Prepare an injection from an ampule and a vial.
Conditions:	Given the following: medication ordered by the physician, needle and syringe, antiseptic wipe, and medication tray.
Standards:	Time: 10 minutes. Student completed procedure in _____ minutes.
	Accuracy: Satisfactory score on the Performance Evaluation Checklist.

Performance Evaluation Checklist

Trial 1	Trial 2	Point Value	Performance Standards
		•	Sanitized hands.
		•	Assembled equipment.
		•	Worked in a quiet, well-lit atmosphere.
		✶	Selected the proper medication from its storage location.
		•	Checked the drug label.
		•	Compared the medication with the physician's instructions.
		•	Checked the expiration date.
		✶	Calculated the correct dose to be given, if needed.
		•	Opened syringe and needle packages.
		•	Assembled the needle and syringe if necessary.
		•	Made sure that the needle is attached firmly to the syringe and moved the plunger back and forth.
		•	Checked the drug label a second time.
		•	If required, mixed the medication.
			Withdrew medication from a vial
		•	Removed the metal or plastic cap if vial is new.
		•	Cleansed the rubber stopper of the vial with an antiseptic wipe and allowed it to dry.
		•	Placed the vial in an upright position on a flat surface.
		•	Removed the needle guard.
		•	Drew air into the syringe equal to the amount of medication to be withdrawn.
		•	Inserted the needle through the rubber stopper until it reached the empty space between the stopper and the fluid level.
		•	Pushed down on the plunger to inject air into the vial.
		•	Kept the needle above the fluid level.

Trial 1	Trial 2	Point Value	Performance Standards
		▷	Explained why air must be injected into the vial.
		•	Inverted the vial while holding onto the syringe and plunger.
		✷	Held the syringe at eye level and withdrew the proper amount of medication.
		•	Kept the needle opening below the fluid level.
		▷	Explained why the needle opening must be kept below the fluid level.
		•	Removed any air bubbles in the syringe by tapping the barrel with the fingertips.
		▷	Explained why air bubbles should be removed from the syringe.
		•	Removed any air remaining at the top of the syringe by pushing the plunger forward.
		•	Removed the needle from the rubber stopper and replaced the needle guard.
		•	If required, removed the needle and replaced it with a new needle.
		•	Checked the drug label for a third time and returned the medication to its storage location.
			Withdrew medication from an ampule
		•	Removed the regular needle from the syringe and attached a filter needle.
		▷	Stated the purpose of a filter needle.
		•	Cleansed the neck of the vial with an antiseptic wipe.
		•	Tapped the stem of the ampule lightly to remove any medication in the neck of ampule.
		•	Checked the medication label a second time.
		•	Placed a piece of gauze around the neck of ampule.
		•	Broke off the stem by snapping it quickly and firmly away from the body.
		•	Discarded the stem and gauze in a biohazard sharps container.
		•	Placed the ampule on a flat surface.
		•	Removed the needle guard.
		•	Inserted the needle opening below the fluid level.
		✷	Withdrew the proper amount of medication.
		•	Kept the needle opening below the fluid level.
		▷	Explained why the needle opening must be kept below the fluid level.
		•	Removed the needle from the ampule and replaced the needle guard.
		•	Checked the drug label for a third time.
		•	Discarded the ampule in a biohazard sharps container.
		•	Removed the filter needle and reapplied the regular needle (and guard) to the syringe.
		•	Tapped the syringe to remove air bubbles.
		•	Removed the needle guard and expelled air remaining at the top of syringe.
		•	Replaced the needle guard.
		✷	Completed the procedure within 10 minutes.
			Totals

Evaluation of Student Performance

EVALUATION CRITERIA			COMMENTS
Symbol	**Category**	**Point Value**	
∗	Critical Step	16 points	
•	Essential Step	6 points	
▷	Theory Question	2 points	

Score calculation: 100 points

  − _____ points missed

  _____ Score

Satisfactory score: 85 or above

CAAHEP Competencies Achieved

Psychomotor (Skills)

☑ II. 1. Prepare proper dosages of medication for administration.

Affective (Behavior)

☑ II. 1. Verify ordered doses or dosages before administration.

ABHES Competencies Achieved

☑ 9. j. Prepare and administer oral and parenteral medications as directed by physician.

Notes

Procedure 11-3: Reconstituting Powdered Drugs

Name: _____   Date: _____

Evaluated by: _____   Score: _____

Performance Objective

Outcome:	Reconstitute a powdered drug for parenteral administration.
Conditions:	Given the following: vial containing the powdered drug, reconstituting liquid, and a needle and syringe.
Standards:	Time: 5 minutes. Student completed procedure in _____ minutes.
	Accuracy: Satisfactory score on the Performance Evaluation Checklist.

Performance Evaluation Checklist

Trial 1	Trial 2	Point Value	Performance Standards
		•	Sanitized hands.
		•	Assembled equipment.
		✶	Selected the proper medication from its storage location.
		•	Checked the drug label.
		•	Compared the medication with the physician's instructions.
		•	Checked the expiration date.
		✶	Calculated the correct dose to be given, if needed.
		•	Opened the syringe and needle packages.
		•	Assembled the needle and syringe, if necessary.
		•	Made sure that the needle is attached firmly to the syringe and moved the plunger back and forth.
		•	Checked the drug label a second time.
		•	Withdrew an amount of air equal to the amount of liquid to be injected into the vial from the vial containing the powdered drug.
		•	Injected the air into the vial of diluent.
		✶	Inverted the diluent vial and withdrew the proper amount of liquid into the syringe.
		•	Removed air bubbles from the syringe and removed the needle from the vial.
		•	Inserted the needle into the powdered drug vial.
		•	Injected the diluent into the vial.
		•	Removed the needle from the vial and replaced the needle guard.
		•	Rolled the vial between hands to mix it.
		•	Labeled multiple-dose vials with the date of preparation and your initials.
		•	Administered the medication.
		•	Stored multiple-dose vials as indicated in the manufacturer's instructions.

Trial 1	Trial 2	Point Value	Performance Standards
		▷	Explained the importance of checking the date of preparation of a reconstituted multiple-dose vial before administering it.
		✴	Completed the procedure within 5 minutes.
			Totals

Evaluation of Student Performance

EVALUATION CRITERIA			COMMENTS
Symbol	**Category**	**Point Value**	
✴	Critical Step	16 points	
•	Essential Step	6 points	
▷	Theory Question	2 points	

Score calculation: 100 points

− _____ points missed

_____ Score

Satisfactory score: 85 or above

CAAHEP Competencies Achieved

Psychomotor (Skills)

☑ II. 1. Prepare proper dosages of medication for administration.

Affective (Behavior)

☑ II. 1. Verify ordered doses/dosages prior to administration.

ABHES Competencies Achieved

☑ 9. j. Prepare and administer oral and parenteral medications as directed by physician.

Procedure 11-4: Administering a Subcutaneous Injection

Name: _____   Date: _____

Evaluated by: _____   Score: _____

Performance Objective

Outcome:	Administer a subcutaneous injection.
Conditions:	Given the following: appropriate medication, appropriate needle and syringe, antiseptic wipe, 2 × 2 gauze pad, disposable gloves, and a biohazard sharps container.
Standards:	Time: 5 minutes. Student completed procedure in _____ minutes.
	Accuracy: Satisfactory score on the Performance Evaluation Checklist.

Performance Evaluation Checklist

Trial 1	Trial 2	Point Value	Performance Standards
		•	Sanitized hands.
		•	Prepared the injection.
		•	Greeted the patient and introduced yourself.
		•	Identified the patient and explained the procedure and purpose of the injection.
		•	Selected an appropriate subcutaneous injection site.
		▷	Stated the sites that can be used to administer a subcutaneous injection.
		•	Cleansed the area with an antiseptic wipe and allowed it to dry completely.
		▷	Explained why the site should be allowed to dry.
		•	Applied gloves.
		•	Removed the needle guard.
		•	Properly positioned the hand on the area surrounding the injection site.
		▷	Explained when the area should be grasped and when it should be held taut.
		•	Inserted needle to the hub at a 45-degree or 90-degree angle (depending on the length of the needle) with a quick, smooth motion.
		▷	Explained how needle length determines the angle of insertion for a subcutaneous injection.
		•	Removed the hand from the skin.
		▷	Explained why the hand should be removed from the skin.
		✶	Aspirated to make sure that the needle was not in a blood vessel.
		▷	Explained what should be done if the needle is in a blood vessel.
		•	Injected the medication slowly and steadily.
		▷	Described what would happen if the medication were injected rapidly.
		•	Placed an antiseptic wipe or gauze pad gently over the injection site and removed the needle quickly at the same angle as insertion.

543

Trial 1	Trial 2	Point Value	Performance Standards
		▷	Explained why the needle should be removed at the angle of insertion.
		•	Applied gentle pressure to the injection site.
		▷	Stated why the site should not be vigorously massaged.
		•	Activated the safety shield on the needle.
		•	Properly disposed of the needle and syringe.
		•	Removed gloves and sanitized hands.
		•	Charted the procedure correctly.
		•	Remained with the patient to make sure there were no unusual reactions.
		▷	Stated the steps to follow if the patient has been given an allergy injection.
		✷	Completed the procedure within 5 minutes.
			Totals

CHART	
Date	

Evaluation of Student Performance

EVALUATION CRITERIA			COMMENTS
Symbol	**Category**	**Point Value**	
✷	Critical Step	16 points	
•	Essential Step	6 points	
▷	Theory Question	2 points	

Score calculation: 100 points

    − _____ points missed

    _____ Score

Satisfactory score: 85 or above

CAAHEP Competencies Achieved

Psychomotor (Skills)

☑ I. 7. Select proper sites for administering parenteral medication.

☑ I. 9. Administer parenteral (excluding IV) medications.

☑ IX. 7. Document accurately in the patient record.

☑ XI. 5. Demonstrate proper use of the following equipment: c. Sharps disposal containers.

Affective (Behavior)

☑ III. 3. Show awareness of patients' concerns regarding their perceptions related to the procedure being performed.

ABHES Competencies Achieved

☑ 4. a. Document accurately.

☑ 9. j. Prepare and administer oral and parenteral medications as directed by physician.

Notes

Procedure 11-5: Administering an Intramuscular Injection

Name: _____   Date: _____

Evaluated by: _____   Score: _____

Performance Objective

Outcome:	Administer an intramuscular injection.
Conditions:	Given the following: appropriate medication, appropriate needle and syringe, antiseptic wipe, 2 × 2 gauze pad, disposable gloves, and a biohazard sharps container.
Standards:	Time: 5 minutes. Student completed procedure in _____ minutes.
	Accuracy: Satisfactory score on the Performance Evaluation Checklist.

Performance Evaluation Checklist

Trial 1	Trial 2	Point Value	Performance Standards
		•	Sanitized hands.
		•	Prepared the injection.
		•	Greeted the patient and introduced yourself.
		•	Identified the patient and explained the procedure and purpose of the injection.
			Located the intramuscular injection sites
		✳	Dorsogluteal
		✳	Deltoid
		✳	Vastus lateralis
		✳	Ventrogluteal
		▷	Stated what tissue layer of the body the medication will be injected into.
		•	Cleansed area with an antiseptic wipe and allowed it to dry completely.
		•	Applied gloves.
		•	Removed the needle guard.
		•	Stretched the skin taut over the injection site.
		▷	Explained why the skin should be stretched taut.
		•	Held the barrel of syringe like a dart and inserted the needle quickly at a 90-degree angle to the patient's skin with a firm motion.
		•	Inserted the needle to the hub.
		▷	Explained why the needle should be inserted at a 90-degree angle and to the hub.
		✳	Aspirated to make sure that the needle was not in a blood vessel.
		▷	Described what would happen if the medication was injected into a blood vessel.
		•	Injected the medication slowly and steadily.

Trial 1	Trial 2	Point Value	Performance Standards
		•	Placed an antiseptic wipe or gauze pad gently over the injection site and removed the needle quickly at the same angle as insertion.
		•	Applied gentle pressure to the injection site.
		▷	Stated the reason for applying pressure to the injection site.
		•	Activated the safety shield on the needle.
		•	Properly disposed of the needle and syringe.
		•	Removed gloves and sanitized hands.
		•	Charted the procedure correctly.
		▷	Stated the purpose of the lot number on the medication vial.
		•	Remained with the patient to make sure there were no unusual reactions.
		✳	Completed the procedure within 5 minutes.
			Totals

CHART

Date	

Evaluation of Student Performance

EVALUATION CRITERIA			COMMENTS
Symbol	**Category**	**Point Value**	
✳	Critical Step	16 points	
•	Essential Step	6 points	
▷	Theory Question	2 points	

Score calculation: 100 points

−_____ points missed

_____ Score

Satisfactory score: 85 or above

CAAHEP Competencies Achieved

Psychomotor (Skills)

☑ I. 7. Select proper sites for administering parenteral medication.

☑ I. 9. Administer parenteral (excluding IV) medications.

☑ IX. 7. Document accurately in the patient record.

☑ XI. 5. Demonstrate proper use of the following equipment: c. Sharps disposal containers.

Affective (Behavior)

☑ III. 3. Show awareness of patients' concerns regarding their perceptions related to the procedure being performed.

ABHES Competencies Achieved

☑ 4. a. Document accurately.

☑ 9. j. Prepare and administer oral and parenteral medications as directed by physician.

Notes

Procedure 11-6: Z-Track Intramuscular Injection Technique

Name: _____ Date: _____

Evaluated by: _____ Score: _____

Performance Objective

Outcome:	Administer an intramuscular injection using the Z-track method.
Conditions:	Given the following: appropriate medication, appropriate needle and syringe, antiseptic wipe, disposable gloves, and a biohazard sharps container.
Standards:	Time: 5 minutes. Student completed procedure in _____ minutes.
	Accuracy: Satisfactory score on the Performance Evaluation Checklist.

Performance Evaluation Checklist

Trial 1	Trial 2	Point Value	Performance Standards
		•	Sanitized hands.
		•	Prepared the injection.
		•	Greeted the patient and introduced yourself.
		•	Identified the patient and explained the procedure and purpose of the injection.
		•	Selected and properly located the intramuscular injection site.
		•	Cleansed the area with an antiseptic wipe and allowed it to dry completely.
		•	Applied gloves.
		•	Removed the needle guard.
		•	Pulled the skin away laterally from the injection site with the nondominant hand approximately 1 to 1½ inches.
		•	Inserted the needle quickly and smoothly at a 90-degree angle.
		✳	Aspirated to make sure that the needle was not in a blood vessel.
		•	Injected the medication slowly and steadily.
		•	Waited 10 seconds before withdrawing the needle.
		▷	Explained why there should be a 10-second waiting period.
		•	Withdrew the needle quickly at the same angle as that of insertion.
		•	Released the traction on the skin.
		▷	Described what occurs when the skin traction is released.
		•	Did not apply pressure to the injection site.
		▷	Stated why pressure should not be applied to the injection site.
		•	Activated the safety shield on the needle.
		•	Properly disposed of the needle and syringe.

Trial 1	Trial 2	Point Value	Performance Standards
		•	Removed gloves and sanitized hands.
		•	Charted the procedure correctly.
		•	Remained with the patient to make sure there were no unusual reactions.
		✳	Completed the procedure within 5 minutes.
			Totals

CHART	
Date	

Evaluation of Student Performance

EVALUATION CRITERIA			COMMENTS
Symbol	**Category**	**Point Value**	
✳	Critical Step	16 points	
•	Essential Step	6 points	
▷	Theory Question	2 points	

Score calculation: 100 points

−　　　　　points missed

　　　　Score

Satisfactory score: 85 or above

CAAHEP Competencies Achieved

Psychomotor (Skills)

☑ I. 7. Select proper sites for administering parenteral medication.

☑ I. 9. Administer parenteral (excluding IV) medications.

☑ IX. 7. Document accurately in the patient record.

☑ XI. 5. Demonstrate proper use of the following equipment: c. Sharps disposal containers.

Affective (Behavior)

☑ III. 3. Show awareness of patients' concerns regarding their perceptions related to the procedure being performed.

ABHES Competencies Achieved

☑ 4. a. Document accurately.

☑ 9. j. Prepare and administer oral and parenteral medications as directed by physician.

EVALUATION OF COMPETENCY

Procedure Procedure 11-7: Administering an Intradermal Injection

Name: _____ Date: _____

Evaluated by: _____ Score: _____

Performance Objective

Outcome:	Administer an intradermal injection and read the test results.
Conditions:	Given the following: skin testing solution, appropriate needle and syringe, antiseptic wipe, 2 × 2 gauze pad, disposable gloves, millimeter ruler, TB skin test record card, and a biohazard sharps container.
Standards:	Time: 5 minutes. Student completed procedure in _____ minutes.
	Accuracy: Satisfactory score on the Performance Evaluation Checklist.

Performance Evaluation Checklist

Trial 1	Trial 2	Point Value	Performance Standards
		•	Sanitized hands.
		•	Prepared the injection.
		•	Greeted the patient and introduced yourself.
		•	Identified the patient and explained the procedure and purpose of the injection.
		•	Selected an appropriate intradermal injection site.
		▷	Stated the recommended sites for an intradermal injection.
		•	Cleansed the area with an antiseptic wipe and allowed it to dry completely.
		•	Applied gloves.
		•	Removed the needle guard.
		•	Stretched the skin taut at the site of administration.
		▷	Explained why the skin is held taut.
		•	Inserted the needle at an angle of 10 to 15 degrees and with the bevel upward.
		•	The bevel of the needle just penetrated the skin.
		▷	Stated why the bevel should face upward.
		•	Injected the medication slowly and steadily, ensuring that a wheal formed (approximately 6 to 10 mm in diameter).
		▷	Explained what to do if a wheal does not form.
		•	Placed an antiseptic wipe or gauze pad gently over the injection site and removed the needle quickly at the same angle as that of insertion.
		•	Did not apply pressure to the injection site.
		▷	Explained why pressure should not be applied to the site.
		•	Activated the safety shield on the needle.
		•	Properly disposed of the needle and syringe.

553

Trial 1	Trial 2	Point Value	Performance Standards
		•	Removed gloves and sanitized hands.
		•	Remained with the patient to make sure that there were no unusual reactions.
			Allergy skin tests
		•	Read the test results within 20 to 30 minutes.
		•	Inspected and palpated the site of the skin tests.
		•	Interpreted the skin test results.
		•	Charted the procedure correctly.
			Mantoux tuberculin test
		•	Informed the patient to return in 48 to 72 hours to have the results read.
		▷	Stated what must be done if the patient does not return to have the results read.
		•	Instructed the patient in the care of the test site.
		▷	Stated the instructions that must be relayed to the patient.
		•	Charted the procedure correctly.
			Reading Mantoux test results
		•	Greeted the patient and introduced yourself.
		•	Identified the patient and explained the procedure.
		•	Worked in a quiet, well-lit atmosphere.
		•	Checked the patient's chart to determine the site of administration of the test.
		•	Sanitized hands and applied gloves.
		•	Positioned the patient's arm on a firm surface with the arm flexed at the elbow.
		•	Located the application site.
		•	Gently rubbed the fingertip over the test site.
		•	If induration is present, rubbed the area lightly, going from the area of normal skin to the indurated area to assess the size of the indurated area.
		•	Measured the diameter of the induration with a millimeter ruler.
		✻	The measurement was recorded in mm and was identical to the evaluator's measurement.
		•	Removed gloves and sanitized hands.
		•	Charted the results correctly.
		•	Completed a TB test record card and gave it to the patient.
		✻	Completed the procedure within 10 minutes.
			Totals
			CHART
Date			

Chapter **11 Administration of Medication and Intravenous Therapy**

Evaluation of Student Performance

EVALUATION CRITERIA			COMMENTS
Symbol	**Category**	**Point Value**	
✳	Critical Step	16 points	
•	Essential Step	6 points	
▷	Theory Question	2 points	

Score calculation: 100 points

− _____ points missed

_____ Score

Satisfactory score: 85 or above

CAAHEP Competencies Achieved

Psychomotor (Skills)

☑ I. 7. Select proper sites for administering parenteral medication.

☑ I. 9. Administer parenteral (excluding IV) medications.

☑ IX. 7. Document accurately in the patient record.

☑ XI. 5. Demonstrate proper use of the following equipment: c. Sharps disposal containers.

Affective (Behavior)

☑ III. 3. Show awareness of patients' concerns regarding their perceptions related to the procedure being performed.

ABHES Competencies Achieved

☑ 4. a. Document accurately.

☑ 9. j. Prepare and administer oral and parenteral medications as directed by physician.

Notes

DRUG DOSAGE CALCULATION: SUPPLEMENTAL EDUCATION FOR CHAPTER 11

This section is designed as supplemental education for Chapter 11 (Administration of Medication) in your textbook. Completion of these exercises will enable you to calculate drug dosage effectively and accurately, which is essential for administering the proper amount of medication to patients and preventing medication errors. Because each unit builds on the next one, you should become completely familiar with each step before proceeding to the next.

LEARNING OBJECTIVES

After completing this chapter, you should be able to:
1. Identify metric abbreviations.
2. Indicate dose quantity using metric notation guidelines.
3. Identify apothecary abbreviations.
4. Indicate dose quantity using apothecary notations.
5. Identify common medical abbreviations used in writing medication orders.
6. Interpret medication orders.
7. Convert units of measurement within the following systems: metric, apothecary, and household.
8. Convert units of measurement using ratio and proportion.
9. Convert units of measurement between the metric, apothecary, and household systems.
10. Determine oral drug dosage.
11. Determine parenteral drug dosage.

UNIT 1: THE METRIC SYSTEM

A. Units of Measurement: Practice Problems

The basic units of measurement in the metric system are the gram, liter, and meter. The gram is a unit of weight used to measure solids, the liter is a unit volume used to measure liquids, and the meter is a unit of length used to measure distance. In the space provided, indicate whether each of the following metric units of measurement is a unit of weight (W), volume (V), or length (L).

_____ 1. milligram

_____ 2. cubic centimeter

_____ 3. meter

_____ 4. kilogram

_____ 5. liter

_____ 6. milliliter

_____ 7. kiloliter

_____ 8. millimeter

_____ 9. microgram

_____ 10. gram

B. Metric Abbreviations: Practice Problems

Review the metric abbreviations in your textbook before completing these problems. In the space provided, indicate the correct abbreviation for each of the metric units of measurement.

_____ 1. milligram

_____ 2. gram

_____ 3. kilogram

_____ 4. liter

_____ 5. cubic centimeter

_____ 6. microgram

_____ 7. milliliter

557

C. Metric Notation: Practice Problems

To read prescriptions and medication orders, to record medication administration, and to avoid medication errors, the medical assistant must be able to use metric notation guidelines. Review the Metric Notation Guidelines on page 435 of your textbook before completing the following practice problems. In the space provided, use metric notation guidelines to indicate the dose quantities.

_____ 1. 25 milligrams

_____ 2. 5 grams

_____ 3. 1½ liters

_____ 4. 1 cubic centimeter

_____ 5. 10 milliliters

_____ 6. ½ gram

_____ 7. 50 milligrams

_____ 8. ½ cubic centimeter

_____ 9. 4 milliliters

_____ 10. 2 kilograms

_____ 11. 120 milliliters

_____ 12. 3 cubic centimeters

_____ 13. ¼ gram

_____ 14. 250 milligrams

_____ 15. ½ liter

_____ 16. 500 milliliters

_____ 17. 1 cubic centimeter

_____ 18. 5 kilograms

_____ 19. 2½ grams

_____ 20. 10 milligrams

UNIT 2: THE APOTHECARY SYSTEMS

A. Units of Measurement: Practice Problems

The basic units of measurement in the apothecary system are the grain, minim, and inch. The grain is a unit of weight used to measure solids, the minim is a unit of volume used to measure liquids, and the inch is a unit of length used to measure distance. In the space provided, indicate whether each of the following units of measurement is a unit of weight (W), volume (V), or length (L).

_____ 1. grain

_____ 2. inch

_____ 3. minim

_____ 4. fluid dram

_____ 5. foot

_____ 6. quart

_____ 7. ounce

Chapter **11** **Administration of Medication and Intravenous Therapy**

_____ 8. gallon

_____ 9. yard

_____ 10. fluid ounce

_____ 11. pound

_____ 12. pint

_____ 13. dram

_____ 14. mile

B. Apothecary Abbreviations: Practice Problems

Review the apothecary abbreviations in your textbook before completing these problems. In the space provided, indicate the correct abbreviation or symbol for each of the apothecary units of measurement listed below.

_____ 1. grain

_____ 2. dram

_____ 3. ounce

_____ 4. minim

_____ 5. fluid dram

_____ 6. fluid ounce

_____ 7. pint

_____ 8. quart

_____ 9. gallon

_____ 10. inch

C. Apothecary Notation: Practice Problems

Although the apothecary system is used less frequently than the metric system, the medical assistant must still be able to use apothecary notation guidelines. Review the Apothecary Notation Guidelines on page 437 of your textbook before completing the practice problems. In the space provided, use apothecary notations to indicate the following dose quantities.

_____ 1. 4 ounces

_____ 2. 10 grains

_____ 3. 5 drams

_____ 4. ½ ounce

_____ 5. 6 fluid drams

_____ 6. 7½ grains

_____ 7. 3½ ounces

_____ 8. 10 minims

_____ 9. 3 fluid ounces

_____ 10. 2 drams

_____ 11. ¼ grain

_____ 12. 16 ounces

_____ 13. 12 minims

_____ 14. 1 dram

_____ 15. 9 fluid drams

_____ 16. 4 grains

_____ 17. 8 drams

_____ 18. 32 fluid ounces

_____ 19. 30 minims

_____ 20. 8 ounces

UNIT 3: THE HOUSEHOLD SYSTEM

The household system is more complicated and less accurate for administering medication than the metric and apothecary systems. However, most individuals are familiar with this system because of its frequent use in the United States. This system of measurement may be the only one the patient can fully relate to and therefore may safely use to administer liquid medication at home.

A. Units of Measurement: Practice Problems

Volume is the only household unit of measurement used to administer medication. The basic unit of liquid volume is the drop. The remaining units, in order of increasing volume, are the teaspoon, tablespoon, ounce, cup, and glass. In the space provided, indicate the correct abbreviation for each of the household units of measurement listed.

_____ 1. drop

_____ 2. teaspoon

_____ 3. tablespoon

_____ 4. ounce

UNIT 4: MEDICATION ORDERS

A. Medical Abbreviations: Practice Problems

To safely administer medication, the medical assistant must be completely familiar with common medical abbreviations. Review Table 11-5 in your textbook before completing the following practice problems. In the space provided, write the meaning of the following medical abbreviations.

_____ 1. NPO

_____ 2. prn

_____ 3. hs

_____ 4. tab

_____ 5. ac

_____ 6. pc

_____ 7. qid

_____ 8. $\bar{c}$

_____ 9. $\bar{s}$

_____ 10. bid

_____ 11. tid

_____ 12. qh

_____ 13. gtts

_____ 14. q4h

_____ 15. qs

_____ 16. IM

_____ 17. caps

_____ 18. po

_____ 19. ad lib

_____ 20. $\overline{aa}$

B. Interpreting Medication Orders: Practice Problems

To safely administer medication and instruct patients on administering medication at home, the medical assistant must be able to interpret medication orders. Interpret the following medication orders and, using a drug reference, indicate the drug category based on action and a brand name for each medication.

1. Tetracycline 250 mg po qid × 10 days

   _____

   Drug category: _____

   Brand name: _____

2. Lansoprazole 30 mg po every day ac

   _____

   Drug category: _____

   Brand name: _____

3. Alprazolam 0.25 mg po tid

   _____

   Drug category: _____

   Brand name: _____

4. Diltiazem 50 mg po q4h

   _____

   Drug category: _____

   Brand name: _____

5. Ciprofloxacin 500 mg q12h

   _____

   Drug category: _____

   Brand name: _____

6. Hydrocodone/acetaminophen 5 mg q4h prn

   _____

   Drug category: _____

   Brand name: _____

7. Furosemide 40 mg po q AM

   _____

   Drug category: _____

   Brand name: _____

8. Paroxetine 20 mg po every day in AM

   _____

   Drug category: _____

   Brand name: _____

9. Cetirizine 5 mg po every day

   _____

   Drug category: _____

   Brand name: _____

10. Cyclobenzaprine 10 mg po tid × 1 wk

    _____

    Drug category: _____

    Brand name: _____

UNIT 5: CONVERTING UNITS OF MEASUREMENT

A. Using Conversion Tables

Changing from one unit of measurement to another is known as *conversion*. Conversion is required when medication is ordered in one unit of measurement and the medication label expresses the drug strength in a different unit. The dose quantity must be mathematically translated or converted to the unit of measurement of the medication on hand. For example, if the physician orders 5 grams of an oral solid medication and the medication label expresses the drug strength in milligrams, the medical assistant must convert the grams into milligrams to know how much medication to administer. Converting units of measurement can be classified as follows:

1. Conversion of units within a measurement system
2. Conversion of units from one measurement system to another

Converting units within a measurement system allows a quantity to be expressed in a different but equal unit of measurement within the same system. An example of converting between units of weight within the metric system is as follows: 1 gram is equal to 1000 milligrams.

Converting from one measurement system to another allows a quantity to be expressed in a unit of measurement of another system. An example of a conversion between the apothecary and metric systems is as follows: 1 grain (apothecary system) is equivalent to 60 milligrams (metric system). Methods used to convert units of measurement are presented in this unit and in Unit 6.

Conversion requires the use of a conversion table to indicate the equivalent values between units of measurement. The practice problems that follow can assist you in attaining competency in using conversion tables.

Conversion Tables: Practice Problems

Refer to the conversion tables at the end of this chapter. Locate and record the equivalent value for each of the units of measurement listed. In the space provided, indicate the conversion table you used to locate the equivalent value (e.g., metric, apothecary, metric to apothecary).

		ANSWER	CONVERSION TABLE
1. 1 g	=	_____ mg	_____
2. 1 ounce	=	_____ drams	_____
3. 1 tablespoon	=	_____ teaspoons	_____
4. 1 grain	=	_____ mg	_____
5. 1 liter	=	_____ mL	_____
6. 1 dram	=	_____ grains	_____
7. 1 pint	=	_____ fluid ounces	_____
8. 1 teaspoon	=	_____ drops	_____
9. 1 mL	=	_____ cc	_____
10. 1 mL	=	_____ minims	_____
11. 1 fluid ounce	=	_____ mL	_____
12. 1 kg	=	_____ g	_____
13. 1 fluid dram	=	_____ minims	_____
14. 1 gallon	=	_____ quarts	_____
15. 1 ounce	=	_____ tablespoons	_____
16. 1 quart	=	_____ pints	_____
17. 1 fluid dram	=	_____ mL	_____
18. 1 g	=	_____ grains	_____
19. 1 quart	=	_____ mL	_____
20. 1 drop	=	_____ minims	_____
21. 1 fluid ounce	=	_____ tablespoons	_____
22. 1 fluid dram	=	_____ teaspoons	_____
23. 1 tablespoon	=	_____ fluid drams	_____
24. 1 kg	=	_____ pounds	_____
25. 1 glass	=	_____ mL	_____

B. Converting Units within the Metric System

Drug administration often requires conversion within the metric system to prepare the correct dosage. Metric conversion involves converting a larger unit to a smaller unit (e.g., grams to milligrams) or converting a smaller unit to a larger unit (e.g., milliliters to liters). Methods used to convert one metric unit to another are described in the next sections.

Converting a Larger Unit to a Smaller Unit

Converting a larger unit to a smaller unit within the metric system can be accomplished using one of three methods. The method chosen is based on personal preference and the level of difficulty of the conversion problem. For example, more difficult problems require the use of ratio and proportion as the method of conversion. Examples of converting a larger unit to a smaller unit are as follows:
1. Grams to milligrams
2. Liters to milliliters
3. Kilograms to grams

METHODS OF CONVERSION: To convert a larger unit to a smaller unit within the metric system, use one of the following:

Method 1: Multiply the unit to be changed by 1000.

Method 2: Move the decimal point of the unit to be changed three places to the right.

Method 3: Ratio and proportion (see Unit 6).

GUIDELINE: When converting a larger unit to a smaller unit, expect the quantity to become larger. Use this guideline to assist in making accurate conversions. The problems illustrate this guideline.

EXAMPLES

PROBLEM	2 L = _____ mL
Method 1:	Multiply the unit to be changed by 1000.
	2 × 1000 = 2000 mL
Method 2:	Move the decimal point of the unit to be changed three places to the right.
	2.0 0 0. = 2000 mL

Answer	2 L = 2000 mL

PROBLEM	4 g = _____ mg
Method 1:	Multiply the unit to be changed by 1000.
	4 × 1000 = 4000 mg
Method 2:	Move the decimal point of the unit to be changed three places to the right.
	4.0 0 0. = 4000 mg

Answer	4 g = 4000 mg

Converting a Smaller Unit to a Larger Unit

Converting a smaller unit to a larger unit within the metric system can be accomplished using one of three methods of conversion as outlined below. Examples of converting a smaller unit to a larger unit are as follows:

1. Milligrams to grams
2. Milliliters to liters
3. Grams to kilograms

METHOD OF CONVERSION: To convert a smaller unit to a larger unit within the metric system, use one of the following:

Method 1: Divide the unit to be changed by 1000.

Method 2: Move the decimal point of the unit to be changed three places to the left.

Method 3: Ratio and proportion (see Unit 6).

GUIDELINE: When converting a smaller unit to a larger unit, expect the quantity to become smaller. The problems illustrate this guideline.

EXAMPLES

PROBLEM	250 mg = _____ g
Method 1:	Divide the unit to be changed by 1000.
	250 ÷ 1000 = 0.25 g
Method 2:	Move the decimal point of the unit to be changed three places to the left.
	.2 5 0. = 0.25 g

Answer	250 mg = 0.25 g

PROBLEM   1500 mL = _____ L
Method 1:   Divide the unit to be changed by 1000.
                1500 ÷ 1000 = 1.5 L
Method 2:   Move the decimal point of the unit to be changed three places to the left.
                1.5 0 0. = 1.5 L

Answer	1500 mL = 1.5 L

Converting Units within the Metric System: Practice Problems

Directions: Convert the following metric units of measurement using Method 1 or Method 2. In the space provided, indicate whether the conversion is going from a larger to smaller unit (L→S) or smaller to larger unit (S→L), and indicate the conversion table you used.

		ANSWER	**CONVERSION TABLE**
1. 1 g	=	_____ mg	_____
2. 750 mg	=	_____ g	_____
3. 2 kg	=	_____ g	_____
4. 1000 g	=	_____ kg	_____
5. 1.5 L	=	_____ mL	_____
6. 250 mL	=	_____ L	_____
7. 5 g	=	_____ mg	_____
8. 0.25 kg	=	_____ g	_____
9. 1000 mg	=	_____ g	_____
10. 2.5 g	=	_____ mg	_____
11. 475 mL	=	_____ L	_____
12. 0.05 g	=	_____ mg	_____
13. 0.5 L	=	_____ mL	_____
14. 1000 mL	=	_____ L	_____
15. 500 g	=	_____ kg	_____
16. 50 mg	=	_____ g	_____
17. 1 L	=	_____ mL	_____
18. 40 g	=	_____ mg	_____
19. 50 mL	=	_____ L	_____
20. 1 kg	=	_____ g	_____

C. Converting Units within the Apothecary System

Drug administration may sometimes require conversion within the apothecary system to prepare the correct dosage. Apothecary conversion involves converting a larger unit to a smaller unit (e.g., drams to grains) or converting a smaller unit to a larger unit (e.g., ounces to pounds). Methods used to convert one apothecary unit to another are described below.

Converting a Larger Unit to a Smaller Unit

Converting a larger unit to a smaller unit within the apothecary system is accomplished through either the equivalent value method or the ratio and proportion method. Examples of converting a larger unit to a smaller unit follow:

Weight	*Volume*
drams to grains	fluid drams to minims
ounces to drams	fluid ounces to fluid drams
pounds to ounces	pints to fluid ounces
	quarts to pints
	gallons to quarts

565

METHOD OF CONVERSION: To convert a larger unit to a smaller unit within the apothecary system, use one of the following:

Method 1:
a. Look at Table 11-2 (apothecary conversion) at the end of this chapter to determine the equivalent value between the two units of measurement.
b. Multiply the equivalent value by the number next to the larger unit of measurement.

Method 2: Ratio and proportion (see Unit 6).

EXAMPLES

PROBLEM   4 drams = _____ grains
Method 1:
a. Look at the conversion table to determine the equivalent value:
   1 dram = 60 grains
   60 = the equivalent value
b. Multiply the equivalent value by the number next to the larger unit of measurement:
   4 × 60 = 240 grains

Answer	4 drams = 240 grams

PROBLEM   1½ pints = ____ fluid ounces
Method 1:
a. Look at the conversion table to determine the equivalent value:
   1 pint = 16 fluid ounces
   16 = the equivalent value
b. Multiply the equivalent value by the number next to the larger unit of measurement:
   1.5 × 16 = 24 fluid ounces

Answer	1½ pints = 24 fluid ounces

Converting a Smaller Unit to a Larger Unit

Converting a smaller unit to a larger unit within the apothecary system also can be accomplished using the equivalent value method or the ratio and proportion method. Examples of converting from a smaller unit to a larger unit follow:

Weight	*Volume*
grains to drams	minims to fluid drams
drams to ounces	fluid drams to fluid ounces
ounces to pounds	fluid ounces to pints
	pints to quarts
	quarts to gallons

METHOD OF CONVERSION: To convert a smaller unit to a larger unit within the apothecary system, use one of the following:

Method 1:
a. Look at Table 11-2 (apothecary conversion) at the end of this chapter to determine the equivalent value between the two units of measurement.
b. Divide the equivalent value into the number next to the smaller unit of measurement.

Method 2: Ratio and proportion (see Unit 6).

566

Chapter **11 Administration of Medication and Intravenous Therapy**

EXAMPLES
PROBLEM   30 grains = _____ drams
Method 1:
   a. Look at the conversion table to determine the equivalent value:
      60 grains = 1 dram
      60 = the equivalent value
   b. Divide the equivalent value into the number next to the smaller unit of measurement:
      30 ÷ 60 = ½ dram

Answer   30 grains = ½ dram

PROBLEM   16 fluid drams = _____ fluid ounces
Method 1:
   a. Look at the conversion table to determine the equivalent value:
      8 fluid drams = 1 fluid ounce
      8 = the equivalent value
   b. Divide the equivalent value into the number next to the smaller unit of measurement:
      16 ÷ 8 = 2 fluid ounces

Answer   16 fluid drams = 2 fluid ounces

Converting Units within the Apothecary: Practice Problems

Convert the apothecary units of measurement using the equivalent value method of conversion. In the space provided, indicate the equivalent value for each problem.

		ANSWER	EQUIVALENT VALUE
1. 2 quarts	=	_____ pints	_____
2. 4 drams	=	_____ grains	_____
3. ½ ounce	=	_____ drams	_____
4. 300 grains	=	_____ drams	_____
5. 2 fluid drams	=	_____ minims	_____
6. 8 pints	=	_____ quarts	_____
7. 16 drams	=	_____ ounces	_____
8. 24 fluid drams	=	_____ fluid ounces	_____
9. 18 ounces	=	_____ pounds	_____
10. 32 fluid ounces	=	_____ pints	_____
11. ½ quart	=	_____ pints	_____
12. ½ dram	=	_____ grains	_____
13. 3 ounces	=	_____ drams	_____
14. 210 grains	=	_____ drams	_____
15. 4½ fluid drams	=	_____ minims	_____
16. 3 pints	=	_____ quarts	_____
17. 4 drams	=	_____ ounces	_____
18. 24 ounces	=	_____ pounds	_____
19. 8 fluid ounces	=	_____ pints	_____
20. 2 quarts	=	_____ gallons	_____

Chapter **11 Administration of Medication and Intravenous Therapy**

21. 120 minims ＝ _____ fluid drams _____

22. 2 fluid ounces ＝ _____ fluid drams _____

23. ½ pound ＝ _____ ounces _____

24. 4 pints ＝ _____ fluid ounces _____

25. 2 gallons ＝ _____ quarts _____

D. Converting Units within the Household System

Household system conversion involves converting a larger unit to a smaller unit (e.g., tablespoons to teaspoons) or converting a smaller unit to a larger unit (e.g., tablespoons to ounces). Methods used to convert one unit to another are described.

Converting a Larger Unit to a Smaller Unit

Converting a larger unit to a smaller unit within the household system is accomplished using the equivalent value method or the ratio and proportion method. The method chosen is based on personal preference and on the level of difficulty of the conversion problem. Examples of converting a larger unit to a smaller unit follow:

Volume
teaspoons to drops
tablespoons to teaspoons
ounces to teaspoons
ounces to tablespoons
teacup to ounces
glass to ounces

METHOD OF CONVERSION: To convert a larger unit to a smaller unit within the household system, use one of the following:

Method 1:
a. Look at Table 11-3 (household conversion) at the end of this chapter to determine the equivalent value between the two units of measurement.
b. Multiply the equivalent value by the number next to the larger unit of measurement.

Method 2: Ratio and proportion (see Unit 6).

EXAMPLES
PROBLEM   2 tablespoons = _____ teaspoons
Method 1:
a. Look at the conversion table to determine the equivalent value:
   1 tablespoon = 3 teaspoons
   3 = the equivalent value
b. Multiply the equivalent value by the number next to the larger unit of measurement:
   2 × 3 = 6 teaspoons

   | *Answer*   2 tablespoons = 6 teaspoons |

PROBLEM   ½ teaspoon = _____ drops
Method 1:
a. Look at the conversion table to determine the equivalent value:
   1 teaspoon = 60 drops
   60 = the equivalent value
b. Multiply the equivalent value by the number next to the larger unit of measurement:
   ½ × 60 = 30 drops

   | *Answer*   ½ tablespoon = 30 drops |

Converting a Smaller Unit to a Larger Unit

Converting a smaller unit to a larger unit within the household system is accomplished using the equivalent value method or the ratio and proportion method. Examples of converting from a smaller unit to a larger unit follow:

Volume
drops to teaspoons
teaspoons to tablespoons
teaspoons to ounces
tablespoons to ounces
ounces to teacups
ounces to glasses

METHOD OF CONVERSION: To convert a smaller unit to a larger unit within the household system, use one of the following:

Method 1:
a. Look at Table 11-3 (household conversion) at the end of this chapter to determine the equivalent value between the two units of measurement.
b. Divide the equivalent value into the number next to the smaller unit of measurement.

Method 2: Ratio and proportion (see Unit 6).

EXAMPLES

PROBLEM   4 tablespoons = _____ ounces
Method 1:
   a. Look at the conversion table to determine the equivalent value:
     1 ounce = 2 tablespoons
     2 = the equivalent value
   b. Divide the equivalent value into the number next to the smaller unit of measurement:
     $4 \div 2 = 2$ ounces

Answer   4 tablespoon = 2 ounces

PROBLEM   24 ounces = ____ glasses
Method 1:
   a. Look at the conversion table to determine the equivalent value:
     1 glass = 8 ounces
     8 = the equivalent value
   b. Divide the equivalent value into the number next to the smaller unit of measurement:
     $24 \div 8 = 3$ glasses

Answer   24 ounces = 3 glasses

Converting Units within the Household System: Practice Problems

Directions: Convert the following household units of measurement using the equivalent value method of conversion. In the space provided, indicate the equivalent value for each problem.

		ANSWER	EQUIVALENT VALUE
1. 12 teaspoons	=	_____ ounces	_____
2. 4 ounces	=	_____ glasses	_____
3. 90 drops	=	_____ teaspoons	_____
4. ½ ounce	=	_____ tablespoons	_____

5. 6 teaspoons	=	_____ tablespoons	_____
6. 3 tablespoons	=	_____ ounces	_____
7. 18 ounces	=	_____ teacups	_____
8. ½ ounce	=	_____ teaspoons	_____
9. 3 tablespoons	=	_____ teaspoons	_____
10. ½ teaspoon	=	_____ drops	_____

UNIT 6: RATIO AND PROPORTION

Ratio and proportion are used to convert units of measurement. This method of conversion has the advantage of clarifying the mathematical rationale for the methods of conversion previously presented. It is also useful in converting units of measurement that are more difficult to calculate, such as converting between systems, such as when converting an apothecary unit of measurement to a metric unit of measurement.

A. Ratio and Proportion Guidelines

Some guidelines must be followed when using ratio and proportion:

1. A **ratio** is composed of two related numbers separated by a colon. It indicates the relationship between two quantities or numbers. The ratio example shows a relationship between milligrams and grams (i.e., 1000 mg = 1 g).

   EXAMPLE   1000 mg : 1 g

2. A **proportion** shows the relationship between two equal ratios. The proportion consists of two ratios separated by an equal sign (=), which indicates that the two ratios are equal. This proportion example shows the relationship between two equal ratios of milligrams and grams.

   EXAMPLE   1000 mg : 1 g = 2000 mg : 2 g

3. The units of measurement in the two ratios of a proportion must be expressed in the same sequence. The correct sequencing in the proportion example is mg : g = mg : g, *not* mg : g = g : mg.

   EXAMPLE   *Correct:*   1000 mg : 1 g = 2000 mg : 2 g
              Incorrect: 1000 mg : 1 g = 2 g : 2000 mg

4. The numbers on the ends of a proportion are called the **extremes**, and the numbers in the middle of the proportion are known as the **means**. In this example, the means consist of 1 g and 2000 mg, and the extremes are 1000 mg and 2 g.

   EXAMPLE   1000 mg : 1 g = 2000 mg : 2g

5. The product of the means equals the product of the extremes. The calculation of the product of the means in the example is $1 \times 2000 = 2000$. The calculation of the product of the extremes is $1000 \times 2 = 2000$. The product of the means equals the product of the extremes or 2000 = 2000.

   EXAMPLE   1000 mg : 1 g = 2000 mg : 2 g
              $1 \times 2000 = 1000 \times 2$
              2000 = 2000

6. In setting up a proportion, one side of the equation consists of the known quantities, and the other side of the equation consists of the unknown quantity. The letter x is commonly used to express the unknown quantity. To be consistent, the known quantities are indicated on the left side of the equation, and the unknown quantity is indicated on the right side of the equation. Using the previous proportion example, but inserting an unknown quantity, or x, the equation is set up as follows:

   EXAMPLE   1000 mg : 1 g x mg : 2 g
                  (known quantities)   (unknown quantity)

Ratio and Proportion: Practice Problems

Answer the following questions.

1. What is a ratio? _____

_____

2. In the space provided, place a check mark next to each correct example of a ratio.

_____ a. 15 drops : 15 minims : 1 mL

_____ b. 1000 mL = 1 L

_____ c. 1 ounce : 8 drams

_____ d. 60 minims/1 fluid dram

_____ e. 1 dram : 60 grains

_____ f. 1 mL : 1 cc

3. What is a proportion?

_____

_____

_____

4. In the space provided, place a check mark next to each correct example of a proportion.

_____ a. 1 mL : 1 cc

_____ b. 1 grain : 60 mg = 4 grains : 240 mg

_____ c. $2x$ = 60 mg

_____ d. 1000 mL : 1 L = 500 mL : 0.5 L

_____ e. 1000 mg : 1 grain = 1000 mL : 1 L

5. In the space provided, place a check mark next to each proportion that has correct sequencing for the units of measurement.

_____ a. 1000 g : 1 kg = 1500 g : 1.5 kg

_____ b. 60 grains : 1 dram = 2 drams : 120 grains

_____ c. 1000 mg : 1 g = 2000 mg : x g

6. Circle the means and underline the extremes in each of the following proportions:

a. 1000 mg : 1 g = 500 mg : 0.5 g
b. 2 pints : 1 quart = 4 pints : 2 quarts
c. 1 mL : 1 cc = 2 mL : 2 cc

7. In each of the following proportions, what is the product of the means, and what is the product of the extremes?

a. 1000 g : 1 kg = 1500 g : 1.5 kg

_____ product of the means

_____ product of the extremes

b. 60 minims : 1 fluid dram = 120 minims : 2 fluid drams

_____ product of the means

_____ product of the extremes

c. 60 mg : 1 grain = 300 mg : 5 grains

_____ product of the means

_____ product of the extremes

8. In each of the following proportions, circle the known quantities and underline the unknown quantity.

a. 1000 mg : 1 g = 500 mg : x g

b. 1 g : 15 grains = 2 g : x grains

c. 8 drams : 1 ounce = x drams : 4 ounces

B. Converting Units Using Ratio and Proportion

Units can be converted using ratio and proportion.

METHOD OF CONVERSION: To convert a unit of measurement using ratio and proportion, use the following steps:
  a. Look at the appropriate conversion table at the end of this chapter to determine
     what is known about the two units of measurement (equivalent value).
  b. State the known quantities as a ratio.
  c. Determine the unknown quantity.
  d. State the unknown quantity as a ratio.
  e. Set up the proportion with the known quantities on the left side and the unknown
     quantity on the right side of the equation.
  f. To solve the equation, multiply the product of the means and the product of the
     extremes. Divide the equation by the numbers before the x.
  g. Include the unit of measure corresponding to x in the original equation with the
     answer.

EXAMPLES
PROBLEM   2 g = _____ mg
  a. Look at Table 11-1 (metric conversion) to determine what is known about the two units of measurement:
     1000 mg = 1 g
  b. State the known quantities as a ratio:
     1000 mg : 1 g
  c. Determine the unknown quantity:
     2 g = x mg
  d. State the unknown quantity as a ratio using the correct unit of measurement sequencing:
     x mg : 2 g
  e. Set up the proportion with the known quantities on the left side and the unknown quantity on the right side of the
     equation:
     1000 mg : 1 g = x mg : 2 g
  f. Solve the equation by multiplying the product of the means and the product of the extremes and dividing the equa-
     tion by the number before the x:
     1000 mg : 1 g = x mg : 2 g
     $1 \times x = 1000 \times 2$
     $1x = 2000$
     $x = 2000$

Chapter **11 Administration of Medication and Intravenous Therapy**

Copyright © 2015, 2012, 2008, 2004, 2000, 1995, 1990 by Saunders, an imprint of Elsevier Inc.
All rights reserved.

g. Include the unit of measure corresponding to x in the original equation with the answer:
$x = 2000$ mg

> **Answer**   2 g = 2000 mg

PROBLEM
300 mg = _____ grains

The steps previously outlined are followed here. However, they are combined as they would be in working an actual conversion problem.

60 mg : 1 grain = 300 mg : x grains
$1 \times 300 = 60 \times x$
$300 = 60\ x$
$300 \div 60 = 60\ x \div 60$
$x = 5$ grains

> **Answer**   300 mg = 5 grains

Converting Units Using Ratio and Proportion: Practice Problems
Directions: Use ratio and proportion to convert among the apothecary, metric, and household systems by completing the problems below. In the space at the right, indicate what is known regarding the two units of measurement.

		ANSWER	KNOWN QUANTITIES
1. 30 minims	=	_____ mL	_____
2. 4 kg	=	_____ pounds	_____
3. 90 mL	=	_____ fluid ounces	_____
4. 30 mg	=	_____ grains	_____
5. 60 mg	=	_____ ounces	_____
6. 250 mL	=	_____ pints	_____
7. 6 g	=	_____ drams	_____
8. 1½ quarts	=	_____ mL	_____
9. 3 g	=	_____ grains	_____
10. 5 fluid drams	=	_____ mL	_____
11. 80 pounds	=	_____ kg	_____
12. 500 mL	=	_____ quarts	_____
13. 8 mL	=	_____ teaspoons	_____
14. 4 grains	=	_____ mg	_____
15. 32 mL	=	_____ fluid drams	_____
16. 120 mg	=	_____ grains	_____
17. 30 mL	=	_____ tablespoons	_____
18. 60 drops	=	_____ mL	_____
19. 1½ fluid ounces	=	_____ tablespoons	_____
20. ½ fluid ounce	=	_____ mL	_____

A. Oral Administration

Dosage refers to the amount of medication to be administered to the patient. Each medication has a certain dosage range or range of quantities that produce therapeutic effects. It is important to administer the exact drug dosage. If the dose is too small, it will not produce a therapeutic effect, whereas too large a dose could harm or even kill the patient. The steps to follow in determining drug dosage depend on the unit of measurement in which the drug is ordered and the unit of measurement of the drug you have available, or the dose on hand.

1. If the dose on hand is the same as that ordered, no calculation is required. In this example, the dose ordered and the dose on hand are in the same unit of measurement, and one tablet is administered to the patient.

    EXAMPLE   The physician orders 50 mg of a medication po.
    The drug label reads 50 mg/tablet.

2. If the dosage ordered is in the same unit of measurement as that indicated on the medication label, only one calculation step is required. In this example, the dose ordered and the dose on hand are in the same unit of measurement, or grains. The calculation determines the number of tablets to administer to the patient.

    EXAMPLE   The physician orders gr $\bar{v}$ of a medication po.
    The drug label reads gr $\bar{x}$ tablet.

3. If the dosage ordered is in a different unit of measurement than indicated on the drug label, two calculation steps are required to determine the amount of medication to administer to the patient. In this example, the dose ordered and the dose on hand are stated in different units of measurement, or in grams and milligrams. The first step requires conversion of the dose ordered to the unit of measurement of the dose on hand; in this example, grams must be converted to milligrams. The second step is to determine the number of tablets to administer to the patient.

    EXAMPLE   The physician orders 1 g of a medication po.
    The drug label reads 500 mg/tablet.

A detailed discussion of determining drug dosage for administration of oral medication follows. The method used to calculate drug dosage when the units of measurement are the same is presented first, followed by the method used when the units of measurement are different.

Determining Drug Dosage with the Same Units of Measurement

Determining the correct drug dosage to be administered when the units of measurement are the same requires the use of a drug dosage formula.

DRUG DOSAGE FORMULA

$$\frac{D \text{ (dose ordered)}}{H \text{ (on hand)}} \times V \text{ (vehicle)} = x \text{ (Amount of medication to be administered)}$$

D (*dose ordered*): This is the amount of medication ordered by the physician.

H (*drug strength on hand*): This is the dosage strength available as indicated on the medication label or the dose on hand.

V (*vehicle*): The vehicle refers to the type of preparation containing the dose on hand (e.g., tablet, capsule, liquid).

x: The letter *x* is used to express the unknown quantity or the amount of medication to be administered.

GUIDELINES
1. The units of measurement must be included when setting up the problem.
2. The values for D and H must be in the same unit of measurement.
3. The value of *x* is expressed in the same unit as V.
4. When determining the drug dosage for oral liquid medication, the vehicle must also include the amount of liquid in which the available drug is contained. For example, if the medication label reads 250 mg/5 mL, the value of V is 5 mL.

The method to follow to determine drug dosage using this formula is outlined in the following examples. The first problem illustrates determining dosage for solid medication taken orally.

EXAMPLES

PROBLEM   *Oral solid medication*:
                 The physician orders 50 mg of a medication po.
                 The medication label reads 25 mg/tablet.
                 How much medication should be administered to the patient?

Drug dosage formula:

$$\frac{D}{V} \times V = x$$

a. Identify the dose ordered.
   D = 50 mg

b. Identify the strength of the drug on hand.
   H = 25 mg

c. Determine the vehicle containing the dose on hand.
   V = 1 tablet

d. Calculate the amount of medication to administer to the patient. The units of measurement must be included when setting up the problem, and the values for D and H must be in the same unit of measurement. The value of *x* is expressed in the same unit as V; in this problem V = 1 tablet.

$$\frac{50 \text{ mg}}{25 \text{ mg}} \times 1 \text{ tablet} = x$$

$(50 \div 25 = 2) \times 1$ tablet $= x$
2×1 tablet $= x$
$x = 2$ tablets

Answer   2 tablets administered to the patient

The next problem illustrates the determination of drug dosage for liquid medication taken orally. The steps previously outlined are followed; however, they are combined as should be done when working out drug dosage problems. Remember, with oral liquid medication, the vehicle must also include the amount of liquid in which the available drug is contained; in the following problem, V = 5 mL.

PROBLEM   *Oral liquid medication:*
                           The physician orders 500 mg of a medication.
                           The medication label reads 250 mg/5 mL.
                           How much medication should be administered to the patient?

$$\frac{D}{V} \times 1 \text{ tablet} = x$$

$$\frac{500 \text{ mg}}{250 \text{ mg}} \times 1 \text{ tablet} = x$$

$(500 \div 250 = 2) \times 5$ mL $= x$
2×5 mL $= x$
$x = 10$ mL

Answer   A dose of 10 mL of medication is administered to the patient.

Determining Drug Dosage with Different Units of Measurement

Sometimes, the medication ordered is in a different unit of measurement than indicated on the drug label. In this case, the desired dose quantity must be converted to the unit of measurement of the dose on hand before the drug dosage is determined. The method chosen to convert a unit of measurement is based on personal preference. Refer to Units 5 and 6 to review methods of conversion before completing this section.

The following steps are required to determine drug dosage when the units of measurement are different:

Step 1: Convert the dose quantities to the same unit of measurement. For consistency, it is best to convert to the unit of measurement of the drug on hand.

Step 2: Determine the amount of medication to administer to the patient, by using the drug dosage formula.

EXAMPLES

PROBLEM   *Oral solid medication:*
             The physician orders gr $\bar{x}$ of medication po.
             The medication label reads 300 mg/tablet.
             How much medication should be administered to the patient?

Step 1: The dosage ordered must be converted to the unit of measurement of the medication on hand. In this problem, 10 grains must be converted to milligrams. The ratio and proportion method of conversion is used to make the conversion.

gr x = mg

1 grain : 60 mg = 10 grains : x mg
600 = 1 x
x = 600 mg

Answer   gr $\bar{x}$ = 600 mg

The medication ordered is in the same unit of measurement as the medication on hand.

Step 2: Determine the amount of medication to administer to the patient using the drug dosage formula.

$$\frac{D}{H} \times V = x$$

$$\frac{600 \text{ mg}}{300 \text{ mg}} \times 1 \text{ tablet}$$

(600 ÷ 300 = 2) × 1 tablet = x
2 × 1 tablet = x
x = 2 tablets

Answer   A dose of 2 tablets is administered to the patient.

PROBLEM   *Oral liquid medication:*
             The physician orders gr $\overline{xv}$ of a medication po.
             The medication label reads 300 mg/fluid dram.
             How much medication should be administered to the patient?

Step 1: Convert 15 grains to milligrams using ratio and proportion:

gr $\overline{xv}$ = _____ mg
60 mg : 1 grain = x mg : 15 grains
1 x = 900 mg
x = 900 mg

Answer   gr $\overline{xv}$ = 900 mg

Step 2: Determine the amount of medication to administer to the patient using the drug dosage formula.

$$\frac{D}{H} \times V = x$$

$$\frac{900 \text{ mg}}{300 \text{ mg}} \times 1 \text{ fluid dram} = x$$

$(900 \div 300 = 3) \times 1 \text{ fluid dram} = x$

$3 \times 1 \text{ fluid dram} = x$

$x = 3 \text{ fluid drams}$

Answer	A dose of 3 fluid drams of medication is administered to the patient.

Oral Administration: Practice Problems

Directions: Determine the drug dosage to be administered for each of the following oral medication orders, and record your answer below. In the space provided, indicate the drug category based on action for each medication using a drug reference.

Oral Solid Medications

1. The physician orders Inderal 160 mg po.
   Medication label:

   > Inderal
   >
   > propranolol
   >
   > 80 mg/capsule

   How much medication should be administered? _____

   Drug category: _____

2. The physician orders Tagamet gr v̄ po.
   Medication label:

   > Tagamet
   >
   > cimetidine
   >
   > 300 mg/tablet

   How much medication should be administered? _____

   Drug category: _____

3. The physician orders Amoxil 0.5 g po.
   Medication label:

   > Amoxil
   >
   > amoxicillin
   >
   > 250 mg/capsule

   How much medication should be administered? _____

   Drug category: _____

4. The physician orders Lasix 80 mg po.
   Medication label:

Lasix
furosemide
40 mg/tablet

   How much medication should be administered? _____

   Drug category: _____

5. The physician orders Lomotil 5 mg po.
   Medication label:

Lomotil
diphenoxylate/atropine
2.5 mg/tablet

   How much medication should be administered? _____

   Drug category: _____

6. The physician orders Zithromax 0.5 g po.
   Medication label:

Zithromax
azithromycin
250 mg/tablet

   How much medication should be administered? _____

   Drug category: _____

7. The physician orders Calan gr ii po.
   Medication label:

Calan
verapamil
40 mg/tablet

   How much medication should be administered? _____

   Drug category: _____

8. The physician orders Xanax 0.5 mg po.
   Medication label:

Xanax
alprazolam
0.25 mg/tablet

   How much medication should be administered? _____

   Drug category: _____

9. The physician orders Phenergan 25 mg po.
   Medication label:

   | Phenergan |
   | promethazine |
   | 12.5 mg/tablet |

   How much medication should be administered? _____

   Drug category: _____

10. The physician orders Procardia XL 30 mg po.
    Medication label:

    | Procardia |
    | nifedipine |
    | 10 mg/tablet |

    How much medication should be administered? _____

    Drug category: _____

Oral Liquid Medications

1. The physician orders Sumycin Suspension 250 mg po.
   Medication label:

   | Sumycin Suspension |
   | tetracycline |
   | 125 mg/5 mL |

   How much medication should be administered? _____

   Drug category: _____

2. The physician orders Tagamet liquid 300 mg po.
   Medication label:

   | Tagamet |
   | Cimetidine liquid |
   | 300 mg/5 mL |

   How much medication should be administered? _____

   Drug category: _____

3. The physician orders Tylenol Elixir 60 mg po.
   Medication label:

   | Tylenol Elixir |
   | acetaminophen |
   | 120 mg/5 mL |

   How much medication should be administered? _____

   Drug category: _____

4. The physician orders Amoxil Suspension 0.5 g po.
   Medication label:

Amoxil Suspension
amoxicillin
125 mg/5 mL

   How much medication should be administered? _____

   Drug category: _____

5. The physician orders Gantanol Suspension 1 g po.
   Medication label:

Gantanol Suspension
sulfamethoxazole
500 mg/5 mL

   How much medication should be administered? _____

   Drug category: _____

B. Parenteral Administration

Medications for parenteral administration must be suspended in solution. The medication label indicates the amount of the drug contained in each milliliter of solution. For example, if a medication label reads 10 mg/mL, there are 10 mg of medication for each 1 mL of liquid volume. Some medications, such as penicillin, insulin, and heparin, are ordered and measured in *units* (e.g., 300,000 units/mL). This refers to their biologic activity in animal tests or the amount of the drug that is required to produce a particular response.

Parenteral medication is available in several dispensing forms, including ampules, single-dose vials, and multiple-dose vials. After the proper drug dosage has been determined, the medication is drawn into a syringe from the dispensing unit. Most syringes are calibrated in milliliters (mL).

Determining drug dosage for parenteral administration is calculated in a similar manner as that for oral liquid medication. The first problem illustrates the determination of drug dosage when the medication is ordered in a different unit of measurement from the dose on hand, thus requiring two calculation steps.

EXAMPLES

PROBLEM   The physician orders 0.5 g of a medication IM.
The medication label reads 250 mg/2 mL.
How much medication should be administered?

Step 1: Convert 0.5 gram to milligrams.

0.5 g = mg

1000 mg : 1 g = x mg : 0.5 g

1 x = 500

x = 500 mg

Answer	0.5 mg = 500 mg

Step 2: Determine the amount of medication to administer to the patient:

$$\frac{D}{H} \times V = x$$

$$\frac{500 \text{ mg}}{250 \text{ mg}} \times 2 \text{ mL} = x$$

$(500 \div 250 = 2) \times 2 \text{ mL} = x$

$2 \times 2 \text{ mL} = x$

$x = 4 \text{ mL}$

> ***Answer***   A dose of 4 mL of medication is administered to the patient.

The next problem illustrates the determination of drug dosage with a medication ordered in units. Notice that the dose ordered and the dose on hand are in the same unit of measurement; therefore, conversion of units of measurement is not necessary.

PROBLEM   The physician orders 600,000 units of a medication IM.
The medication label reads 300,000 units/mL.
How much medication should be administered?

$$\frac{D}{H} \times V = x$$

$$\frac{600,000 \text{ units}}{300,000 \text{ units}} \times 1 \text{ mL} = x$$

$(600,000 \div 300,000 = 2) \times 1 \text{ mL} = x$

$x = 2 \text{ mL}$

> ***Answer***   A dose of 2 mL of medication is administered to the patient.

Parenteral Administration: Practice Problems

Determine the drug dosage to be administered for each of the following parenteral medication orders, and record your answer. In the space provided, indicate the drug category based on action using a drug reference.

1. The physician orders Vistaril 75 mg IM.
   Medication label:

Vistaril
hydroxyzine injection
50 mg/mL

   How much medication should be administered? _____

   Drug category: _____

2. The physician orders Cobex (vitamin B_{12}) 200 mcg IM.
   Medication label:

Cobex
cyanocobalamin injection
100 mcg/mL

   How much medication should be administered? _____

   Drug category: _____

3. The physician orders Depo-Medrol 40 mg IM.
   Medication label:

Depo-Medrol
methylprednisolone injection
80 mg/mL

   How much medication should be administered? _____

   Drug category: _____

4. The physician orders Wycillin 600,000 units IM.
   Medication label:

Wycillin
porcine penicillin G injection
300,000 units/mL

   How much medication should be administered? _____

   Drug category: _____

5. The physician orders Rocephin 1000 mg IM.
   Medication label:

Rocephin
ceftriaxone injection
1 g/mL

   How much medication should be administered? _____

   Drug category: _____

6. The physician orders INFeD 100 mg IM.
   Medication label:

INFeD
iron dextran injection
50 mg/mL

   How much medication should be administered? _____

   Drug category: _____

7. The physician orders Bicillin 1.2 million units IM.
   Medication label:

   > Bicillin
   >
   > benzathine penicillin G injection
   >
   > 600,000 units/mL

   How much medication should be administered? _____

   Drug category: _____

8. The physician orders Depo-Provera 150 mg IM.
   Medication label:

   > Depo-Provera
   >
   > medroxyprogesterone
   >
   > 150 mg/mL

   How much medication should be administered? _____

   Drug category: _____

9. The physician orders Pronestyl 0.25 g IM.
   Medication label:

   > Pronestyl
   >
   > procainamide injection
   >
   > 500 mg/mL

   How much medication should be administered? _____

   Drug category: _____

10. The physician orders Compazine 7 mg IM.
    Medication label:

    > Compazine
    >
    > prochlorperazine injection
    >
    > 5 mg/mL

    How much medication should be administered? _____

    Drug category: _____

Table 11-1. Metric System Conversion of Equivalent Values
WEIGHT
1000 micrograms = 1 milligram
1000 milligrams = 1 gram
1000 grams = 1 kilogram
VOLUME
1000 milliliters = 1 liter
1000 liters = 1 kiloliter
1 milliliter = 1 cubic centimeter

Chapter **11** Administration of Medication and Intravenous Therapy

Table 11-2. Apothecary System: Conversion of Equivalent Values

WEIGHT
60 grains = 1 dram
8 drams = 1 ounce
12 ounces = 1 pound

VOLUME
60 minims = 1 fluid dram
8 fluid drams = 1 fluid ounce
16 fluid ounces = 1 pint
2 pints = 1 quart
4 quarts = 1 gallon

Table 11-3. Household System: Conversion of Equivalent Values

ABBREVIATIONS
drop: gtt
teaspoon: tsp
tablespoon: T
ounce: oz
cup: c

VOLUME
60 drops = 1 teaspoon
3 teaspoons = 1 tablespoon
6 teaspoons = 1 ounce
2 tablespoons = 1 ounce
6 ounces = 1 teacup
8 ounces = 1 glass
8 ounces = 1 cup

Table 11-4. Conversion Chart for Metric and Apothecary Systems (Commonly Used Approximate Equivalents)

Metric System to Apothecary System	Apothecary System to Metric System
WEIGHT	**WEIGHT**
60 mg = 1 grain	15 grains = 1000 mg (1 g)
1 g = 15 grains	10 grains = 600 mg
4 g = 1 dram	7.5 grains = 500 mg
30 mg = 1 ounce	5 grains = 300 mg
1 kg = 2.2 pounds	3 grains = 200 mg
	1.5 grains = 100 mg
	1 grain = 60 mg
VOLUME	¾ grain = 50 mg
0.06 mL = 1 minim	½ grain = 30 mg
1 mL (cc) = 15 minims	¼ grain = 15 mg
4 mL = 1 fluid dram	⅙ grain = 10 mg
30 mL = 1 fluid ounce	⅛ grain = 8 mg
500 mL = 1 pint	$\frac{1}{12}$ grain = 5 mg
1000 mL (1 L) = 1 quart	$\frac{1}{15}$ grain = 4 mg
	$\frac{1}{20}$ grain = 3 mg
	$\frac{1}{30}$ grain = 2 mg
	$\frac{1}{40}$ grain = 1.5 mg
	$\frac{1}{50}$ grain = 1.2 mg
	$\frac{1}{60}$ grain = 1 mg
	$\frac{1}{100}$ grain = 0.6 mg
	$\frac{1}{120}$ grain = 0.5 mg
	$\frac{1}{150}$ grain = 0.4 mg
	$\frac{1}{200}$ grain = 0.3 mg
	$\frac{1}{300}$ grain = 0.2 mg
	$\frac{1}{600}$ grain = 0.1 mg

Table 11-5. Conversion Chart for Apothecary and Metric Equivalents of Household Measures (Volume)

Household	Apothecary	Metric
1 drop	= 1 minim	= 0.06 mL
15 drops	= 15 minims	= 1 mL (cc)
1 teaspoon	= 1 fluid dram	= 5 (4) mL
1 tablespoon	= 4 fluid drams	= 15 mL
2 tablespoons	= 1 fluid ounce	= 30 mL
1 ounce	= 1 fluid ounce	= 30 mL
1 teacup	= 6 fluid ounces	= 180 mL
1 glass	= 8 fluid ounces	= 240 mL

Notes

12 Cardiopulmonary Procedures

√ After Completing	Date Due	Textbook Pages	TEXTBOOK ASSIGNMENTS	Possible Points	Points You Earned
		491–450	Read Chapter 12: Cardiopulmonary Procedures		
		501 536–537	Read Case Study 1 Case Study 1 questions	5	
		521 537	Read Case Study 2 Case Study 2 questions	5	
		522 537	Read Case Study 3 Case Study 3 questions	5	
			Total points		

√ After Completing	Date Due	Study Guide Pages	STUDY GUIDE ASSIGNMENTS (CTA = Critical Thinking Activity)	Possible Points	Points You Earned
		591	Pretest	10	
		592 593	Term Key Term Assessment A. Definitions B. Word Parts (Add 1 point for each medical term)	21 14	
		594–601	Evaluation of Learning questions	60	
		602	CTA A: Chest Leads	5	
			Evolve Activity: Chapter 12 Find That Lead: ECG Chest Leads (Record points earned)		
		602	CTA B: ECG Cycle	10	
		603–608	CTA C: GO TO! Game (Record points earned)		
			Evolve Site: Chapter 12 It's a Cycle: ECG Cycle (Record points earned)		
			Evolve Site: Chapter 12 Nutrition Nugget: Congestive Heart Failure	10	

√ After Completing	Date Due	Study Guide Pages	STUDY GUIDE ASSIGNMENTS (CTA = Critical Thinking Activity)	Possible Points	Points You Earned
			Evolve Site: Chapter 12 It's an Artifact: ECG Artifacts (Record points earned)		
		609	CTA D: ECG Artifacts (10 points each)	30	
		609–612	CTA E: Myocardial Infarction	20	
		613	CTA F: Peak Flow Chart	10	
		614	CTA G: Crossword Puzzle	29	
			Evolve Site: Chapter 12 Animations (2 points each)	38	
			Evolve Site: Apply Your Knowledge questions	12	
		615–616	Video Evaluation	33	
		591	Posttest	10	
			ADDITIONAL ASSIGNMENTS		
			Total points		

√ When Assigned by Your Instructor	Study Guide Pages	Practices Required	LABORATORY ASSIGNMENTS (Procedure Number and Name)	Score*
	617–618	3	Practice for Competency 12-1: Running a 12-Lead, Three-Channel Electrocardiogram Textbook reference: pp. 506–509	
	621–623		Evaluation of Competency 12-1: Running a 12-Lead, Three-Channel Electrocardiogram	*
	617–618	3	Practice for Competency 12-2: Applying a Holter Monitor Textbook reference: pp. 513–516	
	625–627		Evaluation of Competency 12-2: Applying a Holter Monitor	*
	618–619	3	Practice for Competency 12-3: Spirometry Testing Textbook reference: pp. 524–525	
	629–631		Evaluation of Competency 12-3: Spirometry Testing	*
	618–619	3	Practice for Competency 12-4: Measuring Peak Flow Rate Textbook reference: pp. 530–531	
	633–635		Evaluation of Competency 12-4: Measuring Peak Flow Rate	*
			ADDITIONAL ASSIGNMENTS	

Notes

Name: _____ Date: _____

True or False

_____ 1. Blood enters the right atrium from the superior and inferior vena cava.

_____ 2. The cardiac cycle represents one complete heartbeat.

_____ 3. A standard electrocardiogram consists of 10 leads.

_____ 4. An electrolyte facilitates the transmission of electrical impulses.

_____ 5. Leads V_1 through V_6 are known as the *augmented leads*.

_____ 6. Electrodes that are too loose can cause a 60-cycle interference artifact.

_____ 7. An electrocardiographic (ECG) result that is within normal limits is said to indicate normal sinus rhythm.

_____ 8. The most serious cardiac dysrhythmia is atrial fibrillation.

_____ 9. The purpose of a pulmonary function test is to assess cardiac functioning.

_____ 10. During an asthma attack, the bronchial tubes constrict, swell, and become clogged with mucus.

📑 **POSTTEST**

True or False

_____ 1. An electrocardiogram is a recording of the electrical activity of the heart.

_____ 2. The AV node sets the pace of the heart.

_____ 3. The P wave represents the contraction of the ventricles.

_____ 4. If the electrocardiograph is standardized, the standardization mark will be 20 mm high.

_____ 5. A muscle artifact can be identified by its fuzzy, irregular baseline.

_____ 6. The patient is permitted to shower while wearing a Holter monitor.

_____ 7. A patient with a PAT dysrhythmia often experiences weakness and acute apprehension.

_____ 8. A spirometer measures how much air is exhaled from the lungs and how fast it is exhaled.

_____ 9. Spirometry can be used to assess a patient with emphysema.

_____ 10. A nasal cannula interferes with a patient's ability to talk, eat, and drink.

A. Definitions

Directions: Match each medical term (numbers) with its definition (letters).

_____ 1. Artifact

_____ 2. Atherosclerosis

_____ 3. Baseline

_____ 4. Cardiac cycle

_____ 5. Dysrhythmia

_____ 6. ECG cycle

_____ 7. Electrocardiogram

_____ 8. Electrocardiograph

_____ 9. Flow rate

_____ 10. Electrode

_____ 11. Electrolyte

_____ 12. Hypoxemia

_____ 13. Hypoxia

_____ 14. Interval

_____ 15. Ischemia

_____ 16. Normal sinus rhythm

_____ 17. Oxygen therapy

_____ 18. Peak flow rate

_____ 19. Segment

_____ 20. Spirometer

_____ 21. Wheezing

A. A chemical substance that promotes conduction of an electrical current

B. The flat, horizontal line that separates the various waves of the ECG cycle

C. The instrument used to record the electrical activity of the heart

D. Additional electrical activity picked up by the electrocardiograph that interferes with the normal appearance of the ECG cycles

E. Refers to an electrocardiogram that is within normal limits

F. One complete heartbeat

G. The graphic representation of the electrical activity of the heart

H. The length of a wave or the length of a wave with a segment

I. The graphic representation of a heartbeat

J. A conductor of electricity, which is used to promote contact between the body and the electrocardiograph

K. The portion of the ECG between two waves

L. Deficiency of blood in a body part

M. An instrument for measuring air taken into and expelled from the lungs

N. Buildup of fibrous plaques of fatty deposits and cholesterol on the inner walls of an artery that causes narrowing, obstruction, and hardening of the artery

O. An irregular heart rate or rhythm

P. The number of liters of oxygen per minute that come out of an oxygen delivery system

Q. A decrease in the oxygen saturation of the blood

R. A reduction in the oxygen supply to the tissues of the body

S. The administration of supplemental oxygen at concentrations greater than room air to treat or prevent hypoxemia

T. The maximum volume of air that can be exhaled when a patient blows into a peak flow meter as forcefully and as rapidly as possible

U. A continuous, high-pitched whistling musical sound heard particularly during exhalation and sometimes during inhalation

B. Word Parts

Directions: Indicate the meaning of each word part in the space provided. List as many medical terms as possible that incorporate the word part in the space provided.

Word Part	Meaning of Word Part	Medical Terms That Incorporate Word Part
1. ather/o		
2. -sclerosis		
3. cardi/o		
4. electr/o		
5. -gram		
6. -graph		
7. hypo-		
8. ox/i		
9. -emia		
10. -ia		
11. isch/o		
12. spir/o		
13. -meter		
14. -metry		

Directions: Fill in each blank with the correct answer.

1. What is the purpose of electrocardiography?

   _____

   _____

   _____

2. Trace the path blood takes through the heart, starting with the right atrium.

   _____

   _____

   _____

3. What is the function of the coronary arteries?

   _____

   _____

4. What is the function of the SA node?

   _____

   _____

5. Why is the impulse initiated by the SA node delayed momentarily by the AV node?

   _____

6. What is the cardiac cycle?

   _____

7. Label the following on the ECG cycle:
P wave	P-R segment
QRS complex	S-T segment
T wave	P-R interval
Q-T interval	

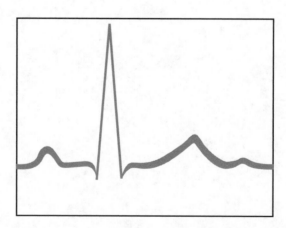

8. Explain what each component of the ECG cycle represents.

P wave _____

QRS complex _____

T wave _____

P-R segment _____

S-T segment _____

P-R interval _____

Q-T interval _____

9. Why is the R wave taller than the P wave on the ECG graph cycle?

_____

_____

10. Why does atrial repolarization not appear as a separate wave on the ECG cycle?

_____

_____

11. Why is the baseline flat following the U wave?

_____

_____

12. What changes can occur on an ECG as a result of the following?

a. Coronary artery disease:

b. Myocardial infarction:

13. What is the purpose of standardizing the electrocardiograph?

_____

_____

_____

14. How high should the standardization mark be when the electrocardiograph is standardized?

_____

_____

15. What is a lead, and what information does it provide?

_____

_____

16. What is the function of an electrode?

_____

_____

17. Why must an electrolyte be used when recording an electrocardiogram?

_____

_____

_____

18. Diagram the bipolar leads on the following illustration:

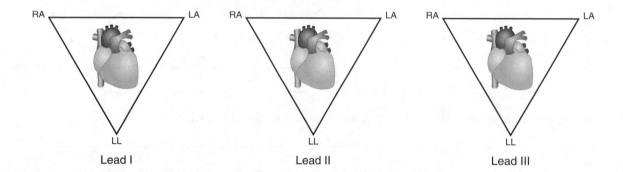

| Lead I | Lead II | Lead III |

19. Locate and label the location of the chest electrodes on the following illustration:

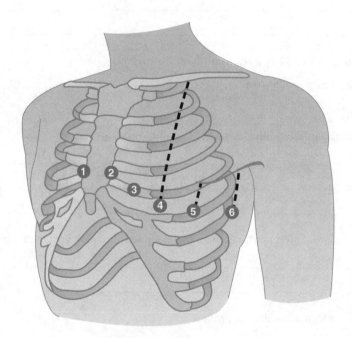

20. At what speed does the paper move while recording a normal electrocardiogram?

_____

21. What is the difference between a three-channel and a single-channel electrocardiograph?

_____

_____

_____

22. What is the purpose of each of the following electrocardiograph capabilities?

a. Interpretive capability

_____

_____

b. EMR connectivity

_____

_____

c. Teletransmission

_____

_____

23. Why should artifacts be eliminated if they occur in an ECG recording?

_____

_____

_____

24. What is the function of an artifact filter?

_____

25. List three possible causes of muscle artifacts.

_____

_____

_____

26. List three possible causes of wandering baseline.

_____

_____

27. List three possible causes of 60-cycle interference artifacts.

_____

_____

_____

28. List four uses of Holter monitor electrocardiography.

_____

_____

_____

_____

29. Explain the use of the patient diary in Holter monitor electrocardiography.

_____

_____

_____

30. List five guidelines that should be relayed to the patient undergoing Holter monitor electrocardiography.

_____

_____

_____

_____

_____

31. List the distinguishing characteristics of each of the following cardiac arrhythmias.

a. Paroxysmal atrial tachycardia

_____

_____

b. Atrial fibrillation

_____

_____

c. Premature ventricular contraction

_____

_____

d. Ventricular fibrillation

_____

_____

32. What is the purpose of a pulmonary function test?

_____

33. What are the indications for performing spirometry?

_____

_____

_____

34. What is forced vital capacity?

_____

_____

35. What patient preparation is required for spirometry?

_____

_____

_____

36. What is the purpose of postbronchodilator spirometry?

_____

_____

37. What are the characteristics of asthma?

_____

_____

38. What are five examples of allergens that may trigger an asthma attack?

_____

_____

39. What are five examples of environmental irritants, activities, or events that may trigger an asthma attack?

_____

_____

40. What happens to the bronchial tubes during an asthma attack?

_____

_____

41. What is the purpose of long-term-control asthma medication?

_____

_____

42. What is the purpose of quick-relief asthma medication?

_____

_____

43. What is the purpose of a peak flow meter?

_____

_____

44. What is the difference between a low-range and full-range peak flow meter?

_____

_____

45. What is the purpose of peak flow measurements?

_____

_____

_____

_____

46. Why is oxygen needed by the body?

_____

_____

47. What occurs when the body cannot maintain an adequate oxygen level?

_____

_____

48. What conditions may require home oxygen therapy?

_____

_____

49. What information is included on a prescription for home oxygen therapy?

_____

_____

50. What are the advantages and disadvantages of compressed oxygen gas?
    a. Advantages:

    _____

    _____

    b. Disadvantages:

    _____

    _____

51. What is liquid oxygen?

_____

_____

52. What are the advantages and disadvantages of liquid oxygen?
    a. Advantages:

    _____

    _____

    b. Disadvantages:

    _____

    _____

53. What is an oxygen concentrator?

_____

_____

54. What are the advantages and disadvantages of an oxygen concentrator?

    a. Advantages:

    _____

    _____

    b. Disadvantages:

    _____

    _____

55. What is the primary advantage of using a nasal cannula to administer oxygen?

_____

_____

56. List two reasons for using a face mask to administer oxygen therapy.

_____

_____

57. What are the symptoms of a low oxygen level in the body?

_____

_____

58. How much tubing should be used with an oxygen delivery system and why?

_____

_____

59. What occurs if oxygen comes in contact with a fire?

_____

_____

60. How should oxygen be stored?

_____

_____

CRITICAL THINKING ACTIVITIES

A. Chest Leads

Practice locating the six chest leads on five individuals. Select individuals of both sexes and of various ages and body contours. Record each person's name here after you have successfully located the chest leads. Record any problems you encountered locating the leads.

1. _____

2. _____

3. _____

4. _____

5. _____

B. ECG Cycle

Attach part of an ECG from a recording. Identify and label the various waves, intervals, and segments making up an ECG cycle on two of the leads.

C. GO TO! Game

Object: To demonstrate your knowledge of locating the waves, intervals, and segments on an ECG cycle and to answer questions relating to the ECG cycle

Needed: **GO TO!** game board

Game cards

A small token for each player (e.g., button, coin)

Score card

Directions:

1. Cut out the **GO TO!** game cards.
2. Review the components of the ECG cycle.
3. Form a group of three players.
4. Place one complete set of the game cards on the game board with the **GO TO!** question facing up and the answer facing down.
5. In turn, a player selects a game card and goes to the site indicated on the card.
6. If the player goes to the correct site, he or she is awarded 5 points. If there is a question regarding the correct site, consult the instructor.
7. The player then answers the question on the game card. If the question is answered correctly, the player is awarded another 5 points.
8. Keep track of your points on the score card provided.
9. Continue playing until all the game cards have been used.
10. Calculate your points, and determine the knowledge level you attained.
11. If time permits, shuffle the game cards, and play the game again.

GO TO!
SCORE CARD

Name: _____

Recording Points:
Cross off a number each time you go to a site correctly. Cross off another number each time you answer a question correctly. Your total points will be equal to the last number you crossed off. Record this number in the space provided, and determine the knowledge level you attained.

Points:	
5	75
10	80
15	85
20	90
25	95
30	100
35	105
40	110
45	115
50	120
55	125
60	130
65	135
70	140

Total points: _____

LEVEL: _____

☐ 95 points and above: **Sheer genius!**

☐ 75 to 90 points: **Shows great promise**

☐ 55 to 70 points: **Time to study**

☐ 50 points and under: **Brain freeze**

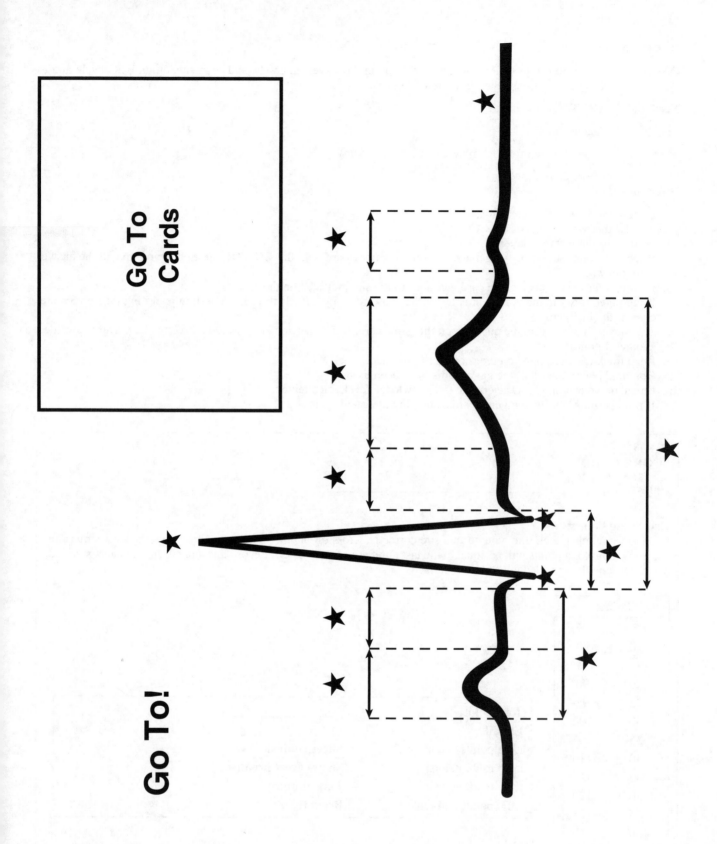

Go To
Cards

Go To!

GO TO:
P WAVE

Q: What are the cuspid valves doing right now?

GO TO:
Q WAVE

Q: Which heart chamber pumps blood
from the heart and out into the body?

GO TO:
R WAVE
You are on top of the world.
Answer your question and
take another turn.

Q: Why is the R wave taller than the
P wave?

GO TO:
S WAVE

Q: State the location of V_2.

GO TO:
T WAVE

Q: What is happening in the heart
during this time?

GO TO:
U WAVE

Q: State the location of V_1.

GO TO:
P-R SEGMENT

Q: What does this time lapse represent?

GO TO:
P-R INTERVAL

Q: What does this time lapse represent?

A: Left ventricle

A: The cuspid valves are open.

A: Fourth intercostal space at left
margin of sternum

A: At horizontal level of V_4 at left
anterior axillary line

A: Fourth intercostal space at right
margin of sternum

A: The ventricles are larger than the
atria and therefore require a stronger
electrical stimulus to depolarize.

A: The time interval from the
beginning of the atrial depolarization
to the beginning of ventricular
depolarization

A: The time interval from the end of the
atrial depolarization to the beginning of
ventricular depolarization

GO TO:
QRS COMPLEX

Q: What are the atria doing right now?

GO TO:
S-T SEGMENT

Q: What does this time interval represent?

GO TO:
Q-T INTERVAL

Q: What does this time interval represent?

GO TO:
WHERE THE ATRIA ARE CONTRACTING

Q: What are the semilunar valves doing right now?

GO TO:
WHERE THE IMPULSE IS BEING DELAYED AT THE AV NODE

Q: Why is the impulse being delayed at the AV node?

GO TO:
WHERE THE VENTRICLES ARE CONTRACTING

Q: What are the cuspid valves doing right now?

GO TO:
VENTRICLES ARE RECOVERING

Q: State the location of V_3.

GO TO:
WHERE THE HEART RESTS TAKE A REST. ANSWER THIS QUESTION, BUT YOU LOSE YOUR NEXT TURN.

Q: State the location of V_4.

A: The time interval from the end of the
ventricular depolarization to
the beginning of repolarization
of the ventricles

A: The atria are resting.

A: The semilunar valves are closed.

A: The time interval from the beginning
of the ventricular depolarization
to the end of repolarization
of the ventricles

A: The cuspid valves are closed.

A: To allow for complete contraction of the
atria and the filling of the ventricles with
blood from the atria

A: Fifth intercostal space at
junction of the left midclavicular line

A: Midway between
V_2 and V_4

D. ECG Artifacts

If possible, attach examples of the following types of artifacts here:

1. Muscle artifact

2. Wandering baseline artifact

3. 60-cycle interference artifact

E. Myocardial Infarction

You are working for a cardiologist. Your physician is concerned about the increase in the numbers of patients having heart attacks. He asks you to design a colorful, creative, and informative brochure on heart attacks using the brochure provided on the following page. This brochure will be published and placed in the waiting room to provide patients with education about heart attacks. The heart disease Internet sites listed under "On the Web" at the end of Chapter 12 in your textbook can be used to complete this activity.

609

FAQ ON:

Q: A:

Q: A:

Q: A:

Q: A:

Q:

A:

Q:

A:

Illustration

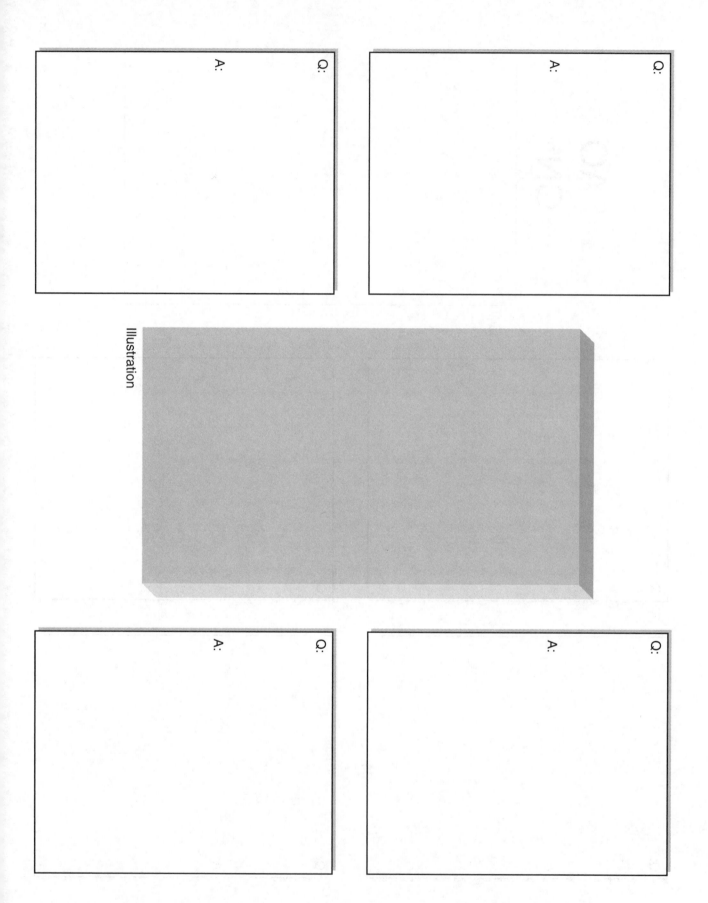

Q:

A:

Q:

A:

612

Chapter **12** **Cardiopulmonary Procedures**

F. Peak Flow Chart

Chart the following peak flow measurements in the peak flow chart provided. "Connect the dots" after entering the measurement on the chart.

Date	Time	Peak Flow Measurement
4/1	9:00	550
4/2	9:15	540
4/3	9:10	500
4/4	9:30	480
4/5	8:45	510
4/6	9:00	530
4/7	9:10	520
4/8	9:15	560
4/9	9:30	570
4/10	9:15	550

G. Crossword Puzzle: Cardiopulmonary Procedures

Directions: Complete the crossword puzzle using the clues provided.

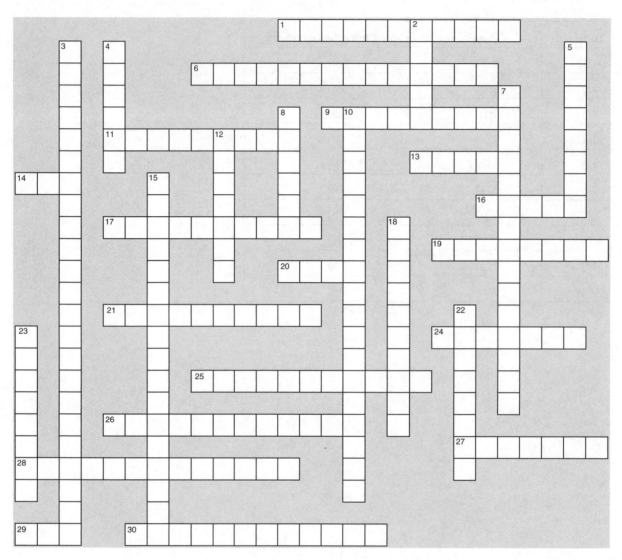

Across

1 Rhythm not normal
6 Drug that opens air passages
9 Asthma allergen trigger
11 Damaged alveoli disease
13 Atria contract
14 Take a deep breath and blow it all out!
16 Mighty big artery
17 Lower heart chambers
19 Keep this blanket away from a Holter
20 Fourth intercostal to the left
21 "How well can you breathe" test
24 Leads I, II, III
26 O_2 administration device
27 Delivers asthma med
28 Drug for angina
29 ECG std mark in mm
30 Inflammation of heart's lining

Down

2 The ventricles are recovering
3 Serious rhythm disturbance
4 Not with a Holter on
5 Not enough blood
7 Coronary artery plaque condition
8 Pacemaker of the heart
10 Separates O_2 out of air
12 Primary cause of COPD
15 "Too loose" electrodes cause this
18 Heart muscle layer
22 Left-side heart valve
23 High-pitched whistling sound

614

Chapter **12 Cardiopulmonary Procedures**

Name: _____

Directions:

a. Watch the indicated videos.
b. Mark each true statement with a T and each false statement with an F. For each false statement, change the wording of the question so that it becomes a true statement.

Video: Procedure 12-1: Running a 12-Lead, Three-Channel Electrocardiogram

_____ 1. The electrocardiograph is an instrument used to record the electrical activity of the heart.

_____ 2. The most common reason for running an ECG in the medical office is to diagnose the presence of a myocardial infarction.

_____ 3. Patient movement when running an electrocardiogram can cause 60-cycle interference artifacts to appear on the ECG recording.

_____ 4. The arms and legs should be well supported to prevent the occurrence of muscle artifacts on the ECG recording.

_____ 5. If the patient is uncomfortable or cold, a wandering baseline artifact may appear on the ECG recording.

_____ 6. The power cord should point away from the patient and not pass under the table, to reduce the occurrence of 60-cycle interference artifacts on the recording.

_____ 7. That patient's skin must be dry and free of oil and body hair for the adhesive backing of the electrode to stick to the patient's skin and stay on during the procedure.

_____ 8. The electrode tabs of the arms should point downward, and the electrode tabs of the legs should point upward.

_____ 9. If the electrodes pull away from the patient's skin, a wandering baseline artifact may result on the recording.

_____ 10. Chest lead V_2 is located at the fourth intercostal space at the right margin of the sternum.

_____ 11. The lead wires should be arranged to follow body contour to prevent 60-cycle interference artifacts on the recording.

_____ 12. The patient's data entered into an interpretive electrocardiograph are used to perform a computer analysis of the recording.

_____ 13. The standardization mark should be 20 mm high.

_____ 14. The R wave on lead 1 should have a negative deflection.

_____ 15. If an artifact is present on the recording, correct the problem and run another ECG.

Video: Procedure 12-3: Spirometry Testing

_____ 1. Spirometry is a noninvasive screening test for pulmonary function.

_____ 2. A spirometer measures how much air is pushed out of the lungs and how fast it is pushed out.

_____ 3. Spirometry is often performed on patients exhibiting urinary tract infections.

_____ 4. The spirometer is calibrated by injecting 3 liters of air into the spirometer from a calibration syringe.

_____ 5. For 24 hours before spirometry, the patient must not eat a heavy meal or smoke.

_____ 6. Heavy or constricting clothing can make it difficult to perform the procedure.

_____ 7. The patient's data must be entered into the spirometer for the accurate calculation of predicted values.

_____ 8. Nose clips must be placed on the patient's nose to prevent air from escaping from the nostrils.

_____ 9. The patient should be instructed to blow out as hard as possible and for as long as possible until the lungs are completely empty.

_____ 10. Fear and anxiety can lead to unreliable results.

Video: Procedure 12-4: Measuring Peak Flow Rate

_____ 1. A peak flow meter is used to measure a breathing maneuver performed by the patient.

_____ 2. A peak flow meter is most frequently used by patients with diabetes.

_____ 3. The sliding indicator must be moved to the bottom of the numbered scale to make it easier for the patient to perform the breathing maneuver.

_____ 4. The purpose of the disposable mouthpiece is to prevent the spread of microorganisms from one patient to another.

_____ 5. The peak flow procedure is repeated until three acceptable efforts have been obtained.

_____ 6. If the patient performs the breathing maneuver correctly, the numbers from the three tests should be about the same.

_____ 7. The mouthpiece should be discarded in a biohazard waste container.

_____ 8. The patient's test results are determined by calculating an average of the three breathing maneuvers.

Procedure 12-1: 12-Lead Electrocardiogram.

Practice the procedure for running a 12-lead electrocardiogram and record the procedure in the chart provided.

Procedure 12-2: Holter Monitor

1. Activity diary. Complete the patient information section on the Holter Activity Diary below.
2. Holter monitor. Practice the procedure for applying the Holter monitor, and record the procedure in the chart provided.

HOLTER MONITOR

PATIENT ACTIVITY DIARY

☐ 10 Hr.   ☐ 12 Hr.   ☐ 24 Hr.   ☐ 26 Hr.

Patient's Name: _____

Patient's Address: _____

_____

Age: ____ Sex: ____ Phone: _____

Date of Birth: _____ Soc. Sec. #: _____

Medication: _____

Doctor: _____ Phone: _____

Hospital: _____ Room: _____

Date of Recording: _____ Started: _____ AM PM

Serial Numbers
  Recorder: _____

  Battery: _____

Connected by: _____

_____

Procedure 12-3: Spirometry. Practice the procedure for performing a spirometry test, and record the procedure in the chart provided.

Procedure 12-4: Peak Flow Rate Measurement. Practice the procedure for measuring peak flow rate, and record the procedure in the chart provided.

	CHART
Date	

CHART	
Date	

PEAK FLOW CHART

Name _____

DATE																	
TIME																	
800																	
750																	
700																	
650																	
600																	
550																	
500																	
450																	
400																	
350																	
300																	
250																	
200																	
150																	
100																	
50																	
Peak Flow Number																	

Procedure 12-1: Running a 12-Lead, Three-Channel Electrocardiogram

Name: _____   Date: _____

Evaluated by: _____   Score: _____

Performance Objective

Outcome:	Record a 12-lead electrocardiogram.
Conditions:	Using a three-channel electrocardiograph.
	Given ECG paper and disposable electrodes.
Standards:	Time: 15 minutes. Student completed procedure in _____ minutes.
	Accuracy: Satisfactory score on the Performance Evaluation Checklist.

Performance Evaluation Checklist

Trial 1	Trial 2	Point Value	Performance Standards
		•	Worked in a quiet atmosphere away from sources of electrical interference.
		•	Sanitized hands.
		•	Checked the expiration date of the electrodes.
		▷	Explained what may occur if the electrodes are outdated.
		•	Greeted the patient and introduced yourself.
		•	Identified the patient and explained the procedure.
		•	Instructed the patient that he or she will need to lie still, breathe normally, and not talk during the procedure.
		▷	Explained why the patient should lie still and not talk.
		•	Asked the patient to remove appropriate clothing.
		•	Assisted the patient into a supine position on the table.
		•	Made sure that the patient's arms and legs were adequately supported on the table.
		•	Draped the patient properly.
		•	Positioned the electrocardiograph with the power cord pointing away from the patient and not passing under the table.
		•	Worked on the left side of the patient.
		•	Prepared the patient's skin for application of the disposable electrodes.
		▷	Explained why the patient's skin must be prepared properly.
		•	Applied the limb electrodes.
		•	Properly located each chest position and applied the chest electrodes.
		▷	Explained why the tabs of the electrodes should be positioned correctly.
		•	Connected the lead wires to the electrodes.
		•	Arranged the lead wires to follow body contour.
		▷	Explained why the lead wires should follow body contour.

Trial 1	Trial 2	Point Value	Performance Standards
		•	Plugged the patient's cable into machine and properly supported the cable.
		•	Turned on the electrocardiograph.
		•	Entered the patient's data using the soft-touch keypad.
		▷	Stated the purpose of entering the patient's data.
		•	Reminded the patient to lie still, and pressed the AUTO button to run the recording.
		•	Checked to make sure the standardization mark is 10 mm high.
		•	Checked to make sure the R wave has a positive deflection.
		▷	Stated what would cause the R wave to have a negative deflection.
		•	Checked the recording for artifacts and corrected them if they occurred.
		•	Informed the patient that he or she can move and talk.
		•	Turned off the electrocardiograph.
		•	Disconnected the lead wires.
		•	Removed and discarded the disposable electrodes.
		•	Assisted the patient from the table.
		•	Sanitized hands.
		•	Charted the procedure correctly.
		•	Placed the recording in the appropriate place to be reviewed by the physician.
		•	Returned equipment to the proper place.
		✶	Completed the procedure within 15 minutes.
			Totals

CHART

Date	

Evaluation of Student Performance

EVALUATION CRITERIA			COMMENTS
Symbol	**Category**	**Point Value**	
✶	Critical Step	16 points	
•	Essential Step	6 points	
▷	Theory Question	2 points	

Score calculation: 100 points

   − _____ points missed

   _____ Score

Satisfactory score: 85 or above

CAAHEP Competencies Achieved
Psychomotor (Skills)
☑ I. 5. Perform electrocardiography.
Affective (Behavior)
☑ I. 2. Use language/verbal skills that enable patients' understanding.
☑ XI. 1. Recognize the effects of stress on all persons involved in emergency situations.

ABHES Competencies Achieved
☑ 8. cc. Communicate on the recipient's level of comprehension.
☑ 9. o. Perform: (1) Electrocardiograms.

Notes

Procedure 12-2: Applying a Holter Monitor

Name: _____   Date: _____

Evaluated by: _____   Score: _____

Performance Objective

Outcome:	Apply a Holter monitor.
Conditions:	Using a Holter monitor with an internal memory card.
	Given the following: battery, disposable pouch and lanyard or a belt clip, disposable electrodes, razor, antiseptic wipes, gauze pads, abrasive pad, nonallergenic tape, and a patient diary.
Standards:	Time: 20 minutes. Student completed procedure in _____ minutes.
	Accuracy: Satisfactory score on the Performance Evaluation Checklist.

Performance Evaluation Checklist

Trial 1	Trial 2	Point Value	Performance Standards
		•	Assembled equipment.
		•	Installed a new battery.
		•	Checked the expiration date of the electrodes.
		•	Connected the Holter monitor to the computer.
		•	Entered the patient's demographic data into the computer and downloaded this information to the monitor.
		•	Sanitized hands.
		•	Greeted the patient and introduced yourself.
		•	Identified the patient and explained the procedure.
		•	Instructed the patient in the guidelines for wearing a Holter monitor.
		•	Asked the patient to remove clothing from the waist up.
		•	Positioned the patient in a sitting position.
		•	Located the chest electrode placement sites.
		•	Shaved the patient's chest at each electrode site, if needed.
		•	Rubbed the patient's skin with an alcohol wipe and allowed it to dry.
		•	Slightly abraded the skin.
		▷	Explained why the skin should be abraded.
		•	Attached a lead wire to the snap of each electrode.
		•	Properly applied the electrodes with an attached lead wire.
		▷	Explained why the electrodes should be firmly attached.
		•	Plugged the patient cable into the monitor and turned on the monitor.
		•	Checked the ECG signal quality.

Trial 1	Trial 2	Point Value	Performance Standards
		▷	Stated why the signal quality should be clear and strong.
		•	Placed tape over each electrode.
		•	Checked to make sure the date and time displayed on the monitor are accurate.
		•	Started the monitor.
		•	Placed the pouch around the patient's neck and inserted the monitor in the pouch.
		•	Instructed the patient to get dressed.
		•	Completed the patient information section of the diary.
		•	Recorded the starting time in the patient diary.
		•	Provided the patient with instructions on completing the diary.
		•	Instructed the patient when to return for removal of the monitor.
		•	Sanitized hands.
		•	Charted the procedure correctly.
		✶	Completed the procedure within 20 minutes.
			Totals
CHART			
Date			

Evaluation of Student Performance

EVALUATION CRITERIA			COMMENTS
Symbol	**Category**	**Point Value**	
✶	Critical Step	16 points	
•	Essential Step	6 points	
▷	Theory Question	2 points	

Score calculation: 100 points

− _____ points missed

_____ Score

Satisfactory score: 85 or above

CAAHEP Competencies Achieved
Psychomotor (Skills)
☑ I. 5. Perform electrocardiography.
Affective (Behavior)
☑ I. 2. Use language/verbal skills that enable patients' understanding.

ABHES Competencies Achieved
☑ 8. cc. Communicate on the recipient's level of comprehension.
☑ 9. o. Perform: (1) Electrocardiograms.

Notes

Procedure 12-3: Spirometry Testing

Name: _____   Date: _____

Evaluated by: _____   Score: _____

Performance Objective

Outcome:	Perform a spirometry test.
Conditions:	Using a spirometer.
	Given the following: disposable tubing, disposable mouthpiece, disposable nose clips, waste container.
Standards:	Time: 20 minutes. Student completed procedure in _____ minutes.
	Accuracy: Satisfactory score on the Performance Evaluation Checklist.

Performance Evaluation Checklist

Trial 1	Trial 2	Point Value	Performance Standards
		•	Sanitized hands.
		•	Assembled and prepared equipment.
		•	Calibrated the spirometer.
		▷	Stated the reason for calibrating the spirometer.
		•	Applied a disposable mouthpiece to the mouthpiece holder.
		•	Greeted the patient and introduced yourself.
		•	Identified the patient and explained the procedure.
		•	Asked the patient whether he or she had prepared properly.
		•	Asked the patient to remove heavy or restrictive clothing, to loosen tight clothing, and to discard gum.
		▷	Explained why tight clothing should be loosened.
		•	Measured the patient's weight and height.
		▷	Explained the reason for measuring weight and height.
		•	Asked the patient to sit near the machine.
		•	Entered the patient's data into the computer database of the spirometer.
			Described and demonstrated the breathing maneuver:
		•	Relax and take the deepest breath possible.
		•	Place the mouthpiece in your mouth and seal your lips tightly around it.
		•	Blow out as hard as you can for as long as possible.
		•	Do not block the opening of the mouthpiece with your tongue.
		•	Remove the mouthpiece from your mouth.
		▷	Explained why the lips should be tightly sealed around the mouthpiece.

Trial 1	Trial 2	Point Value	Performance Standards
		•	Told the patient the instructions would be repeated during the test.
		•	Encouraged the patient to remain calm.
		•	Gently applied the nose clips.
		▷	Stated the purpose of the nose clips.
		•	Handed the mouthpiece to the patient.
		•	Began the test and actively coached the patient.
		•	Informed the patient of modifications needed if the breathing maneuver was not performed correctly.
		•	Continued the test until three acceptable efforts were obtained.
		•	Gently removed the nose clips from the patient's nose.
		•	Removed the mouthpiece from its holder.
		•	Disposed of the nose clips and mouthpiece in a waste container.
		•	Allowed the patient to remain seated for a few minutes.
		•	Sanitized your hands.
		•	Printed the report and labeled it.
		•	Charted the procedure correctly.
		•	Placed the spirometry report in an appropriate location for review by the physician.
		•	Cleaned the spirometer according to the manufacturer's instructions.
		✱	Completed the procedure within 20 minutes.
			Totals

CHART	
Date	

Evaluation of Student Performance

EVALUATION CRITERIA			COMMENTS
Symbol	**Category**	**Point Value**	
✱	Critical Step	16 points	
•	Essential Step	6 points	
▷	Theory Question	2 points	
Score calculation: 100 points			
− _____ points missed			
_____ Score			
Satisfactory score: 85 or above			

CAAHEP Competencies Achieved

Psychomotor (Skills)

☑ I. 4. Perform pulmonary function testing.

☑ I. 11. Perform quality control measures.

Affective (Behavior)

☑ I. 2. Use language/verbal skills that enable patients' understanding.

ABHES Competencies Achieved

☑ 8. cc. Communicate on the recipient's level of comprehension.

☑ 9. o. Perform: (2) Respiratory testing.

Notes

Procedure 12-4: Measuring Peak Flow Rate

Name: _____   Date: _____

Evaluated by: _____   Score: _____

Performance Objective

Outcome:	Measure a patient's peak flow rate.
Conditions:	Using a spirometer.
	Given the following: disposable mouthpiece, waste container.
Standards:	Time: 15 minutes. Student completed procedure in _____ minutes.
	Accuracy: Satisfactory score on the Performance Evaluation Checklist.

Performance Evaluation Checklist

Trial 1	Trial 2	Point Value	Performance Standards
		•	Sanitized hands.
		•	Assembled and prepared equipment.
		•	Moved the sliding indicator to the bottom of the scale.
		▷	Stated why the indicator must be moved to the bottom of the scale.
		•	Applied a disposable mouthpiece to the mouthpiece holder.
		▷	Stated the purpose of the disposable mouthpiece.
		•	Greeted the patient and introduced yourself.
		•	Identified the patient and explained the procedure.
		•	Asked the patient to remove heavy or restrictive clothing, to loosen tight clothing, and to discard gum.
			Described and demonstrated the breathing maneuver:
		•	Relax and take the deepest breath possible.
		•	Place the mouthpiece in your mouth and seal your lips tightly around it.
		•	Blow out as hard and fast as you can.
		•	Try to move the marker as high as you can on the scale.
		•	Do not block the opening of the mouthpiece with your tongue.
		•	Remove the mouthpiece from your mouth.
		•	Told the patient the instructions would be repeated during the test.
		•	Encouraged the patient to remain calm during the procedure.
		▷	Explained why the patient should remain calm.
		•	Placed a new disposable mouthpiece on the peak flow meter.
		•	Slid the marker to the bottom of the numbered scale.
		•	Handed the peak flow meter to the patient.

Trial 1	Trial 2	Point Value	Performance Standards
		•	Instructed the patient to stand up straight and look straight ahead.
		•	Began the test and actively coached the patient.
		•	Noted the number where the indicator stopped on the scale and jotted it down on a piece of paper.
		•	Informed the patient of modifications needed if the breathing maneuver was not performed correctly.
		•	Continued the test until three acceptable efforts were obtained.
			Explained why three acceptable efforts must be obtained.
		•	The numbers from the three tests were about the same.
		▷	Stated the significance of the three numbers being about the same.
		•	Took the peak flow meter from the patient.
		•	Removed the mouthpiece from its holder and discarded it in a waste container.
		•	Sanitized your hands.
		•	Noted the highest of the three peak flow measurements.
		•	Charted the procedure correctly.
		•	Cleaned the peak flow meter.
		▷	Explained how to clean the peak flow meter.
		✶	Completed the procedure within 15 minutes.
			Totals

CHART	
Date	

Evaluation of Student Performance

EVALUATION CRITERIA			COMMENTS
Symbol	**Category**	**Point Value**	
✶	Critical Step	16 points	
•	Essential Step	6 points	
▷	Theory Question	2 points	

Score calculation: 100 points

          −_____ points missed

          _____ Score

Satisfactory score: 85 or above

CAAHEP Competencies Achieved
Psychomotor (Skills)
☑ I. 4. Perform pulmonary function testing.
Affective (Behavior)
☑ I. 2. Use language/verbal skills that enable patients' understanding.

ABHES Competencies Achieved
☑ 8. cc. Communicate on the recipient's level of comprehension.
☑ 9. o. Perform: (2) Respiratory testing.

Notes

13 Colon Procedures and Male Reproductive Health

√ After Completing	Date Due	Textbook Pages	TEXTBOOK ASSIGNMENTS	Possible Points	Points You Earned
	541–578		Read Chapter 13: Colon Procedures and Male Reproductive Health		
	564 576		Read Case Study 1 Case Study 1 questions	5	
	571 576		Read Case Study 2 Case Study 2 questions	5	
	573 576		Read Case Study 3 Case Study 3 questions	5	
			Total points		
√ After Completing	**Date Due**	**Study Guide Pages**	**STUDY GUIDE ASSIGNMENTS (CTA = Critical Thinking Activity)**	**Possible Points**	**Points You Earned**
	641		Pretest	10	
	647 647		Key Term Assessment A. Definitions B. Word Parts (Add 1 point for each medical term)	10 10	
	643–647		Evaluation of Learning questions	40	
	647		CTA A: FOBT Patient Preparation	10	
	648		CTA B: Capsule Endoscopy	25	
	649		CTA C: Dear Gabby	10	
	650		CTA D: Crossword Puzzle	24	
			Evolve Site: Chapter 13 Animations (2 points each)	14	
			Evolve Site: Chapter 13 Nutrition Nugget: Gastrointestinal Disorders	10	

√ After Completing	Date Due	Study Guide Pages	STUDY GUIDE ASSIGNMENTS (CTA = Critical Thinking Activity)	Possible Points	Points You Earned
			e Evolve Site: Apply Your Knowledge questions	12	
		651	*e* Video Evaluation	18	
		641	[?] Posttest	10	
			ADDITIONAL ASSIGNMENTS		
			Total points		

638

Chapter **13** **Colon Procedures and Male Reproductive Health**

Copyright © 2015, 2012, 2008, 2004, 2000, 1995, 1990 by Saunders, an imprint of Elsevier Inc.
All rights reserved.

√ When Assigned by Your Instructor	Study Guide Pages	Practices Required	LABORATORY ASSIGNMENTS (Procedure Number and Name)	Score*
	653	5	Practice for Competency 13-1 and 13-2: Fecal Occult Blood Testing: Guaiac Slide Test Method and Developing the Hemoccult Slide Test Textbook reference: pp. 547–551	
	655–657		Evaluation of Competency 13-1 and 13-2: Fecal Occult Blood Testing: Guaiac Slide Test Method and Developing the Hemoccult Slide Test	*
	653–654	3	Practice for Competency 13-3: Assisting with a Sigmoidoscopy Textbook reference: pp. 555–556	
	659–660		Evaluation of Competency 13-3: Assisting with a Sigmoidoscopy	*
	653–654	5	Practice for Competency 13-A: Testicular Self-Examination Instructions Textbook reference: p. 558	
	661–662		Evaluation of Competency 13-A: Testicular Self-Examination Instructions	*
			ADDITIONAL ASSIGNMENTS	

Notes

Name: _____ Date:_____

True or False

_____ 1. Hemorrhoids can cause visible red blood to appear on the outside of the stool.

_____ 2. Nonvisible blood in the stool is called *occult blood*.

_____ 3. Colorectal cancer is a common form of cancer in individuals older than 50 years.

_____ 4. A blue color appearing on a Hemoccult test result is interpreted as a negative result.

_____ 5. If a Hemoccult test result is positive, the physician may order a colonoscopy.

_____ 6. The patient is placed in the prone position for a colonoscopy.

_____ 7. The function of the prostate gland is to produce sperm.

_____ 8. Most prostate cancers are slow growing.

_____ 9. A normal prostate gland feels firm and hard.

_____ 10. The most common sign of testicular cancer is a small, hard, painless lump on the testicle.

?≡ **POSTTEST**

True or False

_____ 1. Melena means that the stool appears hard and dry.

_____ 2. Consuming red meat may cause a false-positive result on a fecal occult guaiac slide test.

_____ 3. Ibuprofen should be avoided for 7 days before beginning a fecal occult guaiac slide test.

_____ 4. The Hemoccult test should be stored at room temperature after applying a stool specimen to it.

_____ 5. Patient preparation for a sigmoidoscopy includes partial bowel preparation.

_____ 6. After use, a sigmoidoscope must be autoclaved for 20 minutes.

_____ 7. Colonoscopy is performed for the early detection of colorectal cancer.

_____ 8. There are often no symptoms in the early stages of prostate cancer.

_____ 9. A prostate-specific antigen (PSA) level of 20 is within normal range.

_____ 10. Testicular cancer occurs most commonly between the ages of 15 and 34.

A. Definitions

Directions: Match each medical term (numbers) with its definition (letters).

_____ 1. Biopsy

_____ 2. Colonoscope

_____ 3. Colonoscopy

_____ 4. Endoscope

_____ 5. Insufflate

_____ 6. Melena

_____ 7. Occult blood

_____ 8. Peroxidase

_____ 9. Sigmoidoscope

_____ 10. Sigmoidoscopy

A. The visualization of the rectum and the entire colon using a colonoscope

B. Blood occurring in such a small amount that it is not visually detectable by the unaided eye

C. The surgical removal and examination of tissue from the living body

D. The visual examination of the rectum and sigmoid colon using a sigmoidoscope

E. The darkening of the stool caused by the presence of blood in an amount of 50 mL or more

F. An instrument that consists of a tube and an optical system that is used for direct visual inspection of organs or cavities

G. A substance that is able to transfer oxygen from hydrogen peroxide to oxidize guaiac, causing the guaiac to turn blue

H. An endoscope that is specially designed for passage through the anus to permit visualization of the rectum and sigmoid colon

I. To blow a powder, vapor, or gas (such as air) into a body cavity

J. An endoscope that is specially designed for passage through the anus to permit visualization of the rectum and the entire length of the colon

B. Word Parts

Directions: Indicate the meaning of each word part in the space provided. List as many medical terms as possible that incorporate the word part in the space provided.

Word Part	Meaning of Word Part	Medical Terms That Incorporate Word Part
1. bi/o		
2. -opsy		
3. colon/o		
4. -scopy		
5. -scope		
6. endo-		
7. -oxia		
8. -ase		
9. ox/i		
10. sigmoid/o		

Chapter **13 Colon Procedures and Male Reproductive Health**

Fill in each blank with the correct answer.

1. What are the three parts of the large intestine?

   _____

2. What are the functions of the large intestine?

   _____

   _____

3. What is the function of the anal sphincter muscles?

   _____

   _____

4. What is the function of the mucus secreted by the large intestine?

   _____

   _____

5. List five causes of blood in the stool.

   _____

   _____

   _____

   _____

   _____

6. Define the term *melena,* and explain what causes it.

   _____

   _____

   _____

   _____

7. What is the primary reason for screening patients for the presence of fecal occult blood?

   _____

   _____

8. Why must three stool specimens be obtained for the fecal occult guaiac slide test?

   _____

   _____

   _____

9. List two reasons for placing the patient on a high-fiber diet when testing for fecal occult blood.

   _____

   _____

10. What medications and vitamin supplements must be discontinued before guaiac slide testing?

_____

_____

11. List two factors that could cause false-positive test results on a guaiac slide test.

_____

_____

12. List three examples of diagnostic tests that may be performed if the guaiac slide test result is positive.

_____

_____

_____

13. Why is it important to perform quality-control methods when developing the guaiac slide test?

_____

_____

14. How should the guaiac slide test be stored?

_____

_____

15. What factors can cause a failure of the expected control results to occur on a guaiac slide test?

_____

_____

16. List the advantages of the fecal immunochemical test (FIT) compared with the guaiac slide test.

_____

_____

_____

17. How does a fecal DNA test function to detect colorectal cancer?

_____

_____

18. What is the purpose of performing a sigmoidoscopy?

_____

_____

_____

19. Describe the following patient preparation required for a sigmoidoscopy:

    a. The day before the procedure and continuing until the examination is completed:

    _____

    _____

    b. The evening before the procedure:

    _____

    _____

    c. The day of the procedure:

    _____

    _____

20. What is the purpose of the digital rectal examination (DRE)?

_____

_____

_____

21. What is the purpose of insufflating air into the colon during a sigmoidoscopy?

_____

_____

22. What is the purpose of suctioning during sigmoidoscopy?

_____

_____

23. What is the recommended position of the patient during flexible fiberoptic sigmoidoscopy?

_____

24. How can the medical assistant help the patient relax during the sigmoidoscopy?

_____

_____

25. What parts of the colon are viewed during a colonoscopy?

_____

_____

26. What is the purpose of a full bowel preparation before a colonoscopy?

_____

_____

Chapter **13** **Colon Procedures and Male Reproductive Health**

27. How should a patient consume the liquid laxative solution when preparing the bowel for a colonoscopy?

_____

_____

28. Where is the prostate gland located?

_____

_____

29. What are the symptoms of prostate cancer?

_____

_____

_____

30. How is the digital rectal examination used for the early detection of prostate cancer?

_____

_____

31. What conditions can cause an elevated PSA level?

_____

_____

32. What is the PSA level for each of the following?
    a. Normal range _____
    b. Slightly elevated range _____
    c. Moderately elevated range _____
    d. Highly elevated _____

33. What patient preparation is required for a PSA test?

_____

_____

34. What tests may be ordered by the physician if the patient has positive prostate screening results?

_____

_____

35. What is the definition of the term *screening*?

_____

_____

36. What is the American Cancer Society recommendation for the PSA test and the DRE?

_____

_____

_____

37. When does testicular cancer most commonly occur?

_____

38. When is the best time for a male to perform a testicular self-examination (TSE) and why?

_____

_____

39. What are the risk factors for testicular cancer?

_____

_____

_____

40. What is the most common sign of testicular cancer?

_____

_____

CRITICAL THINKING ACTIVITIES

A. FOBT Patient Preparation

Frank Morrison has been given a Hemoccult slide kit for fecal occult blood testing (FOBT). In the space provided, plan breakfast, lunch, and dinner for him following the FOBT patient preparation guidelines on pages 543–544 of your textbook.

_____

_____

_____

_____

_____

_____

B. Capsule Endoscopy

Perform an Internet search for capsule endoscopy. Search for textual information and videos of this procedure. Based on your research, answer the following questions regarding this procedure.

1. What is capsule endoscopy?

_____

_____

_____

_____

_____

2. What conditions can be diagnosed using capsule endoscopy?

_____

_____

_____

3. What patient preparation is required for this procedure?

_____

_____

_____

4. What are the advantages of capsule endoscopy?

_____

_____

_____

5. What are the disadvantages of capsule endoscopy?

_____

_____

_____

_____

C. Dear Gabby

Gabby broke her wrist while ice skating and wants you to fill in for her. In the space provided, respond to the following letter using the knowledge you have acquired in this chapter.

Dear Gabby:

I am 15 years old, and my mom just took me to a new doctor for a sports physical examination. I am going to play football this fall at my high school. Before this, I had always gone to the doctor I had since I was little, but I had to switch because I am getting older. After the doctor did my physical, he told me that I needed to examine my testicles every month and that the medical assistant would be in to explain how this is done.

Gabby, I was totally shocked, and you can bet I got out of that office before she had a chance to do that. I am too embarrassed to ask my parents about this. Gabby, what is going on? I am only 15 years old. Are my parents taking me to a quack, and should I report this to someone?

Signed,

Don't Know What to Do

_____

_____

_____

_____

_____

_____

_____

_____

_____

D. Crossword Puzzle: Colon Procedures and Male Reproductive Health

Directions: Complete the crossword puzzle using the clues provided.

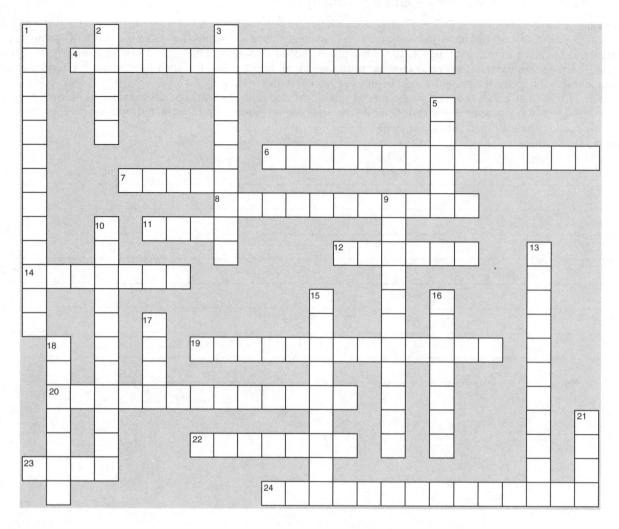

ACROSS
- **4** Normally increases PSA level
- **6** Symptom of CRC
- **7** Majority of large intestine
- **8** Used to visualize entire colon
- **11** Color of positive Hemoccult
- **12** Black and tarlike stool
- **14** Can cause false-positive on FOBT
- **19** Increases risk of CRC
- **20** Secretes fluid that transports sperm
- **22** Age to start TSE
- **23** Patient position for sigmoidoscopy
- **24** Cause of failed FOBT control

DOWN
- **1** Results in an empty colon
- **2** CRC increases after this age
- **3** Leading cause of cancer deaths
- **5** CRC often starts from this
- **9** Colon abnormality detection gold standard
- **10** Can cause blood in the stool
- **13** Hidden blood
- **15** How to clean sigmoidoscope
- **16** Prostrate CA screening test
- **17** Protect FOBT from this
- **18** Med to avoid during FOBT
- **21** May be done after elevated PSA

Name: _____

Directions:

a. Watch the indicated videos.
b. Mark each true statement with a T and each false statement with an F. For each false statement, change the wording of the question so that it becomes a true statement.

Video: Procedures 13-1 and 13-2: Fecal Occult Blood Testing

_____ 1. Colorectal cancer is one of the most common forms of cancer in individuals older than 50 years.

_____ 2. During the early asymptomatic stages, almost all neoplasms of the colon and rectum bleed a small amount on an intermittent basis.

_____ 3. Hidden blood in the stool is known as *melena*.

_____ 4. The stool sample should not be collected if there is visible blood in the stool or urine.

_____ 5. The patient should be instructed to consume foods that are low in fiber starting 3 days before the collection period.

_____ 6. Improper patient preparation for the FOBT can lead to inaccurate test results.

_____ 7. The slides contain filter paper impregnated with guaiac, a chemical necessary for detection of blood in the stool.

_____ 8. The patient should be instructed to store the slides in the refrigerator.

_____ 9. If the Hemoccult slides are exposed to heat, the active reagents impregnated on the filter paper can deteriorate, leading to inaccurate test results.

_____ 10. The patient should be instructed to collect a stool specimen from two different parts of the stool.

_____ 11. A thick smear of the stool specimen should be spread over the filter paper.

_____ 12. The wooden applicators should be flushed down the toilet.

_____ 13. A standard envelope can be used to mail the Hemoccult slides to the medical office.

_____ 14. An outdated solution should not be used to develop the slides because it can lead to inaccurate test results.

_____ 15. Two drops of developing solution should be applied to the guaiac test paper underlying the back of each smear.

_____ 16. The developing solution can cause irritation of the skin and eyes if contact occurs.

_____ 17. Failure of the expected control results to occur indicates an error, and the test results are not valid.

_____ 18. The Hemoccult slides should be discarded in a biohazard waste container.

Chapter **13** **Colon Procedures and Male Reproductive Health**

PRACTICE FOR COMPETENCY

Procedures 13-1 and 13-2: Fecal Occult Blood Testing: Guaiac Slide Test
1. Patient instructions. Instruct the patient in the specimen collection procedure for a fecal occult blood test (e.g., Hemoccult). Record these instructions in the chart provided.
2. Developing the test. Develop a fecal occult blood test, and record the results in the chart provided.

Procedure 13-3: Sigmoidoscopy. Practice the procedure for assisting with a sigmoidoscopy. Record advance patient preparation instructions in the chart provided.

Procedure 13-A: Testicular Self-Examination. Instruct an individual about the procedure for testicular self-examination, and record the procedure in the chart provided.

CHART	
Date	

Chapter **13** Colon Procedures and Male Reproductive Health

CHART	
Date	

Procedures 13-1 and 13-2: Fecal Occult Blood Testing: Guaiac Slide Test Method and Developing the Hemoccult Slide Test

Name: _____ Date: _____

Evaluated by: _____ Score: _____

Performance Objective

Outcome:	Instruct an individual in the specimen collection procedure for a Hemoccult slide test and develop the test.
Conditions:	Given the following: Hemoccult slide testing kit, disposable gloves, developing solution, reference card, and a waste container.
Standards:	Time: 15 minutes. Student completed procedure in _____ minutes.
	Accuracy: Satisfactory score on the Performance Evaluation Checklist.

Performance Evaluation Checklist

Trial 1	Trial 2	Point Value	Performance Standards
			Instructions for the Hemoccult slide test
		•	Obtained the Hemoccult slide testing kit.
		•	Checked the expiration date on the slides.
		▷	Described what may occur if the slides are outdated.
		•	Greeted the patient and introduced yourself.
		•	Identified the patient and explained the purpose of the test.
		•	Informed the patient when the test should not be performed.
		•	Instructed the patient in the proper preparation required for the test.
		•	Encouraged the patient to adhere to the diet modifications.
		▷	Explained why the patient should follow the diet modifications.
		•	Provided the patient with the Hemoccult slide test kit.
		•	Instructed the patient in completion of the information on the front flap of each card.
		•	Provided instructions on the proper care and storage of the slides.
		▷	Explained why the slides must be stored properly.
			Instructed the patient in the initiation of the test
		•	Began the diet modifications.
		•	Collected a stool specimen from the first bowel movement after the 3-day preparatory period.
			Instructed the patient in the collection of the stool specimen
		•	Filled in the collection date on the front flap.
		•	Used a clean, dry container to collect the stool specimen.
		•	Collected the stool sample before it came in contact with toilet bowl water.
		•	Used the wooden applicator to obtain a specimen from one part of the stool.

Trial 1	Trial 2	Point Value	Performance Standards
		•	Opened the front flap of the first cardboard slide.
		•	Spread a thin smear of the specimen over the filter paper in the square labeled A.
		•	Obtained another specimen from a different area of the stool, by using the other end of the applicator.
		•	Spread a thin smear of the specimen over the filter paper in the square labeled B.
		•	Closed the front flap of the cardboard slide and filled in the date.
		•	Discarded the applicator in a waste container.
		▷	Explained why a sample is collected from two different parts of the stool.
		•	Instructed the patient to place the slides in a regular envelope to air-dry overnight.
		•	Instructed the patient to continue the testing period on 3 different days until all three specimens have been obtained.
		•	Instructed the patient to place the cardboard slides in the foil envelope and return them to the medical office.
		•	Provided the patient with an opportunity to ask questions.
		•	Made sure the patient understood the instructions.
		•	Charted the procedure correctly.
			Developing the Hemoccult Slide Test
		•	Assembled equipment.
		•	Checked the expiration date on the developing solution bottle.
		▷	Explained how the solution should be stored.
		•	Sanitized hands and applied gloves.
		•	Opened the back flap of the cardboard slides.
		•	Applied 2 drops of the developing solution to the guaiac test paper underlying the back of each smear.
		•	Did not allow the developing solution to come in contact with skin or eyes.
		•	Read the results within 60 seconds.
		✱	Results were identical to the evaluator's results.
		▷	Explained why the slides should be read within 60 seconds.
		•	Performed the quality-control procedure on each slide.
		•	Read the quality-control results after 10 seconds.
		▷	Described what is observed during a normal positive and negative control reaction.
		▷	Stated the purpose of the quality-control procedure.
		•	Properly disposed of the slides in a regular waste container.
		•	Removed gloves and sanitized hands.
		•	Charted the results correctly.
		✱	Completed the procedure within 15 minutes.
			Totals

CHART		
Date		

Evaluation of Student Performance

EVALUATION CRITERIA			COMMENTS
Symbol	**Category**	**Point Value**	
✳	Critical Step	16 points	
•	Essential Step	6 points	
▷	Theory Question	2 points	

Score calculation: 100 points

$$- \underline{\hspace{3cm}} \text{ points missed}$$

$$\underline{\hspace{2cm}} \text{ Score}$$

Satisfactory score: 85 or above

CAAHEP Competencies Achieved

Psychomotor (Skills)

☑ I. 11. Perform quality-control measures.

☑ IV. 5. Instruct patients according to their needs to promote health maintenance and disease prevention.

Affective (Behavior)

☑ III. 1. Display sensitivity to patient rights and feelings in collecting specimens.

ABHES Competencies Achieved

☑ 8. cc. Communicate on the recipient's level of communication.

☑ 10. b. Perform selected CLIA-waived tests that assist with diagnosis and treatment (6) kit testing.

☑ 10. f. Instruct patients in the collection of a fecal specimen.

Notes

Procedure 13-3: Assisting with a Sigmoidoscopy

Name: _____   Date: _____

Evaluated by: _____   Score: _____

Performance Objective

Outcome:	Assist with a sigmoidoscopy.
Conditions:	Given the following: flexible sigmoidoscope, disposable gloves, lubricant, drape, biopsy forceps, sterile specimen container with a preservative, 4 × 4 gauze, tissues, and a waste container.
Standards:	Time: 15 minutes. Student completed procedure in _____ minutes.
	Accuracy: Satisfactory score on the Performance Evaluation Checklist.

Performance Evaluation Checklist

Trial 1	Trial 2	Point Value	Performance Standards
		•	Sanitized hands.
		•	Assembled equipment.
		•	Checked to make sure that light source is working.
		•	Greeted the patient and introduced yourself.
		•	Identified the patient and explained the procedure.
		•	Asked the patient whether he or she needs to empty his or her bladder.
		▷	Explained why the patient should have an empty bladder.
		•	Instructed and prepared the patient for the examination.
		•	Assisted the patient onto the examining table.
		•	Assisted the patient into Sims' position.
		•	Properly draped the patient.
		•	Reassured the patient and helped him or her to relax during the examination.
			Assisted physician during the examination
		•	Lubricated the physician's gloved finger for the digital rectal examination.
		•	Placed lubricant on the end of the insertion tube of the sigmoidoscope.
		•	Assisted with the suction equipment as required.
		▷	Stated the purpose of the suctioning equipment.
		•	Assisted with the collection of a biopsy.
		•	After the examination, applied gloves and cleaned the patient's anal region of excess lubricant.
		•	Removed gloves and sanitized hands.
		•	Assisted the patient from the examining table and instructed the patient to get dressed.
		•	If a biopsy was obtained, labeled the specimen container.

Trial 1	Trial 2	Point Value	Performance Standards
		•	Prepared the biopsy specimen for transport to the laboratory.
		•	Completed the biopsy request form and inserted it in the specimen bag.
		•	Placed the specimen bag in the appropriate location for pickup by the laboratory.
		•	Charted the date of transport of the specimen to the lab.
		•	Cleaned the examining room.
		•	Sanitized and disinfected the sigmoidoscope according to the manufacturer's instructions.
		✱	Completed the procedure within 15 minutes.
			Totals

Evaluation of Student Performance

EVALUATION CRITERIA			COMMENTS
Symbol	**Category**	**Point Value**	
✱	Critical Step	16 points	
•	Essential Step	6 points	
▷	Theory Question	2 points	

Score calculation: 100 points

− _____ points missed

_____ Score

Satisfactory score: 85 or above

CAAHEP Competencies Achieved

Psychomotor (Skills)

☑ I.10. Assist physician with patient care.

☑ IV. 6. Prepare a patient for procedures and/or treatments.

Affective (Behavior)

☑ III. 2. Explain the rationale for performance of a procedure to the patient.

☑ III. 3. Show awareness of patients' concerns regarding their perceptions related to the procedure being performed.

ABHES Competencies Achieved

☑ 8. bb. Are impartial and show empathy when dealing with patients.

☑ 9. l. Prepare patient for examinations and treatments.

☑ 9. m. Assist physician with routine and specialty examinations and treatments.

Procedure 13-A: Testicular Self-Examination Instructions

Name: _____   Date: _____

Evaluated by: _____   Score: _____

Performance Objective

Outcome:	Instruct an individual in the procedure for performing a testicular self-examination (TSE).
Conditions:	None.
Standards:	Time: 10 minutes. Student completed procedure in _____ minutes.
	Accuracy: Satisfactory score on the Performance Evaluation Checklist.

Performance Evaluation Checklist

Trial 1	Trial 2	Point Value	Performance Standards
		•	Greeted the patient and introduced yourself.
		•	Identified the patient and explained that you will be instructing the patient in a TSE.
		•	Explained the purpose of the examination and when to perform it.
			Instructed the patient as follows:
		•	Take a warm bath or shower.
		•	Stand in front of a mirror.
		•	Inspect for any swelling of the skin of the scrotum.
		•	Place the index and middle fingers of both hands on the underside of one testicle and the thumbs on top of the testicle.
		•	Apply a small amount of pressure, and gently roll the testicle between the thumb and fingers of both hands.
		•	Palpate for lumps, swelling, or any change in the size, shape, or consistency of the testicle.
		▷	Stated the normal characteristics of a testicle.
		•	Locate the epididymis so that you do not confuse it with a lump.
		▷	Stated the characteristics and function of the epididymis.
		•	Repeat the examination on the other testicle.
		•	Report any abnormalities to the physician.
		▷	Stated examples of abnormalities that should be reported.
		•	Charted the procedure correctly.
		✶	Completed the procedure within 10 minutes.
			Totals

CHART	
Date	

Evaluation of Student Performance

EVALUATION CRITERIA			COMMENTS
Symbol	**Category**	**Point Value**	
✳	Critical Step	16 points	
•	Essential Step	6 points	
▷	Theory Question	2 points	

Score calculation: 100 points

$$-\underline{}\ \text{points missed}$$

$$\underline{}\ \text{Score}$$

Satisfactory score: 85 or above

CAAHEP Competencies Achieved

Psychomotor (Skills)

☑ IV. 5. Instruct patients according to their needs to promote health maintenance and disease prevention.

☑ IV. 9. Document patient education.

Affective (Behavior)

☑ I. 2. Use language/verbal skills that enable patients' understanding.

☑ IV. 3. Use appropriate body language and other nonverbal skills in communicating with patients, family, and staff.

ABHES Competencies Achieved

☑ 8. e. Locate resources and information for patients and employers.

☑ 8. cc. Communicate on the recipient's level of comprehension.

☑ 8. ii. Recognize and respond to verbal and nonverbal communication.

☑ 9. r. Teach patients methods of health promotion and disease prevention.

14 Radiology and Diagnostic Imaging

√ After Completing	Date Due	Textbook Pages	TEXTBOOK ASSIGNMENTS	Possible Points	Points You Earned
		562–578	Read Chapter 14: Radiology and Diagnostic Imaging		
		564 576	Read Case Study 1 Case Study 1 questions	5	
		571 576	Read Case Study 2 Case Study 2 questions	5	
		573 576	Read Case Study 3 Case Study 3 questions	5	
			Total points		
√ After Completing	**Date Due**	**Study Guide Pages**	**STUDY GUIDE ASSIGNMENTS (CTA = Critical Thinking Activity)**	**Possible Points**	**Points You Earned**
		667	Pretest	10	
		668 668–669	Term Key Term Assessment A. Definitions B. Word Parts	13 15	
		669–673	Evaluation of Learning questions	42	
		674	CTA A: Lower Gastrointestinal Tract	5	
		674	CTA B: Intravenous Pyelogram	5	
		675	CTA C: Magnetic Resonance Imaging	7	
		676	CTA D: Crossword Puzzle	22	
			Evolve Site: Chapter 14 Animations (2 points each)	14	
			Evolve Site: Chapter 14 Nutrition Nugget: Osteoporosis	10	
			Evolve Site: Chapter 11 Apply Your Knowledge questions	10	
		667	Posttest	10	

√ After Completing	Date Due	Study Guide Pages	STUDY GUIDE ASSIGNMENTS (CTA = Critical Thinking Activity)	Possible Points	Points You Earned
			ADDITIONAL ASSIGNMENTS		
			Total points		

√ When Assigned by Your Instructor	Study Guide Pages	Practices Required	LABORATORY ASSIGNMENTS (Procedure Number and Name)	Score*
	667–678	3	Practice for Competency 14-A: Preparation for Radiology Examinations Textbook reference: pp. 563–569	
	679–680		Evaluation of Competency 14-A: Preparation for Radiology Examinations	*
	677–678	3	Practice for Competency 14-B: Preparation for Diagnostic Imaging Procedures Textbook reference: pp. 569–575	
	681–682		Evaluation of Competency 14-B: Preparation for Diagnostic Imaging Procedures	*
			ADDITIONAL ASSIGNMENTS	

Notes

Name: _____ Date: _____

True or False

_____ 1. A radiologist is a medical doctor specializing in the diagnosis and treatment of disease using radiation and other imaging techniques.

_____ 2. The permanent record of the picture produced on x-ray film is a sonogram.

_____ 3. The purpose of a contrast medium is to make a structure visible on a radiograph.

_____ 4. With an anteroposterior view, x-rays are directed from the back toward the front of the body.

_____ 5. Mammography can be used to detect breast calcifications.

_____ 6. An upper gastrointestinal (GI) examination assists in diagnosing kidney stones.

_____ 7. An IVP is a radiograph of the kidneys, ureters, and bladder.

_____ 8. Ultrasonography allows for continuous viewing of a structure.

_____ 9. Obstetric ultrasound can be used to determine gestational age.

_____ 10. A patient must remove all metal before undergoing MRI.

?🗏 **POSTTEST**

True or False

_____ 1. Wilhelm Roentgen discovered x-rays in 1895.

_____ 2. Bone is an example of a radiolucent structure.

_____ 3. An instrument used to view internal organs directly is a fluoroscope.

_____ 4. The patient should be instructed not to move during a radiographic examination to prevent confusing shadows on the film.

_____ 5. The breasts are compressed during mammography to prevent radiation burns.

_____ 6. After an upper GI study is performed, the barium causes the stool to be loose and watery.

_____ 7. Gas must be removed from the colon before a lower GI study to prevent blurring of the radiograph.

_____ 8. Before performing an IVP, the patient must be asked whether he or she is allergic to penicillin.

_____ 9. Computed tomography produces a series of cross-sectional images.

_____ 10. A radioactive material is introduced into the body before a nuclear medicine imaging procedure is performed.

A. Definitions

Directions: Match each medical term (numbers) with its definition (letters).

_____ 1. Contrast medium

_____ 2. Echocardiogram

_____ 3. Enema

_____ 4. Fluoroscope

_____ 5. Fluoroscopy

_____ 6. Radiograph

_____ 7. Radiography

_____ 8. Radiologist

_____ 9. Radiology

_____ 10. Radiolucent

_____ 11. Radiopaque

_____ 12. Sonogram

_____ 13. Ultrasonography

A. A permanent record of a picture of an internal body organ or structure produced on radiographic film

B. A physician who specializes in the diagnosis and treatment of disease using radiation and other imaging techniques

C. A substance used to make a particular structure visible on a radiograph

D. The record obtained with ultrasonography

E. An injection of fluid into the rectum to aid in the elimination of feces from the colon

F. The branch of medicine that deals with the use of radiation and other imaging techniques in the diagnosis and treatment of disease

G. An instrument used to view internal organs and structures directly

H. Describing a structure that obstructs the passage of x-rays

I. The taking of permanent records of internal body organs and structures by passing x-rays through the body to act on a specially sensitized film

J. Describing a structure that permits the passage of x-rays

K. Examination of a patient with a fluoroscope

L. An ultrasound examination of the heart

M. The use of high-frequency sound waves to produce an image of an organ or tissue

B. Word Parts

Directions: Indicate the meaning of each word part in the space provided. List as many medical terms as possible that incorporate the word part in the space provided.

Word Part	Meaning of Word Part	Medical Terms That Incorporate Word Part
1. ech/o		
2. cardi/o		
3. -gram		
4. fluor/o		
5. -scope		
6. -scopy		
7. radi/o		
8. -graph		
9. -graphy		
10. -ologist		

11. -ology		
12. lucent		
13. opaque		
14. son/o		
15. ultra-		

EVALUATION OF LEARNING

Directions: Fill in each blank with the correct answer.

1. Who discovered x-rays?

   _____

2. What is the function of x-rays?

   _____

   _____

3. What are the two ways in which radiographs can be taken?

   _____

4. Why is it important for a patient to prepare properly for a radiographic examination?

   _____

   _____

5. What is the function of a radiopaque contrast medium?

   _____

   _____

6. What are the various ways in which contrast medium can be administered to a patient?

   _____

   _____

7. How is a patient positioned to obtain an anteroposterior view?

   _____

   _____

8. What is the purpose of mammography?

   _____

   _____

   _____

9. Why should the patient be instructed not to wear lotions, powders, or deodorants when having a mammogram?

_____

_____

10. Why must the breasts be compressed during mammography?

_____

_____

11. What is the purpose of a bone density scan?

_____

_____

12. What is osteoporosis?

_____

_____

13. Who is at particular risk for osteoporosis?

_____

14. What patient preparation is required for a bone density scan?

_____

_____

15. What information is provided by DEXA bone density measurements?

_____

_____

_____

_____

16. What is the purpose of the upper GI radiographic examination?

_____

_____

_____

17. Why must the GI tract be free of food and fluid before an upper GI radiographic examination is performed?

_____

_____

18. How can the patient prevent constipation after an upper GI examination?

_____

_____

19. A lower GI radiographic examination assists in the diagnosis of what conditions?

_____

_____

20. Why is it important to remove gas and fecal material from the colon before a lower GI radiographic examination is performed?

_____

_____

21. What is the advantage of the air used with a double-contrast barium enema?

_____

_____

22. What is an intravenous pyelogram (IVP)?

_____

_____

23. An IVP assists in the diagnosis of what conditions?

_____

_____

24. What may the patient experience during an IVP when the iodine enters the bloodstream?

_____

_____

25. Define the following:

   a. Angiocardiogram

_____

_____

   b. Bronchogram

_____

_____

   c. Cerebral angiogram

_____

_____

   d. Coronary angiogram

_____

_____

   e. Cystogram

_____

_____

26. What are the primary uses of ultrasonography?

_____

_____

27. What are the advantages of ultrasonography?

_____

_____

_____

28. What can be determined during an echocardiogram?

_____

_____

29. What is the purpose of the gel used with ultrasonography?

_____

_____

30. What is the purpose of performing obstetric ultrasound?

_____

_____

_____

31. Doppler ultrasound assists in the diagnosis of what conditions?

_____

_____

32. What type of image is produced by computed tomography?

_____

_____

33. What are the primary uses of computed tomography?

_____

_____

_____

34. What type of patient preparation is required for computed tomography?

_____

_____

_____

_____

35. What are the primary uses of magnetic resonance imaging?

_____

_____

_____

36. What items must the patient remove before having an MRI scan?

_____

_____

37. What material is used with a nuclear medicine diagnostic imaging procedure?

_____

38. What is the function of a gamma camera used in nuclear medicine?

_____

_____

39. What is the purpose of a bone scan?

_____

_____

40. A nuclear cardiac stress test assists in the evaluation of what heart condition?

_____

_____

41. A PET scan is used to assist in the diagnosis of what conditions?

_____

_____

42. What are the advantages of digital imaging technology?

_____

_____

_____

CRITICAL THINKING ACTIVITIES

A. Lower Gastrointestinal Tract

Trent Douglas has been having pain in his lower abdomen and occult blood in his stool. Dr. Hartman tells you to schedule him for a lower GI radiographic examination at Grant Hospital. In the space provided, explain how you would instruct Mr. Douglas to prepare for this examination. Include the patient preparation and the reason for each of the measures.

_____

_____

_____

_____

_____

_____

B. Intravenous Pyelogram

Dr. Tristen instructs you to schedule Ellie Ray for an intravenous pyelogram (IVP) at Grant Hospital. After you have explained to Ms. Ray the instructions for preparing for the examination, she asks you the following questions. Respond to them in the space provided.

1. What body structures will be "x-rayed" during the examination?

_____

_____

2. Why must gas and fecal material be removed from the intestines?

_____

_____

3. Why will iodine be injected into my veins?

_____

_____

4. Will I feel anything when the iodine is injected?

_____

_____

5. What is done if an individual is allergic to iodine?

_____

_____

C. Magnetic Resonance Imaging

Jason Zindra, a college baseball player, has been experiencing pain in his left shoulder joint. Dr. Baker schedules him for magnetic resonance imaging (MRI) of the left shoulder. Jason asks you the following questions regarding this procedure. Respond to them in the space provided.

1. Is this a safe procedure?

_____

_____

2. Will there be any pain involved with this procedure?

_____

_____

3. Will I be exposed to x-rays?

_____

_____

4. What should I wear to the test?

_____

_____

5. May I wear my watch during the procedure to keep track of the time?

_____

_____

6. Does the MRI machine make any noise?

_____

_____

7. Will the technician be in the room with me?

_____

_____

D. Crossword Puzzle: Radiology and Diagnostic Imaging

Directions: Complete the crossword puzzle using the clues provided.

Across
3 Radiograph of the lungs
5 Can tell if it's twins
7 X-rays directed from back to front
8 Radiograph of urinary bladder
12 Detects "presence" of osteoporosis
14 Lower GI contrast medium
16 Produces cross-sectional images
17 Discovered x-rays
18 Obstructs x-rays
19 Used to diagnose kidney stones
20 Color of radiolucent structure
21 US of heart
22 Radiograph of coronary arteries

Down
1 Helps diagnose blood flow blockages
2 Radiograph of uterus and fallopian tubes
4 IVP contrast medium
6 Used to directly view internal organs
9 Radiograph of bile ducts
10 Detects stress fractures
11 Breast radiograph
13 US recording
15 Remove during an MRI

PRACTICE FOR COMPETENCY

Procedure 14-A: Radiology Examinations. Instruct a patient in the proper preparation required for each of the following types of radiographic examinations: mammogram, bone density scan, upper GI, lower GI, and intravenous pyelogram. Record the procedure in the chart provided.

Procedure 14-B: Diagnostic Imaging Procedures. Instruct a patient in the proper preparation required for each of the following types of diagnostic imaging procedures: ultrasonography, computed tomography, magnetic resonance imaging, and nuclear medicine. Record the procedure in the chart provided.

CHART	
Date	

CHART	
Date	

678

Chapter **14 Radiology and Diagnostic Imaging**

EVALUATION OF COMPETENCY

Procedure 14-A: Preparation for Radiology Examinations

Name: ______________________ Date: ______________

Evaluated by: ______________________ Score: ______________

Performance Objective

Outcome:	Instruct a patient in the proper preparation required for each of the following radiographic examinations: mammogram, upper GI, lower GI, and intravenous pyelogram.
Conditions:	Given the following: a patient instruction sheet for each radiographic examination.
Standards:	Time: 15 minutes. Student completed procedure in ______ minutes.
	Accuracy: Satisfactory score on the Performance Evaluation Checklist.

Performance Evaluation Checklist

Trial 1	Trial 2	Point Value	Performance Standards
		•	Greeted and identified the patient.
		•	Introduced yourself.
			Instructed the patient in the proper preparation for each of the following radiographic examinations:
		•	Mammogram
		•	Bone density scan
		•	Upper GI
		•	Lower GI
		•	Intravenous pyelogram
		•	Charted the procedure correctly.
		✶	Completed the procedure within 15 minutes.
			Totals

CHART	
Date	

EVALUATION CRITERIA			COMMENTS
Symbol	**Category**	**Point Value**	
✳	Critical Step	16 points	
•	Essential Step	6 points	
▷	Theory Question	2 points	

Score calculation: 100 points

    −   _____ points missed

        _____ Score

Satisfactory score: 85 or above

CAAHEP Competencies Achieved

Psychomotor (Skills)

☑ IV. 6. Prepare a patient for procedures and/or treatments.

Affective (Behavior)

☑ I. 2. Use language/verbal skills that enable patient's understanding.

Procedure 14-B: Preparation for Diagnostic Imaging Procedures

Name: _____   Date: _____

Evaluated by: _____   Score: _____

Performance Objective

Outcome:	Instruct a patient in the proper preparation required for each of the following diagnostic imaging procedures: ultrasonography, computed tomography, magnetic resonance imaging, and nuclear medicine.
Conditions:	Given the following: a patient instruction sheet for each diagnostic imaging procedure.
Standards:	Time: 15 minutes. Student completed procedure in _____ minutes.
	Accuracy: Satisfactory score on the Performance Evaluation Checklist.

Performance Evaluation Checklist

Trial 1	Trial 2	Point Value	Performance Standards
		•	Greeted and identified the patient.
		•	Introduced yourself.
			Instructed the patient in the proper preparation for each of the following diagnostic imaging procedures:
		•	Ultrasonography
		•	Computed tomography
		•	Magnetic resonance imaging
		•	Nuclear medicine
		•	Charted the procedure correctly.
		✶	Completed the procedure within 15 minutes.
			Totals
CHART			
Date			

Evaluation of Student Performance

EVALUATION CRITERIA			COMMENTS
Symbol	**Category**	**Point Value**	
✶	Critical Step	16 points	
•	Essential Step	6 points	
▷	Theory Question	2 points	

Score calculation: 100 points

— _____ points missed

_____ Score

Satisfactory score: 85 or above

CAAHEP Competencies Achieved

Psychomotor (Skills)

☑ IV. 6. Prepare a patient for procedures and/or treatments.

Affective (Behavior)

☑ I. 2. Use language/verbal skills that enable patient's understanding.

ABHES Competencies Achieved

☑ 8. cc. Communicate on the recipient's level of communication.

☑ 9. l. Prepare patient for examinations and treatments.

15 Introduction to the Clinical Laboratory

√ After Completing	Date Due	Textbook Pages	TEXTBOOK ASSIGNMENTS	Possible Points	Points You Earned
		579–615	Read Chapter 15: Introduction to the Clinical Laboratory		
		591 613	Read Case Study 1 Case Study 1 questions	5	
		595 613	Read Case Study 2 Case Study 2 questions	5	
		597 613	Read Case Study 3 Case Study 3 questions	5	
			Total points		
√ After Completing	**Date Due**	**Study Guide Pages**	**STUDY GUIDE ASSIGNMENTS (CTA = Critical Thinking Activity)**	**Possible Points**	**Points You Earned**
		687	Pretest	10	
		688	Key Term Assessment	22	
		689–694	Evaluation of Learning questions	43	
		694	CTA A: Laboratory Directory Information	10	
		695	CTA B: Specimen Requirements	15	
		695	CTA C: Identifying Abnormal Values	10	
		695–696	CTA D: Laboratory Report	25	
		696–697	CTA E: Laboratory Directory	9	
		697	CTA F: Testing Kit Product Insert (3 points for each section)	42	
		698	CTA G: Crossword Puzzle	29	
			Evolve Site: Chapter 15 Road to Recovery Game: Laboratory Test Categories (Record points earned)		
			Evolve Site: Chapter 15 Nutrition Nugget: Type 1 and 2 Diabetes	10	

683

√ After Completing	Date Due	Study Guide Pages	STUDY GUIDE ASSIGNMENTS (CTA = Critical Thinking Activity)	Possible Points	Points You Earned
			Evolve Site: Apply Your Knowledge questions	10	
		687	Posttest	10	
			ADDITIONAL ASSIGNMENTS		
			Total points		

√ When Assigned by Your Instructor	Study Guide Pages	Practices Required	LABORATORY ASSIGNMENTS (Procedure Number and Name)	Score*
	699–700	3	Practice for Competency 15-1: Collecting a Specimen for Transport to an Outside Laboratory Textbook reference: pp. 601–603	
	701–702		Evaluation of Competency 15-1: Collecting a Specimen for Transport to an Outside Laboratory	*
			ADDITIONAL ASSIGNMENTS	

Notes

Name: _____ Date: _____

True or False

_____ 1. When the body is in homeostasis, an imbalance exists in the body.

_____ 2. A routine test is performed to assist in the early detection of disease.

_____ 3. The laboratory request form provides the outside laboratory with information needed to test the specimen.

_____ 4. The clinical diagnosis is indicated on a laboratory request to correlate laboratory data with the needs of the physician.

_____ 5. The purpose of a laboratory report is to indicate the patient's diagnosis.

_____ 6. A patient who is fasting in preparation for a laboratory test is permitted to drink diet soda.

_____ 7. A small sample taken from the body to represent the nature of the whole is known as a *specimen*.

_____ 8. A laboratory report marked QNS means that the patient did not prepare properly.

_____ 9. Fecal occult blood testing is an example of a CLIA-waived test.

_____ 10. The purpose of quality control is to prevent accidents in the laboratory.

?📄 **POSTTEST**

True or False

_____ 1. Laboratory tests are most frequently ordered by the physician to assist in the diagnosis of pathologic conditions.

_____ 2. A laboratory directory indicates the patient preparation required for laboratory tests.

_____ 3. Laboratory tests called *profiles* contain a number of different tests.

_____ 4. A lipid profile includes a test for glucose.

_____ 5. The purpose of patient preparation for a laboratory test is to ensure the test results fall within the reference range.

_____ 6. A comprehensive metabolic profile requires that the patient fast.

_____ 7. Antibiotics taken by the patient before the collection of a throat specimen for culture may produce a false-positive result.

_____ 8. The purpose of CLIA is to prevent exposure of employees to bloodborne pathogens.

_____ 9. If a POL is performing moderate-complexity tests, CLIA requires that two levels of controls be run daily.

_____ 10. The study of blood and blood-forming tissues is known as *serology*.

A. Definitions

Directions: Match each medical term (numbers) with its definition (letters).

_____ 1. Analyte

_____ 2. Calibration

_____ 3. Clinical diagnosis

_____ 4. Control

_____ 5. Fasting

_____ 6. Homeostasis

_____ 7. In vivo

_____ 8. Laboratory test

_____ 9. Nonwaived test

_____ 10. Plasma

_____ 11. Product insert

_____ 12. Profile

_____ 13. Qualitative test

_____ 14. Quality control

_____ 15. Quantitative test

_____ 16. Reagent

_____ 17. Reference range

_____ 18. Routine test

_____ 19. Serum

_____ 20. Specimen

_____ 21. Test system

_____ 22. Waived test

A. Liquid part of the blood consisting of a clear, yellowish fluid that comprises approximately 55% of the total blood volume

B. State in which body systems are functioning normally and the internal environment of the body is in equilibrium; the body is in a healthy state

C. Array of laboratory tests for identifying a disease state or evaluating a particular organ or organ system

D. Printed document supplied by the manufacturer with a laboratory test product that contains information on the proper storage and use of the product

E. Solution that is used to monitor a test system to ensure the reliability and accuracy of the test results

F. Test that indicates whether a substance is present in the specimen being tested and provides an approximate indication of the amount of the substance present

G. Application of methods to ensure that test results are reliable and valid and that errors are detected and eliminated

H. Occurring in the living body or organism

I. Test that indicates the exact amount of a chemical substance that is present in the body, with the results being reported in measurable units

J. Substance that is being identified or measured in a laboratory test

K. Substance that produces a reaction with a patient specimen that allows detection or measurement of the substance by the test system

L. A certain established and acceptable parameter of reference range within which the laboratory test results of a healthy individual are expected to fall

M. Tentative diagnosis of a patient's condition obtained through the evaluation of the health history and the physical examination, without the benefit of laboratory or diagnostic tests

N. Abstaining from food or fluids (except water) for a specified amount of time before the collection of a specimen

O. Laboratory test that meets the CLIA criteria for being a simple procedure that is easy to perform and has a low risk of erroneous test results

P. Laboratory test performed routinely on apparently healthy patients to assist in the early detection of disease

Q. Clear, straw-colored part of the blood (plasma) that remains after the solid elements and the clotting factor fibrinogen have been separated from it

R. Mechanism to check the precision and accuracy of a test system, such as an automated analyzer

S. Small sample of something taken to show the nature of the whole

T. Clinical analysis and study of materials, fluids, or tissues obtained from patients to assist in diagnosis and treatment of disease

U. Setup that includes all of the test components required to perform a laboratory test such as testing devices, controls, and testing reagents

V. Complex laboratory test that does not meet the CLIA criteria for waiver and is subject to the CLIA regulations

✍️ EVALUATION OF LEARNING

Directions: Fill in each blank with the correct answer.

1. What is the general purpose of a laboratory test?

_____

_____

_____

2. Define each of the following categories of laboratory tests.

   a. Hematology:

   _____

   _____

   b. Clinical chemistry:

   _____

   _____

   c. Immunology and blood banking:

   _____

   _____

   d. Urinalysis:

   _____

   _____

   e. Microbiology:

   _____

   _____

3. List five specific uses of laboratory test results.

   _____

   _____

   _____

   _____

   _____

4. What is the purpose of performing a routine test?

   _____

   _____

5. What is the purpose of CLIA?

   _____

   _____

6. What requirements must be followed regarding a refrigerator used to store specimens and testing components?

_____

_____

7. What temperature is usually required for storing testing materials and performing laboratory tests?

_____

8. What information is included in a laboratory directory?

_____

_____

_____

9. What is the purpose of a laboratory request?

_____

_____

10. What is the reason for indicating the following information on the laboratory request form?

   a. Patient's age and gender:

   _____

   _____

   b. Date and time of collection of the specimen:

   _____

   _____

   c. Source of the specimen:

   _____

   _____

   d. Physician's clinical diagnosis:

   _____

   _____

   e. Medications the patient is taking:

   _____

   _____

11. How does a laboratory report the results when a laboratory request is marked STAT?

_____

_____

_____

12. What tests are included in the following profiles?

    a. Comprehensive metabolic profile:

_____

_____

    b. Hepatic function profile:

_____

_____

    c. Prenatal profile:

_____

_____

13. What information is included on laboratory reports?

_____

_____

_____

_____

14. Why must the test results of specimens tested by an outside laboratory be compared with the reference ranges supplied by the laboratory?

_____

_____

15. How are laboratory reports delivered to the medical office?

_____

_____

16. If a laboratory request form is completed on a computer, how is it transmitted to the laboratory?

_____

_____

_____

17. Why do some laboratory tests require advance patient preparation?

_____

_____

18. Why is it important to explain the reason for the advance preparation to the patient?

_____

19. Why are fasting specimens usually collected in the morning?

_____

_____

_____

20. What is a specimen?

_____

_____

21. List 10 examples of specimens.

_____

_____

_____

_____

_____

22. What reference source should be used to locate the specimen collection and handling requirements for the following?

a. Specimen transported to an outside laboratory:

_____

b. Specimen tested in the medical office:

_____

23. Why must the appropriate container be used to collect a specimen?

_____

_____

24. What is a unique identifier?

_____

_____

25. What two methods can be used to label a specimen?

_____

_____

26. Why is it important to identify a patient properly?

_____

27. Why must a specimen be properly handled and stored?

_____

_____

28. List the CLIA-waived tests that are most frequently performed in the medical office.

_____

_____

_____

_____

29. What is included in a laboratory testing kit?

_____

_____

30. What may occur if a testing kit is outdated?

_____

_____

31. What is a unitized testing device?

_____

_____

32. Describe a CLIA-waived automated analyzer.

_____

_____

33. What is the purpose of quality control?

_____

_____

34. What are the storage requirements for most testing systems?

_____

_____

35. What should be written on the label of a control that is stable for only a certain period of time after opening it?

_____

_____

36. What is an internal control?

_____

37. An internal control checks for what conditions?

_____

_____

38. What is the purpose of an external control?

_____

_____

39. What types of results are produced by the following controls?

a. Low-level control:

_____

b. High-level control:

_____

40. What may cause a control to fail to produce expected results?

_____

_____

41. What may cause invalid test results to occur when testing a specimen with a testing kit?

_____

_____

42. What is the difference between qualitative test results and quantitative test results?

_____

_____

43. List 10 laboratory safety guidelines that should be followed in the medical office to prevent accidents from occurring.

_____

_____

_____

_____

_____

_____

CRITICAL THINKING ACTIVITIES

A. Laboratory Directory Information

Look at a laboratory directory (from an outside medical laboratory), and list the categories of information included in it (e.g., normal range of laboratory tests).

_____

_____

_____

_____

_____

_____

B. Specimen Requirements

Refer to Table 15-2 in your textbook, and list the specimen requirements for each of the following tests:

1. ALT _____

2. Bilirubin, total _____

3. Blood group (ABO) and Rh Type _____

4. BUN, serum _____

5. Calcium _____

6. CBC (with differential) _____

7. CRP _____

8. Glucose, plasma _____

9. LD _____

10. PT/INR _____

11. RPR _____

12. Sedimentation rate (ESR) _____

13. Thyroxine (T_4) _____

14. Triglycerides _____

15. Urinalysis _____

C. Identifying Abnormal Values

Refer to the laboratory report in your textbook (see Fig. 15-5); with a red pen, circle any abnormal values.

D. Laboratory Report

Refer to the laboratory report in your textbook (see Fig. 15-5). Using the normal values listed on this report, determine whether the following test results fall within normal ranges or are high or low. Mark each test according to the following: **N** = normal, **H** = high, **L** = low. Your patient is a woman.

1. Glucose: 140 mg/dL _____

2. BUN: 15 mg/dL _____

3. Creatinine: 1.7 mg/dL _____

4. Calcium: 10.2 mg/dL _____

5. Magnesium: 0.4 mmol/L _____

6. Sodium: 156 mmol/L _____

7. Potassium: 5.5 mmol/L _____

8. Chloride: 84 mmol/L _____

9. Carbon dioxide: 18 mmol/L _____

10. Uric acid: 5.2 mg/dL _____

11. Total protein: 4.0 g/dL _____

12. Albumin: 3.5 g/dL _____

13. Total bilirubin: 0.8 mg/dL _____

14. Alkaline phosphatase: 80 U/L _____

15. LD: 132 U/L _____

16. AST: 24 U/L _____

17. ALT: 44 U/L _____

18. Total cholesterol: 260 mg/dL _____

19. HDL cholesterol: 57 mg/dL _____

20. LDL cholesterol: 165 mg/dL _____

21. WBC: 15.5 ($\times$ 10^3/mm^3) _____

22. Hemoglobin: 10.4 g/dL _____

23. Hematocrit: 34% _____

24. Prothrombin time: 10 seconds _____

25. Neutrophils: 84% _____

E. Laboratory Directory

Your physician has ordered a triglyceride test on a patient that will be analyzed at an outside laboratory. You are required to collect the specimen and prepare it for transport to the outside laboratory. Using Figure 15-9 in your textbook as a reference, respond to the following questions in the space provided.

1. What is the amount and type of specimen required for this test?

_____

2. What patient preparation is required for this test?

_____

_____

3. What collection supplies are required for this test?

_____

4. What collection techniques must be performed after collecting the specimen?

_____

_____

5. How should you store the specimen while awaiting pickup by the laboratory?

_____

_____

6. What would cause the laboratory to reject the specimen?

_____

_____

7. What are the limitations of this test?

_____

_____

_____

8. When would be the best time to collect this specimen (AM or PM)? Explain the reason for your answer.

_____

_____

_____

9. When the laboratory report is returned, the triglyceride test results are 250 mg/dL. How is this interpreted: desirable, borderline high, high, or very high?

_____

F. Testing Kit Product Insert

Obtain a product insert from a CLIA-waived testing kit. The product insert can be obtained from an actual testing kit or from a Google search on the Internet. Provide a brief description of the information included in each section of the product insert in the space provided. Examples of brand names of CLIA-waived testing kits include the following:

Hemoccult fecal occult blood test
ColoScreen fecal occult blood test
Seracult fecal occult blood test
Hemoccult ICT test
QuickVue iFOB test
OSOM mono test
Clearview mono test

Quick-Vue HCG pregnancy test
OSOM HCG urine pregnancy test
ICON HCG urine pregnancy test
Quick-Vue In-Line Strep A test
OSOM Ultra Strep A test
ICON DS Strep A test
Acceava Strep A test

Name of Testing Kit _____

Section	Brief description of information included in this section of the product insert
Intended use	
Summary and explanation	
Principles of the procedure	
Precautions and warnings	
Reagents and materials provided	
Materials not provided	
Storage and stability	
Specimen collection and handling	
Test procedure	
Interpretation and reading results	
Quality control	
Limitations of the procedure	
Expected values	
Performance characteristics	

G. Crossword Puzzle: Introduction to the Clinical Laboratory
Directions: Complete the crossword puzzle using the clues provided.

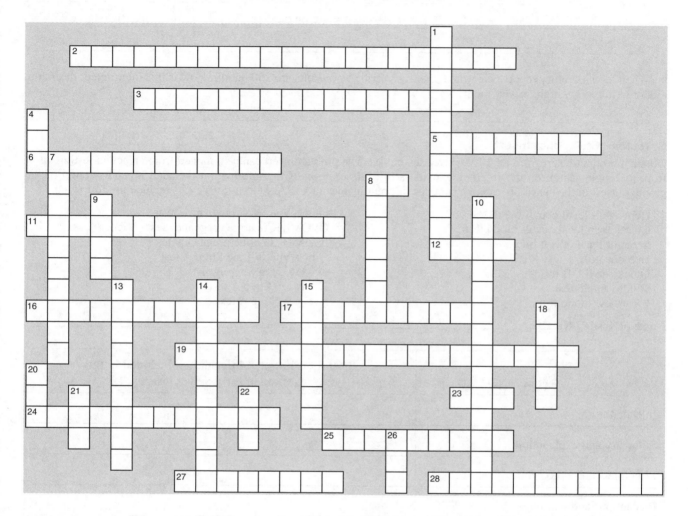

Across
2 Which disease is it?
3 Is that you?
5 Sample of the body
6 Determines CAD risk
8 CLIA requires three times per year
11 Approximate amount of substance present
12 As soon as possible
16 Detects disease early
17 Order a laboratory test
19 Outside lab reference source
23 Not enough specimen?
24 Study of microorganisms
25 What are the results?
27 Pap text (ex)
28 Test system working ok?

Down
1 Healthy body
4 In-house laboratory
7 Study of antigen-antibody reactions
8 More than one laboratory test
9 To improve quality of laboratory testing
10 Accurate and reliable test results
13 Study of tissues
14 Study of blood
15 No food or fluid
18 Plasma minus fibrinogen
20 Microscopic analysis of urine (ex)
21 Hematocrit abbreviation
22 Hemoglobin abbreviation
26 Syphilis test

Procedure 15-1: Collecting Specimen for Transport to an Outside Laboratory

1. Laboratory requisition. Complete the Laboratory Request Form on the following page using a classmate as a patient. The tests that have been ordered by the physician include the following: CBC (with differential), total cholesterol, HDL cholesterol, and plasma glucose.

2. Specimen collection. Practice the procedure for collecting a specimen for transport to an outside laboratory, and record the procedure in the chart provided.

CHART	
Date	

LABORATORY REQUISITION
Biomedical Laboratories, Inc.
100 Main Street
Athens, Georgia 45760

☐ Fax Send additional copy of report to:
☐ Call Client Number/Physician's Name ( ) Phone/Fax number
☐ Mail Physician's Address City, State, Zip

Patient's Name (Last)	(First)	(MI)	Sex	Date of Birth MO | DAY | YEAR	Collection Time : AM PM	Fasting YES NO	Collection Date MO | DAY | YEAR

NPI/UPIN	Physician's ID #	Patient's SS #	Patient's ID #	Urine hrs/vol hrs____ vol____

PATIENT

Physician's Name (Last, First)	Physician's Signature	Patient's Address	Phone
Medicare # (Include prefix/suffix)	☐ Primary ☐ Secondary	City	State ZIP
Medicaid # State	Physician's Provider #		

RESP. PARTY

Name of Responsible Party (if different from patient)

Diagnosis/Signs/Symptoms in ICD-9 Format (Highest Specificity)
R E Q U I R E D

Address of Responsible Party (if different from patient) APT #

City State ZIP

INSURANCE

Patient's Relationship to Responsible Party ■ 1–Self ■ 2–Spouse ■ 3–Child ■ 4–Other

Performance Lab ☐	Carrier	Group #	Employee #	Mem

Insurance Company Name	Plan	Carrier Code
Subscriber/Member #	Location	Group #
Insurance Address	Physician's Provider #	
City	State ZIP	
Employer's Name or Number	Insured SS # (If not patient)	Worker's Comp ☐ Yes ☐ No

I hereby authorize the release of medical information related to the service subscribed herein and authorize payment directed to LabCorp.
X _____
Patient's Signature Date

MEDICARE ADVANCE BENEFICIARY NOTICE
I have read the ABN on the reverse. If Medicare denies payment, I agree to pay for the identified test(s).
X _____
Patient's Signature Date

NOTE: WHEN ORDERING TESTS FOR WHICH MEDICARE OR MEDICAID REIMBURSEMENT WILL BE SOUGHT, PHYSICIANS SHOULD ONLY ORDER TESTS THAT ARE MEDICALLY NECESSARY FOR THE DIAGNOSIS OR TREATMENT OF THE PATIENT. COMPONENTS OF THE ORGAN OR DISEASE PANELS/COMBINATIONS PRINTED BELOW ARE SHOWN ON THE REVERSE SIDE AND MAY ALSO BE ORDERED INDIVIDUALLY BELOW. COMPONENTS MAY BE BILLED SEPARATELY PER CARRIER POLICY.

PROFILES (See reverse for components)

Code	Test		Code	Test		Code	Test	
80049	Basic Metabolic Profile	SST	84520	BUN	SST	83002	LH	SST
80054	Comp Metabolic Profile	SST	82310	Calcium	SST	83690	Lipase	SER
80051	Electrolyte Profile	SST	80156	Carbamazepine (Tegretol®)	SER	80178	Lithium (Eskalith®)	SER
80058	Hepatic Profile	SST	82378	CEA	SST	83735	Magnesium, Serum	SST
80059	Hepatitis Profile	SST	82465	Cholesterol, Total	SST	80184	Phenobarbital (Luminal®)	SER
80061	Lipid Profile	SST	82565	Creatinine	SST	80185	Phenytoin (Dilantin®)	SER
80091	Thyroid Profile	SST	80162	Digoxin	SER	84132	Potassium	SST
80055	Prenatal Profile	RED LAV	82670	Estradiol	SST	84146	Prolactin, Serum	SST
80072	Rheumatoid Profile	SST	82728	Ferritin, Serum	SST	84153	Prostate-Specific Antigen	SST
	HEMATOLOGY		82985	Fructosamine	SST	84066	Prostatic Acid Phos	SST
85025	CBC w Diff	LAV	83001	FSH	SST	84155	Protein, Total	SST
85027	CBC w/o Diff	LAV	83001 83002	FSH and LH	SST	85610	Prothrombin Time (PT)	BLU
85014	Hematocrit	LAV	82977	GGT	SST	85610 85730	PT and PTT Activated	BLU
85018	Hemoglobin	LAV	82947	Glucose, Plasma	GRY	85730	PTT Activated	BLU
85595	Platelet Count	LAV	82947	Glucose, Serum	SST	86431	Rheumatoid Arthritis Factor	SST
85041	RBC Count	LAV	82950	Glucose, 2-hr. PP	SST	86592	RPR	SST
85048	WBC Count	LAV	83036	Glycohemoglobin, Total	LAV	86762	Rubella Antibodies, IgG	SST
85007	WBC Differential	LAV	84703	hCG, Beta Subunit, Qual	SST	85651	Sed Rate	LAV
89190	Nasal Smear, Eosin	Nasal Smear	84702	hCG, Beta Subunit, Quant	SST	84295	Sodium	SST
85060	Pathologist Consult– Peripheral Smear	LAV	83718	HDL Cholesterol	SST	84403	Testosterone	SST
	ALPHABETICAL/COMBINATION TESTS		86677	Helicobacter pylori, IgG	SST	80198	Theophylline	SER
86900 86901	ABO and Rh	LAV	86706	Hep B Surface Antibody	SST	84436	Thyroxine (T₄)	SST
82040	Albumin	SST	87340	Hep B Surface Antigen	SST	84478	Triglycerides	SST
84075	Alkaline Phosphatase	SST	86803	Hep C Antibody	SST	84480	Triiodothyronine (T₃)	SST
84460	ALT (SGPT)	SST	83036	Hemoglobin A₁C	LAV	84443	TSH, High Sensitivity	SST
82150	Amylase, Serum	SST	86701	HIV Antibodies	SST	84550	Uric Acid	SST
86038	Antinuclear Antibodies	SST	83540	Iron, Total	SST	81003	Urinalysis Microscopic on Positives	URN
84450	AST (SGOT)	SST	83540 83550	Iron and IBC	SST	81001	Urinalysis with Microscopic	URN
82607 82746	B₁₂ and Folate	SST	83615	LDH	SST	80164	Valproic Acid (Depakene®)	SER
82250	Bilirubin, Total	SST						

MICROBIOLOGY See Reverse Side

■ENDOCERVICAL ■ THROAT ■ URINE
■STOOL ■ URETHRAL INDICATE SOURCE

Code	Test	
87070	Aerobic Bacterial Culture	Bact Trnspt
87490 87590	Chlamydia/GC DNA Probe w/ Confirmation on Positives	Probe Trnspt
87490 87590	Chlamydia/GC DNA Probe Without Confirmation	Probe Trnspt
87490	Chlamydia DNA Probe	Probe Trnspt
87081	Genital, Beta-Hemolytic Strep Cult, Group B	Bact Trnspt
87070	Genital Culture, Routine	Bact Trnspt
87070	Lower Respiratory Culture	Steril Trnspt
87590	N. gonorrhoeae DNA Probe	Probe Trnspt
87015 87211	Ova and Parasites	O & P Kit
87081 X2 87045	Stool Culture	Fecal Trnspt
87081	Throat, Beta-Hemolytic Strep Cult, Group A	Bact Trnspt
87060	Upper Respiratory Culture, Routine	Bact Trnspt
87086	Urine Culture, Routine	Urn Cult Trnspt

Clinical Information/Comments

OTHER TESTS/INDIVIDUAL COMPONENTS
TEST # TEST NAMES

LAB USE ONLY	STAT	VENIPUNCTURE	TRAVEL	NON LABCORP	VERBAL ORDER	CHART ORDER	HANDWRITTEN	24 HR TUV	PST/PSC #
	☐998074	☐998085	☐998096	☐998239	☐998250	☐998261	☐998272	☐998283	

CONTAINERS RECEIVED →

SST SPUN	USST UNSPUN	SER SERUM TRNSPT	FRZ FRZ TRANS	RED RED	LAV LAVENDER	SLD SLIDE	BLU LT. BLUE	GRY GREY	GRN GREEN	RYB RYL BLU	YEL ACD	PLS PLASMA	URN URINE	24U 24 HR URINE	TA-U TART. ACID	FL FLUID	OT OTHER	BACT TRNSP	O & P KIT	PROBE TRNSP	URN CULT TRNSP	STERIL TRNSP	FECAL TRNSP	VIRAL TRNSP

300-0384

Procedure 15-1: Collecting a Specimen for Transport to an Outside Laboratory

Name: _____

Date: _____

Evaluated by: _____

Score: _____

Performance Objective

Outcome:	Collect a specimen for transport to an outside laboratory.
Conditions:	Given the appropriate supplies for the specimen collection and transport (will be based upon the type of specimen collected).
Standards:	Time: 10 minutes. Student completed procedure in _____ minutes.
	Accuracy: Satisfactory score on the Performance Evaluation Checklist.

Performance Evaluation Checklist

Trial 1	Trial 2	Point Value	Performance Standards
		•	Informed the patient of any advance preparation or special instructions.
		▷	Explained why the patient should prepare properly.
		•	Reviewed the requirements in the laboratory directory for the collection and handling of the specimen.
		•	Completed the laboratory request form.
		•	Sanitized hands.
		•	Assembled equipment and supplies.
		•	Labeled the tubes and containers with the patient's name, date, and initials.
		•	Greeted the patient and introduced yourself. Identified the patient and explained the procedure.
		▷	Stated why it is important to correctly identify the patient.
		•	Determined whether the patient prepared properly for the test.
			Collected the specimen incorporating the following guidelines:
		•	Followed the OSHA Standard.
		•	Collected the specimen using proper technique.
		•	Collected the proper type and amount of specimen required for the test.
		•	Processed the specimen further if required by the outside laboratory.
		•	Placed the lid tightly on the specimen container.
			Prepared specimen for transport:
		•	Placed the specimen in a biohazard specimen bag.
		•	Placed the lab request in the outside pocket of the bag.
		•	Properly handled and stored the specimen.
		•	Charted the procedure correctly.

Trial 1	Trial 2	Point Value	Performance Standards
			Processed laboratory report:
		•	Reviewed the laboratory report when it was returned.
		•	Notified the physician of any abnormal results.
		•	Filed the laboratory report in the patient's chart after review by the physician.
		✳	Completed the procedure within 10 minutes.
			Totals

CHART	
Date	

Evaluation of Student Performance

EVALUATION CRITERIA			COMMENTS
Symbol	**Category**	**Point Value**	
✳	Critical Step	16 points	
•	Essential Step	6 points	
▷	Theory Question	2 points	

Score calculation: 100 points

− _____ points missed

_____ Score

Satisfactory score: 85 or above

CAAHEP Competencies Achieved

Psychomotor (Skills)

☑ I. 11. Perform quality control measures.

☑ I. 16. Screen test results.

☑ II. 2. Maintain laboratory test results using flow sheets.

Affective (Behavior)

☑ III. 1. Display sensitivity to patient rights and feelings in collecting specimens.

ABHES Competencies Achieved

☑ 9. f. Screen and follow up patient test results.

☑ 10. a. Practice quality control.

☑ 10. d. Collect, label, and process specimens.

---

16 Urinalysis

CHAPTER ASSIGNMENTS

√ After Completing	Date Due	Textbook Pages	TEXTBOOK ASSIGNMENTS	Possible Points	Points You Earned
		616–656	Read Chapter 16: Urinalysis		
		619 653	Read Case Study 1 / Case Study 1 questions	5	
		626 653	Read Case Study 2 / Case Study 2 questions	5	
		649 653–654	Read Case Study 3 / Case Study 3 questions	5	
			Total points		

√ After Completing	Date Due	Study Guide Pages	STUDY GUIDE ASSIGNMENTS (CTA = Critical Thinking Activity)	Possible Points	Points You Earned
		707	Pretest	10	
		708 709	Key Term Assessment A. Definitions B. Word Parts (Add 1 point for each medical term)	23 16	
		709–712	Evaluation of Learning questions	36	
		713	CTA A: First-Voided Specimen	2	
		713	CTA B: Clean-Catch Specimen	4	
		713–714	CTA C: Urine Testing Kit Instructions	6	
			Evolve Site: Chapter 16 Chemical Testing of Urine (Record points earned)		
		715	CTA D: Crossword Puzzle	21	
			Evolve Site: Road to Recovery: Urinalysis Terminology (Record points earned)		
			Evolve Site: Chapter 16 Animations (2 points each)	12	

√ After Completing	Date Due	Study Guide Pages	STUDY GUIDE ASSIGNMENTS (CTA = Critical Thinking Activity)	Possible Points	Points You Earned
			e Evolve Site: Chapter 16 Nutrition Nugget: Kidney Stones	10	
			e Evolve Site: Apply Your Knowledge questions	10	
		717–718	*e* Video Evaluation	25	
		707	？ Posttest	10	
			ADDITIONAL ASSIGNMENTS		
			Total points		

√ When Assigned by Your Instructor	Study Guide Pages	Practices Required	LABORATORY ASSIGNMENTS (Procedure Number and Name)	Score*
	719–720	3	Practice for Competency 16-1: Clean-Catch Midstream Specimen Collection Instructions Textbook reference: pp. 621–622	
	725–727		Evaluation of Competency 16-1: Clean-Catch Midstream Specimen Collection Instructions	*
	719–720	3	Practice for Competency 16-2: Collection of a 24-Hour Urine Specimen Textbook reference: pp. 622–623	
	729–731		Evaluation of Competency 16-2: Collection of a 24-Hour Urine Specimen	*
	719–720	5	Practice for Competency 16-A: Assessing Color and Appearance of a Urine Specimen Textbook reference: pp. 623–632	
	733–734		Evaluation of Competency 16-A: Assessing Color and Appearance of a Urine Specimen	*
	719–723	5	Practice for Competency 16-3: Chemical Testing of Urine with the Multistix 10 SG Reagent Strip Textbook reference: pp. 632–634	
	735–737		Evaluation of Competency 16-3: Chemical Testing of Urine with the Multistix 10 SG Reagent Strip	*
	719–720	2	Practice for Competency 16-4: Prepare a Urine Specimen for Microscopic Examination—Kova Method Textbook reference: pp. 644–647	
	739–741		Evaluation of Competency 16-4: Prepare a Urine Specimen for Microscopic Examination—Kova Method	*
	719–720	2	Practice for Competency 16-5: Performing a Rapid Urine Culture Test Textbook reference: pp. 649–651	
	743–744		Evaluation of Competency 16-5: Performing a Rapid Urine Culture Test	*

√ When Assigned by Your Instructor	Study Guide Pages	Practices Required	LABORATORY ASSIGNMENTS (Procedure Number and Name)	Score*
	719–720	2	Practice for Competency 16-6: Performing a Urine Pregnancy Test Textbook reference: pp. 651–652	
	745–746		Evaluation of Competency 16-6: Performing a Urine Pregnancy Test	*
			ADDITIONAL ASSIGNMENTS	

Name: _____ 98^{·'·} (⌣) Date: _____

True or False

_T_ 1. The urinary system regulates the fluid balance of the body.

_T_ 2. The functional unit of the kidney is the nephron.

_T_ 3. An excessive increase in urine output is called *polyuria.*

_T_ 4. A clean-catch midstream urine specimen is required for a urine culture.

_T_ 5. Urinalysis consists of a physical, chemical, and microscopic examination of urine.

_F_ 6. A urine specimen that is light yellow indicates that bacteria are present in the specimen.

_F_ 7. The pH of most urine specimens is neutral.

_T_ 8. Blood may normally be present in the urine due to menstruation.

_T_ 9. Hematuria refers to the presence of blood in the urine.

_T_ 10. HCG is a hormone that is present in the urine and blood of a pregnant woman.

?️ **POSTTEST**

True or False

_F_ 1. The external opening of the urethra is known as the external os.

_F_ 2. A normal adult excretes approximately 250 mL of urine each day.

_T_ 3. Vomiting can result in oliguria.

_T_ 4. The distal urethra normally contains microorganisms.

_T✗_ 5. A 24-hour urine specimen may be collected to assist in the diagnosis of a UTI.

_T✗_ 6. If a urine specimen is allowed to stand for more than 1 hour at room temperature, the pH becomes more acidic.

_T_ 7. If a freshly voided specimen is cloudy, the patient may have a urinary tract infection.

_T_ 8. The normal specific gravity of urine ranges from 1.003 to 1.030.

_F_ 9. Dysuria is the inability to control urination at night.

_F_ 10. Casts are formed in the urinary bladder.

A. Definitions

Directions: Match each medical term (numbers) with its definition (letters).

R · 1. Anuria

D · 2. Bilirubinuria

S · 3. Dysuria

T · 4. Frequency

G · 5. Glycosuria

U · 6. Hematuria

I · 7. Ketonuria

K · 8. Ketosis

J · 9. Micturition

N · 10. Nephron

V · 11. Nocturia

C · 12. Nocturnal enuresis

A · 13. Oliguria

M · 14. pH

E · 15. Polyuria

B · 16. Proteinuria   X B

F · 17. Pyuria

O · 18. Retention

L · 19. Specific gravity

P · 20. Urgency

H · 21. Urinalysis

W · 22. Urinary incontinence

Q · 23. Void

A. Decreased or scant output of urine
B. The presence of protein in the urine
C. Inability of an individual to control urination at night during sleep (bedwetting)
D. The presence of bilirubin in the urine
E. Increased output of urine
F. The presence of pus in the urine
G. The presence of glucose in the urine
H. The physical, chemical, and microscopic analysis of urine
I. The presence of ketone bodies in the urine
J. Act of voiding urine
K. An accumulation of large amounts of ketone bodies in the tissues and body fluids
L. The weight of a substance compared with the weight of an equal volume of a substance known as the standard
M. The unit that describes the acidity or alkalinity of a solution
N. The functional unit of the kidney
O. The inability to empty the bladder; urine is being produced normally but is not being voided
P. The immediate need to urinate
Q. To empty the bladder
R. Failure of the kidneys to produce urine
S. Difficult or painful urination
T. The condition of having to urinate often
U. Blood present in the urine
V. Excessive (voluntary) urination during the night
W. The inability to retain urine

Chapter **16** **Urinalysis**

B. Word Parts

Directions: Indicate the meaning of each word part in the space provided. List as many medical terms as possible that incorporate the word part in the space provided.

Word Part	Meaning of Word Part	Medical Terms That Incorporate Word Part
1. an-	without, absence of	Anuria
2. ur/o	urine	Anuria
3. -ia	cond	Anuria
4. bilirubino/o	bilirubin	bilirubino
5. dys-	difficult, labored, Painful	Dysuria
6. glyc/o	sugar	urine
7. hemato/o	blood	Hematuria
8. keton/o	ketone	Ketonuria
9. -osis	abnormal condition	Ketosis
10. noct/i	night	Nocturia
11. olig/o	scanty few	Oliguria
12. poly	many	Polyuria
13. py/o	PUS	Pyuria
14. supra	above	Suprapubic aspiration
15. pub/o	pubis	Suprapubic aspiration
16. -ic	Pertaining to	Suprapubic aspiration

EVALUATION OF LEARNING

Directions: Fill in each blank with the correct answer.

1. List two functions of the urinary system.

   excretes aqueous waste, maintains fluid balance to regulate fluid and electrolyte balance of the body. To remove waste products

2. What is the function of the urinary bladder?

   to store and expell urine

3. How does the function of the urethra differ in the male and female?

   Male - urine and reproductive secretions
   Female - urine only

4. What is the urinary meatus?

The external opening of the urethra

5. Most of the urine (95%) is composed of what substance?

Water

6. List two conditions that may cause polyuria.

Diabetes mellitus, diabetes insipidus,

7. List two conditions that may cause oliguria.

Vomiting
Dehydration (Decreased fluid consumption)

8. What type of urine specimen is required for the detection of a urinary tract infection (UTI)?

Clean catch, midstream specimen

9. Why is a first-voided morning specimen often preferred for urine testing?

It has the greatest concentration of dissolved substances

10. A 24-hour urine specimen is often used to diagnose what condition?

Kidney stone formation

11. Why should a patient not void directly into a 24-hour urine specimen container that contains a preservative?

The preservative could splash onto the patient, resulting in a chemical burn.

12. List three changes that may take place in a urine specimen if it is allowed to stand at room temperature for more than 1 hour.

Bacteria turn urea to ammonia, changes the PH. May create false positive for protein. Bacteria multiply, makes specimen cloudy, increasing nitrite. Glucose will decrease, Microorgs use it as a source of food. Blood cells break down. Casts Decompose

13. Why does concentrated urine tend to be dark yellow?

Yellow pigment, urochrome, produced by breaking down of hemoglobin. less water, more concentrated, darker urine.

14. List two factors that may cause a urine specimen to become cloudy.

standing to long, or contains bacteria, pus, blood, fat, yeast, sperm mucus, threads, fecal contaminates,

15. A urine specimen that has been allowed to stand at room temperature for a long period of time will have what type of odor?

   Ammonia, from breakdown of urea by bacteria in the specimen

16. What is the purpose of testing the specific gravity of urine?

   Provides info on the ability of the kidneys to dilute or concentrate the urine. Decreased or increase can be sign of Disease.

17. What is the normal range for the specific gravity of urine?

   1.003 to 1.030

18. What is the difference between qualitative and quantitative test results?

   Qualitive, wheter substance is present and approximate amount Quantitative is exact amount of substance present in measureable units.

19. What may cause an increase in the pH of urine?

   Sample at room temperature, to long, over 1hr, may also indicate bacterial infection of urinary tract.

20. Why does urine become more alkaline if it is not preserved?

   Urea is converted to ammonia by bacterial action as urine sits out, Ammonia is alkaline

21. What may cause glycosuria?

   Diabetes mellitus, consumption of large amounts of sugary foods.

22. What conditions may cause proteinuria?

   Stress or strenous exerci. may cause it temporarily, glomerular filtration problems, renal disease, bacterial urinary tract infection.

23. What may cause ketosis?

   Uncontrolled diabetes mellitus, starvation, diet composed entirely of fat

24. What conditions may cause bilirubin to appear in the urine?

   excessive hemolysis of red blood cells, infectious hepatitis, cirrhosis Congestive heart failure, mononucleosis.

25. What may cause blood to appear in the urine?

   Injury or disorders, such as cystitis, bladder tumors, urethritis kidney stones, kidney disorders.

26. Why should a nitrite test not be performed on a urine specimen that has been left standing at room temperature?

Because a false positive results may occur from bacterial contamination from the enviorment.

27. How should urine reagent strips be stored?

In the bottle with cap closed tightly, cool dry area not exposed to sunlight. Room temp 59 to 86 degrees F.

28. What is the purpose of performing a microscopic examination of the urine?

Helps clarify the results of the physical and chemical exams

29. Why is a first-voided urine specimen recommended for a microscopic examination of the urine?

More concentrated, more dissolved substances, small amounts of abnormal substances are more likely to be detected.

30. What effect does concentrated urine have on red blood cells in it?

Cause the red blood cells to become shrunken or crenated, dilute urine swells them.

31. What is a urinary cast?

Clynical structures formed in the lumes of the nephron tubules presence of casts generally indicates disease.

32. What is the name of the vaginal infection caused by yeast?

Candidvasis.

33. List two reasons for performing a urine culture test.

To assist in the diagnosis of a UTI, Asses the effectiveness of antibiotic the therapy for UTI patient

34. List three reasons for performing a pregnancy test.

Early diagnosis for healthy pre-natal care, know before praced that may hurt fetus such as x-ray, know before taking certain medications that may hurt fetus.

35. What is the name of the hormone that is present in the urine and blood only of a pregnant woman?

human chorionic gonadotroppin, or HCG

36. List five guidelines that should be followed when performing a pregnancy test.

Clean disposable urine containers, first morning void, specific gravity test first, may be too dilute for other tests. Specimen at room temp, Kit check expiration, follow manufacture instructions, docuomer internal control.

CRITICAL THINKING ACTIVITIES

A. First-Voided Specimen

You have instructed Jim Pratt to collect a first-voided morning urine specimen, which is to be brought to the medical office for testing. Mr. Pratt asks the following questions. Respond to them in the spaces provided.

1. Why is a first-voided specimen desired?

_____

_____

2. Why must the specimen be preserved until it is brought to the medical office?

_____

_____

B. Clean-Catch Specimen

You have just instructed Ann Berger to obtain a clean-catch midstream specimen at the medical office. Mrs. Berger asks the following questions. Respond to them in the spaces provided.

1. What is the purpose of cleansing the urinary meatus?

_____

_____

2. Why must a front-to-back motion be used to clean the urinary meatus?

_____

_____

3. Why must a small amount of urine first be voided into the toilet?

_____

_____

4. Why should the inside of the specimen cup not be touched?

_____

_____

C. Urine Testing Kit Instructions

Obtain the package insert instructions that come with any type of commercially prepared diagnostic kit for the chemical testing of urine (e.g., Multistix 10 SG). Using the instructions, answer the following questions in the spaces provided. (*Note:* A package insert for Multistix 10 SG can be obtained on the Internet by performing a search for *Multistix 10 SG product insert*).

1. What is the brand name of the test?

_____

2. This test assists in the diagnosis of what conditions?

_____

_____

_____

3. What type of urine specimen is recommended for this test?

_____

_____

_____

4. This test is used to detect the presence of what substances?

_____

_____

_____

5. Explain the proper storage and handling of this test.

_____

_____

_____

6. List any substances or techniques that may interfere with obtaining an accurate reading (e.g., not reading the test at the prescribed time).

_____

_____

_____

D. Crossword Puzzle: Urinalysis

Directions: Complete the crossword puzzle using the clues provided.

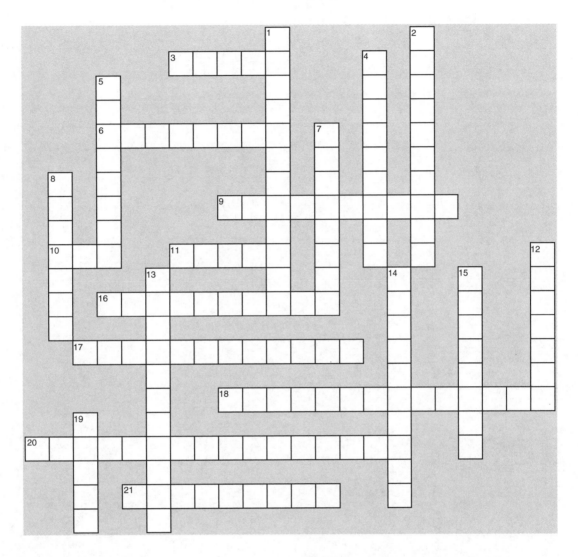

Across
- **3** UTI bacteria
- **6** Deteriorates urine strips
- **9** Tx for UTI
- **10** Makes preg test +
- **11** Neutral pH
- **16** Physical, chemical, and microscopic
- **17** Normal cause of hematuria
- **18** Security for urine drug testing
- **20** Measures exact amount
- **21** Cause of bilirubinuria

Down
- **1** Can be dx by a 24-hour urine spec
- **2** Cause of ketonuria
- **4** Yellow urine pigment
- **5** Cause of oliguria
- **7** Cause of glycosuria
- **8** Kidney unit
- **12** Sym of UTI
- **13** Spec for preg test
- **14** Spec for C & S
- **15** This drug causes polyuria
- **19** Most of urine

Notes

Name: _____

Directions:

a. Watch the indicated videos.
b. Mark each true statement with a T and each false statement with an F. For each false statement, change the wording of the question so that it becomes a true statement.

Video: Procedure 16-1: Clean-Catch Midstream Specimen Collection Instructions

_____ 1. The urinary tract is made up of the kidneys, ureters, urinary bladder, and urethra.

_____ 2. A clean-catch midstream specimen is recommended for identification of the presence of a urinary tract infection.

_____ 3. The kidneys, ureters, and urinary bladder normally harbor microorganisms.

_____ 4. The urinary meatus should be cleansed with a front-to-back motion.

_____ 5. The purpose of cleansing is to remove the normal flora from the urinary meatus.

_____ 6. The first amount of urine should be collected in the specimen container.

_____ 7. The specimen container should be filled about one-half full with urine.

_____ 8. After collection, the urine specimen should be preserved by placing it in a warm, moist area.

Video: Procedure 16-3: Chemical Testing of Urine with the Multistix 10 SG Reagent Strip

_____ 1. Urinalysis includes a physical and chemical examination of a urine specimen.

_____ 2. Freshly voided urine normally has a cloudy appearance.

_____ 3. The chemical testing of urine is an indirect means of detecting abnormal amounts of chemicals in the body.

_____ 4. A quality control procedure should be performed each time a urine test is performed.

_____ 5. Failure of the control to react as expected can be caused by outdated reagent strips.

_____ 6. A first-voided morning specimen is preferred for the Multistix test, but a random specimen is acceptable.

_____ 7. The normal color of urine is dark amber.

_____ 8. The container of testing strips should be recapped immediately to prevent exposing the strips to moisture, light, and heat.

_____ 9. The urine testing strip should be immersed in the urine specimen for 60 seconds.

_____ 10. The urine strip should be held horizontally when reading the test results.

_____ 11. The results for each chemical test must be read at the proper time to prevent inaccurate test results.

Video: Procedure 16-6: Performing a Urine Pregnancy Test

_____ 1. When performed correctly, a urine pregnancy test has a 97% accuracy rate in diagnosing pregnancy.

_____ 2. Pregnancy tests rely on the presence of estrogen for a positive reaction.

_____ 3. The preferred specimen for a urine pregnancy test is a first-voided morning specimen.

_____ 4. An expired pregnancy test may produce inaccurate test results.

_____ 5. External controls are run to ensure that the test results are reliable and valid.

_____ 6. Invalid test results can be caused by an outdated testing kit.

Procedure 16-1: Clean-Catch Midstream Urine Specimen Collection Instructions. Instruct an individual in the procedure for collecting a clean-catch midstream specimen, and record the procedure in the chart provided.

Procedure 16-2: 24-Hour Urine Specimen. Instruct an individual in the procedure for collecting a 24-hour urine specimen, and record the procedure in the chart provided.

Procedure 16-A: Color and Appearance of a Urine Specimen. Assess the color and appearance of a urine specimen, and record the results in the chart provided.

Procedure 16-3: Chemical Testing of Urine Using the Multistix 10 SG Reagent Strip.
   a. Perform a Multistix 10 SG quality control testing procedure, and record the results on the quality control log on the next page.
   b. Perform a chemical assessment of a urine specimen using a Multistix 10 SG reagent strip. Record the results on the laboratory report form provided. Circle any abnormal results.

Procedure 16-4: Prepare a Urine Specimen for Microscopic Examination of Urine. Practice the procedure for preparing a urine specimen for a microscopic analysis of the urine sediment. Examine the specimen, and record the results in the chart provided.

Procedure 16-5: Rapid Urine Culture Test. Perform a rapid urine culture test, and record the results in the chart provided.

Procedure 16-6: Urine Pregnancy Test. Perform a urine pregnancy test, and record the results in the chart provided.

CHART	
Date	

CHART	
Date	

URINALYSIS
QUALITY CONTROL LOG

Name of Test: _____ Date: _____	Name of Control: _____ Lot #: _____ Exp. Date: _____	Technician: _____
TEST	EXPECTED RESULT (specified in product insert accompanying the control)	CONTROL RESULT
Glucose		
Bilirubin		
Ketone		
Specific gravity		
Blood		
pH		
Protein		
Urobilinogen		
Nitrite		
Leukocytes		

Multistix® 10 SG Reagent Strips for Urinalysis

PATIENT

DATE   TIME

Test						
LEUKOCYTES	NEGATIVE ☐		TRACE ☐	SMALL + ☐	MODERATE ++ ☐	LARGE +++ ☐
NITRITE	NEGATIVE ☐		POSITIVE ☐	POSITIVE ☐	(Any degree of uniform pink color is found)	
UROBILINOGEN	NORMAL 0.2 ☐	NORMAL 1 ☐	mg/dL 2 ☐	4 ☐	8 ☐ (1mg = approx. 1 BU)	
PROTEIN	NEGATIVE ☐	TRACE ☐	mg/dL 30 * ☐	100 ++ ☐	300 +++ ☐	2000 OR MORE ☐
pH	5.0 ☐	6.0 ☐	6.5 ☐	7.0 ☐	7.5 ☐	8.0 ☐ 8.5 ☐
BLOOD	NEGATIVE ☐	NON-HEMOLYZED TRACE ☐	NON-HEMOLYZED MODERATE ☐	HEMOLYZED TRACE ☐	SMALL + ☐	MODERATE ++ ☐ LARGE +++ ☐
SPECIFIC GRAVITY	1.000 ☐	1.006 ☐	1.010 ☐	1.015 ☐	1.020 ☐	1.025 ☐ 1.030 ☐
KETONE	NEGATIVE ☐	mg/dL	TRACE 5 ☐	SMALL 15 ☐	MODERATE 40 ☐	LARGE 80 ☐ LARGE 160 ☐
BILIRUBIN	NEGATIVE ☐		SMALL ☐	MODERATE ++ ☐	LARGE +++ ☐	
GLUCOSE	NEGATIVE ☐	g/L (%) mg/dL	1/10 (tr.) + 100 ☐	1/6 250 ☐	1/2 500 ☐	1 1000 ☐ 2 or more 2000 or more ☐

(Modified and printed with permission of Siemens Medical Solutions Diagnostic, Tarrytown, NY 10591.)

Multistix® 10 SG Reagent Strips for Urinalysis

PATIENT

DATE   TIME

Test						
LEUKOCYTES	NEGATIVE ☐		TRACE ☐	SMALL + ☐	MODERATE ++ ☐	LARGE +++ ☐
NITRITE	NEGATIVE ☐		POSITIVE ☐	POSITIVE ☐	(Any degree of uniform pink color is found)	
UROBILINOGEN	NORMAL 0.2 ☐	NORMAL 1 ☐	mg/dL 2 ☐	4 ☐	8 ☐ (1mg = approx. 1 BU)	
PROTEIN	NEGATIVE ☐	TRACE ☐	mg/dL 30 * ☐	100 ++ ☐	300 +++ ☐	2000 OR MORE ☐
pH	5.0 ☐	6.0 ☐	6.5 ☐	7.0 ☐	7.5 ☐	8.0 ☐ 8.5 ☐
BLOOD	NEGATIVE ☐	NON-HEMOLYZED TRACE ☐	NON-HEMOLYZED MODERATE ☐	HEMOLYZED TRACE ☐	SMALL + ☐	MODERATE ++ ☐ LARGE +++ ☐
SPECIFIC GRAVITY	1.000 ☐	1.006 ☐	1.010 ☐	1.015 ☐	1.020 ☐	1.025 ☐ 1.030 ☐
KETONE	NEGATIVE ☐	mg/dL	TRACE 5 ☐	SMALL 15 ☐	MODERATE 40 ☐	LARGE 80 ☐ LARGE 160 ☐
BILIRUBIN	NEGATIVE ☐		SMALL ☐	MODERATE ++ ☐	LARGE +++ ☐	
GLUCOSE	NEGATIVE ☐	g/L (%) mg/dL	1/10 (tr.) + 100 ☐	1/6 250 ☐	1/2 500 ☐	1 1000 ☐ 2 or more 2000 or more ☐

(Modified and printed with permission of Siemens Medical Solutions Diagnostic, Tarrytown, NY 10591.)

Multistix® 10 SG Reagent Strips for Urinalysis

PATIENT

DATE   TIME

LEUKOCYTES	NEGATIVE ☐			TRACE ☐	SMALL ☐ +	MODERATE ☐ ++		LARGE ☐ +++	
NITRITE	NEGATIVE ☐			POSITIVE ☐	POSITIVE ☐	(Any degree of uniform pink color is found)			
UROBILINOGEN	NORMAL ☐ 0.2	NORMAL ☐ 1	mg/dL ☐ 2	4 ☐	8 ☐	(1mg = approx. 1 BU)			
PROTEIN	NEGATIVE ☐	TRACE ☐	mg/dL ☐ 30 *	100 ☐ ++	300 ☐ +++	2000 OR MORE ☐			
pH	5.0 ☐	6.0 ☐	6.5 ☐	7.0 ☐	7.5 ☐		8.0 ☐	8.5 ☐	
BLOOD	NEGATIVE ☐	NON-HEMOLYZED ☐ TRACE	NON-HEMOLYZED ☐ MODERATE	HEMOLYZED ☐ TRACE	SMALL ☐ +	MODERATE ☐ ++		LARGE ☐ +++	
SPECIFIC GRAVITY	1.000 ☐	1.006 ☐	1.010 ☐	1.015 ☐	1.020 ☐	1.025 ☐		1.030 ☐	
KETONE	NEGATIVE ☐	mg/dL	TRACE ☐ 5	SMALL ☐ 15	MODERATE ☐ 40	LARGE ☐ 80		LARGE ☐ 160	
BILIRUBIN	NEGATIVE ☐		SMALL ☐ +	MODERATE ☐ ++	LARGE ☐ +++				
GLUCOSE	NEGATIVE ☐	g/L (%) mg/dL	1/10 (tr.) ☐ 100	1/6 ☐ 250	1/2 ☐ 500	1 ☐ 1000		2 or more ☐ 2000 or more	

(Modified and printed with permission of Siemens Medical Solutions Diagnostic, Tarrytown, NY 10591.)

Multistix® 10 SG Reagent Strips for Urinalysis

PATIENT

DATE   TIME

LEUKOCYTES	NEGATIVE ☐			TRACE ☐	SMALL ☐ +	MODERATE ☐ ++		LARGE ☐ +++	
NITRITE	NEGATIVE ☐			POSITIVE ☐	POSITIVE ☐	(Any degree of uniform pink color is found)			
UROBILINOGEN	NORMAL ☐ 0.2	NORMAL ☐ 1	mg/dL ☐ 2	4 ☐	8 ☐	(1mg = approx. 1 BU)			
PROTEIN	NEGATIVE ☐	TRACE ☐	mg/dL ☐ 30 *	100 ☐ ++	300 ☐ +++	2000 OR MORE ☐			
pH	5.0 ☐	6.0 ☐	6.5 ☐	7.0 ☐	7.5 ☐		8.0 ☐	8.5 ☐	
BLOOD	NEGATIVE ☐	NON-HEMOLYZED ☐ TRACE	NON-HEMOLYZED ☐ MODERATE	HEMOLYZED ☐ TRACE	SMALL ☐ +	MODERATE ☐ ++		LARGE ☐ +++	
SPECIFIC GRAVITY	1.000 ☐	1.006 ☐	1.010 ☐	1.015 ☐	1.020 ☐	1.025 ☐		1.030 ☐	
KETONE	NEGATIVE ☐	mg/dL	TRACE ☐ 5	SMALL ☐ 15	MODERATE ☐ 40	LARGE ☐ 80		LARGE ☐ 160	
BILIRUBIN	NEGATIVE ☐		SMALL ☐ +	MODERATE ☐ ++	LARGE ☐ +++				
GLUCOSE	NEGATIVE ☐	g/L (%) mg/dL	1/10 (tr.) ☐ 100	1/6 ☐ 250	1/2 ☐ 500	1 ☐ 1000		2 or more ☐ 2000 or more	

(Modified and printed with permission of Siemens Medical Solutions Diagnostic, Tarrytown, NY 10591.)

Notes

EVALUATION OF COMPETENCY

Procedure 16-1: Clean-Catch Midstream Specimen Collection Instructions

Name: _____   Date: _____

Evaluated by: _____   Score: _____

Performance Objective

Outcome:	Instruct a patient in the procedure for collecting a clean-catch midstream urine specimen.
Conditions:	Given the following: sterile specimen container, personal antiseptic towelettes, and tissues.
Standards:	Time: 10 minutes. Student completed procedure in _____ minutes.
	Accuracy: Satisfactory score on the Performance Evaluation Checklist.

Performance Evaluation Checklist

Trial 1	Trial 2	Point Value	Performance Standards
		•	Sanitized hands.
		•	Greeted the patient and introduced yourself.
		•	Identified the patient and explained the procedure.
		•	Assembled equipment.
		•	Labeled the specimen container.
			Instructed the female patient by telling her to:
		•	Wash hands and open antiseptic towelettes.
		•	Remove the lid from the specimen container without touching the inside of the container or lid.
		•	Pull down undergarments and sit on the toilet.
		•	Expose the urinary meatus by spreading the labia apart with one hand.
		•	Cleanse each side of the urinary meatus with a front-to-back motion using a separate towelette on each side of the meatus.
		▷	Explained why a front-to-back motion should be used.
		•	After use, discard each towelette in the toilet.
		•	Cleanse directly across the meatus using a third towelette and discard it.
		•	Void a small amount of urine into the toilet while continuing to hold the labia apart.
		▷	Explained the purpose of voiding into the toilet.
		•	Without stopping the urine flow, collect the next amount of urine by voiding into the sterile container.
		•	Fill the container approximately half full with urine without touching the inside of the container.
		▷	Stated why the inside of the container should not be touched.
		•	Void the last amount of urine into the toilet.

Trial 1	Trial 2	Point Value	Performance Standards
		•	Replace the specimen container lid.
		•	Wipe the area dry with a tissue, flush the toilet, and wash hands.
			Instructed the male patient by telling him to:
		•	Wash hands and open antiseptic towelettes, and remove the lid from the specimen container.
		•	Pull down undergarments and stand in front of the toilet.
		•	Retract the foreskin of the penis if uncircumcised.
		•	Cleanse the area around the meatus and the urethral opening by wiping each side of the meatus with a separate antiseptic towelette.
		•	Cleanse directly across the meatus using a third antiseptic towelette.
		•	Discard each towelette in the toilet after use.
		•	Void a small amount of urine into the toilet.
		•	Collect the next amount of urine by voiding into the sterile container without touching the inside of the container.
		•	Fill the container approximately half full with urine.
		•	Void the last amount of urine into the toilet.
		•	Replace the lid on the specimen container.
		•	Wipe the area dry with a tissue, flush the toilet, and wash hands.
			Performed the following:
		•	Provided the patient with instructions on what to do with the specimen.
		•	Charted the procedure correctly.
		•	Tested the specimen or prepared it for transport to an outside laboratory.
		✳	Completed the procedure within 10 minutes.
			Totals
CHART			
Date			

Evaluation of Student Performance

EVALUATION CRITERIA			COMMENTS
Symbol	**Category**	**Point Value**	
✷	Critical Step	16 points	
•	Essential Step	6 points	
▷	Theory Question	2 points	

Score calculation: 100 points

− _____ points missed

_____ Score

Satisfactory score: 85 or above

CAAHEP Competencies Achieved

Psychomotor (Skills)

☑ IV. 2. Report relevant information to others succinctly and accurately.

Affective (Behavior)

☑ III. 1. Display sensitivity to patient rights and feelings in collecting specimens.

☑ III. 2. Explain the rationale for performance of a procedure to the patient.

ABHES Competencies Achieved

☑ 8. cc. Communicate on the recipient's level of comprehension.

☑ 10. e. Instruct patients in the collection of a clean-catch midstream urine specimen.

Notes

📑 **EVALUATION OF COMPETENCY**

Procedure 16-2: Collection of a 24-Hour Urine Specimen

Name: _____   Date: _____

Evaluated by: _____   Score: _____

Performance Objective

Outcome:	Instruct a patient in the procedure for collecting a 24-hour urine specimen.
Conditions:	Given a large urine specimen container, written instructions, and a laboratory requisition.
Standards:	Time: 10 minutes. Student completed procedure in _____ minutes.
	Accuracy: Satisfactory score on the Performance Evaluation Checklist.

Performance Evaluation Checklist

Trial 1	Trial 2	Point Value	Performance Standards
		•	Sanitized hands.
		•	Greeted and introduced yourself.
		•	Identified the patient and explained the procedure.
		•	Assembled equipment.
		•	Labeled the specimen container.
			Instructed the patient in the collection of the specimen:
		•	Empty your bladder when you get up in the morning.
		•	Write the date and start time on the container label.
		•	The next time you need to urinate, void into the collecting container.
		•	Pour the urine into the large specimen container.
		•	Tightly screw the lid onto the container.
		•	Store the container in the refrigerator or in an ice chest.
		•	Repeat these steps each time you urinate.
		•	Collect all of your urine in a 24-hour period, and store it in the designated container.
		•	Urinate in the collection container before having a bowel movement.
		▷	Stated when the patient must start the collection process again from the beginning.
		•	On the following morning, get up at the same time.
		•	Void into the collection container for the last time, and pour the urine into the large specimen container.
		•	Put the lid on the container tightly.
		•	Write the date and time the test ended on the container label.
		•	Return the urine specimen container to the office the same morning as completing the test.

Trial 1	Trial 2	Point Value	Performance Standards
		•	Provided the patient with the 24-hour specimen container, a collecting container, and written instructions.
		•	Provided the patient with a Material Safety Data Sheet (MSDS) if the specimen container contains a preservative.
		▷	Stated the purpose of the MSDS.
		•	Charted instructions given to the patient in his or her medical record.
			Processing the specimen:
		•	Asked the patient whether there were any problems when he or she returned the specimen container.
		▷	Explained what should be done if the specimen was undercollected or overcollected.
		•	Prepared the specimen for transport to the laboratory.
		•	Completed a laboratory request form.
		•	Charted the results correctly.
		✴	Completed the procedure within 5 minutes.
			Totals

CHART

Date	

Evaluation of Student Performance

EVALUATION CRITERIA			COMMENTS
Symbol	**Category**	**Point Value**	
＊	Critical Step	16 points	
•	Essential Step	6 points	
▷	Theory Question	2 points	

Score calculation: 100 points

＿＿＿＿ – ＿＿＿＿＿ points missed

＿＿＿＿ Score

Satisfactory score: 85 or above

CAAHEP Competencies Achieved

Psychomotor (Skills)

☑ IV. 2. Report relevant information to others succinctly and accurately.

Affective (Behavior)

☑ III. 1. Display sensitivity to patient rights and feelings in collecting specimens.

☑ III. 2. Explain the rationale for performance of a procedure to the patient.

ABHES Competencies Achieved

☑ 8. cc. Communicate on the recipient's level of comprehension.

Notes

Procedure 16-A: Assessing Color and Appearance of a Urine Specimen

Name: _____   Date: _____

Evaluated by: _____   Score: _____

Performance Objective

Outcome:	Assess the color and appearance of a urine specimen.
Conditions:	Given a transparent container and a urine specimen.
Standards:	Time: 5 minutes. Student completed procedure in _____ minutes.
	Accuracy: Satisfactory score on the Performance Evaluation Checklist.

Performance Evaluation Checklist

Trial 1	Trial 2	Point Value	Performance Standards
			Color
		•	Sanitized hands and applied gloves.
		•	Transferred the urine specimen to a transparent container.
		•	Assessed the color of the urine specimen.
		✱	The assessment was identical to the evaluator's assessment.
		•	Charted the results correctly.
			Appearance
		•	Assessed the appearance of the urine specimen in the transparent container.
		✱	The assessment was identical to the evaluator's assessment.
		•	Charted the results correctly.
		•	Properly disposed of the urine specimen.
		•	Sanitized hands and removed gloves.
		✱	Completed the procedure within 5 minutes.
			Totals
CHART			
Date			

Evaluation of Student Performance

EVALUATION CRITERIA			COMMENTS
Symbol	**Category**	**Point Value**	
✳	Critical Step	16 points	
•	Essential Step	6 points	
▷	Theory Question	2 points	

Score calculation: 100 points

    − _____ points missed

       ____ Score

Satisfactory score: 85 or above

CAAHEP Competencies Achieved

Psychomotor (Skills)

☑ I. 14. Perform urinalysis.

Affective (Behavior)

☑ II. 2. Distinguish between normal and abnormal test results.

ABHES Competencies Achieved

☑ 10. b. Perform selected CLIA-waived tests that assist with diagnosis and treatment (1) Urinalysis.

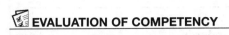
EVALUATION OF COMPETENCY

Procedure 16-3: Chemical Testing of Urine with the Multistix 10 SG Reagent Strip

Name: _____   Date: _____

Evaluated by: _____   Score: _____

Performance Objective

Outcome:	Perform a chemical assessment of a urine specimen.
Conditions:	Given the following: disposable gloves, Multistix 10 SG reagent strips, urine container, laboratory report form, and a waste container.
Standards:	Time: 5 minutes. Student completed procedure in _____ minutes.
	Accuracy: Satisfactory score on the Performance Evaluation Checklist.

Performance Evaluation Checklist

Trial 1	Trial 2	Point Value	Performance Standards
		•	If necessary, performed a quality control testing procedure.
		▷	Stated when a quality control procedure should be performed.
		•	Obtained a freshly voided urine specimen from the patient.
		▷	Explained why the container used to collect specimen should be clean.
		•	Sanitized hands.
		•	Assembled equipment.
		•	Checked the expiration date of the reagent strips.
		▷	Stated why the expiration date should be checked.
		•	Applied gloves.
		•	Removed a reagent strip from the container and recapped immediately.
		▷	Explained why the container should be recapped immediately.
		•	Did not touch the test areas with fingers.
		▷	Explained why the test areas should not be touched with fingers.
		•	Mixed the urine specimen thoroughly.
		•	Removed the lid and completely immersed the reagent strip in the urine specimen.
		•	Removed the strip immediately and ran the edge against the rim of urine container. Started the timer.
		▷	Explained why excess urine should be removed from the strip.
		•	Held the reagent strip in a horizontal position and placed it as close as possible to the corresponding color blocks on the color chart.
		▷	Explained why the strip should be held in a horizontal position.
		•	Read the results at the exact reading times specified on the color chart.
		▷	Explained why the results must be read at specified times.
		✴	The results were identical to the evaluator's results.
		•	Disposed of the strip in a regular waste container.

Trial 1	Trial 2	Point Value	Performance Standards
		•	Removed gloves and sanitized hands.
		•	Charted the results correctly.
		✶	Completed the procedure within 5 minutes.
			Totals

CHART	
Date	

Evaluation of Student Performance

EVALUATION CRITERIA			COMMENTS
Symbol	**Category**	**Point Value**	
✶	Critical Step	16 points	
•	Essential Step	6 points	
▷	Theory Question	2 points	

Score calculation: 100 points

−_____ points missed

_____ Score

Satisfactory score: 85 or above

CAAHEP Competencies Achieved

Psychomotor (Skills)

☑ I. 11. Perform quality control measures.

☑ I. 14. Perform urinalysis.

Affective (Behavior)

☑ II. 2. Distinguish between normal and abnormal test results.

ABHES Competencies Achieved

☑ 10. a. Practice quality control.

☑ 10. b. Perform selected CLIA-waived tests that assist with diagnosis and treatment (1) Urinalysis (6) Kit testing (c) Dip sticks.

Multistix® 10 SG Reagent Strips for Urinalysis

PATIENT _____

DATE _____ TIME _____

LEUKOCYTES	NEGATIVE ☐		TRACE ☐	SMALL + ☐	MODERATE ++ ☐	LARGE +++ ☐	
NITRITE	NEGATIVE ☐		POSITIVE ☐	POSITIVE ☐	(Any degree of uniform pink color is found)		
UROBILINOGEN	NORMAL 0.2 ☐	NORMAL 1 ☐	mg/dL 2 ☐	4 ☐	8 ☐	(1mg = approx. 1 BU)	
PROTEIN	NEGATIVE ☐	TRACE ☐	mg/dL 30 * ☐	100 ++ ☐	300 +++ ☐	2000 OR MORE ☐	
pH	5.0 ☐	6.0 ☐	6.5 ☐	7.0 ☐	7.5 ☐	8.0 ☐	8.5 ☐
BLOOD	NEGATIVE ☐	NON-HEMOLYZED TRACE ☐	NON-HEMOLYZED MODERATE ☐	HEMOLYZED TRACE ☐	SMALL + ☐	MODERATE ++ ☐	LARGE +++ ☐
SPECIFIC GRAVITY	1.000 ☐	1.006 ☐	1.010 ☐	1.015 ☐	1.020 ☐	1.025 ☐	1.030 ☐
KETONE	NEGATIVE ☐	mg/dL	TRACE 5 ☐	SMALL 15 ☐	MODERATE 40 ☐	LARGE 80 ☐	LARGE 160 ☐
BILIRUBIN	NEGATIVE ☐		SMALL + ☐	MODERATE ++ ☐	LARGE +++ ☐		
GLUCOSE	NEGATIVE ☐	g/L (%) mg/dL	1/10 (tr.) 100 ☐	1/6 250 ☐	1/2 500 ☐	1 1000 ☐	2 or more 2000 or more ☐

(Modified and printed with permission of Siemens Medical Solutions Diagnostic, Tarrytown, NY 10591.)

Multistix® 10 SG Reagent Strips for Urinalysis

PATIENT _____

DATE _____ TIME _____

LEUKOCYTES	NEGATIVE ☐		TRACE ☐	SMALL + ☐	MODERATE ++ ☐	LARGE +++ ☐	
NITRITE	NEGATIVE ☐		POSITIVE ☐	POSITIVE ☐	(Any degree of uniform pink color is found)		
UROBILINOGEN	NORMAL 0.2 ☐	NORMAL 1 ☐	mg/dL 2 ☐	4 ☐	8 ☐	(1mg = approx. 1 BU)	
PROTEIN	NEGATIVE ☐	TRACE ☐	mg/dL 30 * ☐	100 ++ ☐	300 +++ ☐	2000 OR MORE ☐	
pH	5.0 ☐	6.0 ☐	6.5 ☐	7.0 ☐	7.5 ☐	8.0 ☐	8.5 ☐
BLOOD	NEGATIVE ☐	NON-HEMOLYZED TRACE ☐	NON-HEMOLYZED MODERATE ☐	HEMOLYZED TRACE ☐	SMALL + ☐	MODERATE ++ ☐	LARGE +++ ☐
SPECIFIC GRAVITY	1.000 ☐	1.006 ☐	1.010 ☐	1.015 ☐	1.020 ☐	1.025 ☐	1.030 ☐
KETONE	NEGATIVE ☐	mg/dL	TRACE 5 ☐	SMALL 15 ☐	MODERATE 40 ☐	LARGE 80 ☐	LARGE 160 ☐
BILIRUBIN	NEGATIVE ☐		SMALL + ☐	MODERATE ++ ☐	LARGE +++ ☐		
GLUCOSE	NEGATIVE ☐	g/L (%) mg/dL	1/10 (tr.) 100 ☐	1/6 250 ☐	1/2 500 ☐	1 1000 ☐	2 or more 2000 or more ☐

(Modified and printed with permission of Siemens Medical Solutions Diagnostic, Tarrytown, NY 10591.)

Notes

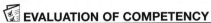

Procedure 16-4: Prepare a Urine Specimen for Microscopic Examination: Kova Method

Name: _____   Date: _____

Evaluated by: _____   Score: _____

Performance Objective

Outcome:	Prepare a urine specimen for microscopic analysis by the physician.
Conditions:	Given the following: disposable gloves; first-voided morning urine specimen; Kova urine centrifuge tube, cap, pipet, slide, and stain; test tube rack; urine centrifuge; mechanical stage microscope; and waste container.
Standards:	Time: 15 minutes. Student completed procedure in _____ minutes.
	Accuracy: Satisfactory score on the Performance Evaluation Checklist.

Performance Evaluation Checklist

Trial 1	Trial 2	Point Value	Performance Standards
		•	Sanitized hands.
		•	Assembled equipment.
		•	Applied gloves.
		•	Mixed the urine specimen with a pipet.
		▷	Stated the purpose of mixing the specimen.
		•	Poured the urine specimen into a urine centrifuge tube to the 12-mL mark.
		•	Capped the tube.
		•	Centrifuged the specimen for 5 minutes.
		▷	Stated the purpose of centrifuging the specimen.
		•	Removed the tube from the centrifuge without disturbing the sediment.
		•	Removed the cap.
		•	Inserted a Kova pipet into the urine tube and seated it firmly.
		•	Poured off the supernatant fluid.
		•	Removed the pipet from the tube.
		•	Added 1 drop of Kova stain to the tube.
		▷	Stated the purpose of the stain.
		•	Placed the pipet back in the tube and mixed the specimen thoroughly.
		•	Placed the urine tube in the test tube rack.
		•	Transferred a sample of the specimen to the Kova slide.
		•	Did not overfill or underfill the well of the Kova slide.
		•	Placed the pipet in the urine tube.
		•	Allowed the specimen to sit for 1 minute.
		▷	Explained the purpose of allowing the specimen to sit 1 minute.

Trial 1	Trial 2	Point Value	Performance Standards
		•	Properly focused the specimen under low power.
		•	Placed the slide on the stage of the microscope.
		•	Properly focused the specimen for the physician.
		•	Removed the slide from the stage when the physician was finished examining the specimen.
		•	Disposed of the slide and pipet in a regular waste container.
		•	Rinsed the remaining urine down the sink.
		•	Capped the empty urine tube and disposed of it in a regular waste container.
		•	Removed gloves and sanitized hands.
		✶	Completed the procedure within 15 minutes.
			Totals
CHART			
Date			

Evaluation of Student Performance

EVALUATION CRITERIA			COMMENTS
Symbol	**Category**	**Point Value**	
✶	Critical Step	16 points	
•	Essential Step	6 points	
▷	Theory Question	2 points	

Score calculation: 100 points

− _____ points missed

_____ Score

Satisfactory score: 85 or above

CAAHEP Competencies Achieved

Psychomotor (Skills)

☑ I. 11. Perform quality control measures.

☑ I. 14. Perform urinalysis.

Affective (Behavior)

☑ III. 2. Explain the rationale for performance of a procedure to the patient.

ABHES Competencies Achieved

☑ 10. a. Practice quality control.

☑ 10. b. Perform selected CLIA-waived tests that assist with diagnosis and treatment (1) Urinalysis.

Notes

Procedure 16-5: Performing a Rapid Urine Culture Test

Name: _____ Date: _____

Evaluated by: _____ Score: _____

Performance Objective

Outcome:	Perform a rapid urine culture test.
Conditions:	Given the following: disposable gloves, rapid urine culture kit, clean-catch midstream urine specimen, incubator and biohazard waste container.
Standards:	Time: 5 minutes. Student completed procedure in _____ minutes.
	Accuracy: Satisfactory score on the Performance Evaluation Checklist.

Performance Evaluation Checklist

Trial 1	Trial 2	Point Value	Performance Standards
			Preparing the specimen
		•	Sanitized hands.
		•	Assembled equipment.
		•	Checked the expiration date on the rapid culture test.
		•	Labeled the vial with the patient's name, date of birth, and date and time of inoculation.
		•	Applied gloves.
		•	Removed the slide from the vial.
		•	Did not touch the culture media.
		•	Completely immersed the slide in the urine specimen.
		•	Allowed the excess urine to drain from the slide.
		•	Immediately replaced the slide in the vial.
		•	Screwed the cap on loosely.
		•	Placed the vial upright in an incubator.
		▷	Explained why the slide should not remain in the incubator for more than 24 hours.
			Reading test results
		•	Applied gloves.
		•	Removed the vial from the incubator.
		•	Removed the slide from the vial.
		•	Compared the slide with the reference chart.
		•	Read and interpreted the results.
		✶	The results were identical to the evaluator's results.
		•	Returned the slide to the vial and screwed on the cap.
		•	Disposed of the test in a biohazard waste container.

Trial 1	Trial 2	Point Value	Performance Standards
		•	Removed gloves and sanitized hands.
		•	Charted the results correctly.
		✶	Completed the procedure within 5 minutes.
			Totals

CHART

Date	

Evaluation of Student Performance

EVALUATION CRITERIA			COMMENTS
Symbol	**Category**	**Point Value**	
✶	Critical Step	16 points	
•	Essential Step	6 points	
▷	Theory Question	2 points	

Score calculation: 100 points

−_____ points missed

_____ Score

Satisfactory score: 85 or above

CAAHEP Competencies Achieved

Psychomotor (Skills)

☑ III. 8. Perform CLIA-waived microbiology testing.

Affective (Behavior)

☑ II. 2. Distinguish between normal and abnormal test results.

ABHES Competencies Achieved

☑ 10. b. Perform selected CLIA-waived tests that assist with diagnosis and treatment (5) Microbiology testing.

Procedure 16-6: Performing a Urine Pregnancy Test

Name: _____   Date: _____

Evaluated by: _____   Score: _____

Performance Objective

Outcome:	Perform a urine pregnancy test.
Conditions:	Given the following: disposable gloves, urine pregnancy testing kit, first-voided morning urine specimen and waste container.
Standards:	Time: 5 minutes. Student completed procedure in _____ minutes.
	Accuracy: Satisfactory score on the Performance Evaluation Checklist.

Performance Evaluation Checklist

Trial 1	Trial 2	Point Value	Performance Standards
		•	Sanitized hands.
		•	Assembled equipment.
		•	Checked the expiration date on the pregnancy test.
		▷	Explained why the expiration date should be checked.
		•	If necessary, ran controls on the pregnancy test.
		▷	Stated when controls should be run.
		•	Applied gloves.
		•	Mixed the urine specimen.
		•	Removed the test cassette from its pouch.
		•	Placed the test cassette on a clean, dry, level surface.
		•	Added 3 drops of urine to the well on the test cassette.
		•	Disposed of the pipet in a regular waste container.
		•	Waited 3 minutes and read the results.
		•	Interpreted the test results.
		✶	The results were identical to the evaluator's results.
		▷	Described the appearance of a positive and a negative test result.
		▷	Explained what should be done if a blue control line does not appear.
		•	Disposed of the test cassette in a regular waste container.
		•	Removed gloves and sanitized hands.
		•	Charted the results correctly.
		✶	Completed the procedure within 5 minutes.
			Totals

CHART	
Date	

Evaluation of Student Performance

EVALUATION CRITERIA			COMMENTS
Symbol	**Category**	**Point Value**	
✶	Critical Step	16 points	
•	Essential Step	6 points	
▷	Theory Question	2 points	

Score calculation: 100 points

          −_____ points missed

          _____ Score

Satisfactory score: 85 or above

CAAHEP Competencies Achieved

Psychomotor (Skills)

☑ I. 11. Perform quality control measures.

☑ I. 16. Screen test results.

Affective (Behavior)

☑ II. 2. Distinguish between normal and abnormal test results.

ABHES Competencies Achieved

☑ 10. a. Practice quality control.

☑ 10. b. Perform selected CLIA-waived tests that assist with diagnosis and treatment (6) Kit testing (a) Pregnancy.

17 Phlebotomy

CHAPTER ASSIGNMENTS

√ After Completing	Date Due	Textbook Pages	TEXTBOOK ASSIGNMENTS	Possible Points	Points You Earned
		657–702	Read Chapter 17: Phlebotomy		
		667 700	Read Case Study 1 Case Study 1 questions	5	
		671 700	Read Case Study 2 Case Study 2 questions	5	
		684 700	Read Case Study 3 Case Study 3 questions	5	
			Total points		

√ After Completing	Date Due	Study Guide Pages	STUDY GUIDE ASSIGNMENTS (CTA = Critical Thinking Activity)	Possible Points	Points You Earned
		751	Pretest	10	
		752 752	Key Term Assessment A. Definitions B. Word Parts (Add 1 point for each medical term)	16 13	
		753–757	Evaluation of Learning questions	42	
		758	CTA A: Antecubital Veins	5	
			Evolve Site: Chapter 17 Got Blood?: Venipuncture Tray Set-Up (Record points earned)		
		758–759	CTA B: Venipuncture Vacuum Tube Method	15	
		759–760	CTA C: Venipuncture Situations	7	
		760–761	CTA D: Separating Serum	6	
		761	CTA E: Skin Puncture	8	
		762	CTA F: Crossword Puzzle	29	
			Evolve Site: Chapter 17 Nutrition Nugget: Eating Disorders	10	

√ After Completing	Date Due	Study Guide Pages	STUDY GUIDE ASSIGNMENTS (CTA = Critical Thinking Activity)	Possible Points	Points You Earned
			e Evolve Site: Apply Your Knowledge questions	10	
		763–764	*e* Video Evaluation	42	
		751	[?] Posttest	10	
			ADDITIONAL ASSIGNMENTS		
			Total points		

√ When Assigned by Your Instructor	Study Guide Pages	Practices Required	LABORATORY ASSIGNMENTS (Procedure Number and Name)	Score*
	765–766	5	*e* Practice for Competency 17-1: Venipuncture—Vacuum Tube Method Textbook reference: pp. 672–677	
	767–770		Evaluation of Competency 17-1: Venipuncture—Vacuum Tube Method	*
	765–766	5	*e* Practice for Competency 17-2: Venipuncture—Butterfly Method Textbook reference: pp. 680–684	
	771–774		Evaluation of Competency 17-2: Venipuncture—Butterfly Method	*
	765–766	3	Practice for Competency 17-3: Separating Serum from a Blood Specimen Textbook reference: pp. 688–690	
	775–776		Evaluation of Competency 17-3: Separating Serum from a Blood Specimen	*
	765–766	3	*e* Practice for Competency 17-4: Skin Puncture—Disposable Semiautomatic Lancet Device Textbook reference: pp. 695–697	
	777–778		Evaluation of Competency 17-4: Skin Puncture—Disposable Semiautomatic Lancet Device	*
	765–766	3	*e* Practice for Competency 17-5: Skin Puncture—Reusable Semiautomatic Lancet Device Textbook reference: pp. 697–699	
	779–780		Evaluation of Competency 17-5: Skin Puncture—Reusable Semiautomatic Lancet Device	*
			ADDITIONAL ASSIGNMENTS	

Notes

Name: _____ Date: _____

True or False

_____ 1. An individual who collects blood specimens is known as a vampire.

_____ 2. The purpose of applying a tourniquet when performing venipuncture is to make the patient's veins stand out.

_____ 3. The tourniquet should be left on the patient's arm for at least 2 minutes before performing a venipuncture.

_____ 4. Serum is obtained from whole blood that has been centrifuged.

_____ 5. A 25-gauge needle is recommended for performing venipuncture.

_____ 6. The size of the evacuated tube used to obtain a venous blood specimen depends on the size of the patient's veins.

_____ 7. A correct order of draw for the vacuum tube method of venipuncture is red, lavender, gray, and green.

_____ 8. Veins are most likely to collapse in patients with large veins and thick walls.

_____ 9. Hemolysis of a blood specimen results in inaccurate test results.

_____ 10. When obtaining a capillary specimen, the first drop of blood should be used for the test.

📝 POSTTEST

True or False

_____ 1. Venous reflux can be prevented by filling the evacuated tube to the exhaustion of the vacuum.

_____ 2. If the tourniquet is applied too tightly, inaccurate test results may occur.

_____ 3. The median cubital vein is the best vein to use for venipuncture.

_____ 4. On standing, a blood specimen to which an anticoagulant has been added separates into plasma, buffy coat, and blood cells.

_____ 5. Whole blood is obtained by using a tube containing an anticoagulant.

_____ 6. An evacuated glass tube with a lavender stopper contains EDTA.

_____ 7. A red-stoppered tube is used to collect a blood specimen for most blood chemistries.

_____ 8. Not filling a tube to the exhaustion of the vacuum can result in hemolysis of the blood specimen.

_____ 9. If the needle is removed from the arm before removing the tourniquet, the evacuated tube will not fill completely.

_____ 10. If a fibrin clot forms in the serum layer of a blood specimen, it will lead to inaccurate test results.

A. Definitions

Directions: Match each medical term (numbers) with its definition (letters).

_____ 1. Antecubital space

_____ 2. Anticoagulant

_____ 3. Buffy coat

_____ 4. Evacuated tube

_____ 5. Hematoma

_____ 6. Hemoconcentration

_____ 7. Hemolysis

_____ 8. Osteochondritis

_____ 9. Osteomyelitis

_____ 10. Phlebotomist

_____ 11. Phlebotomy

_____ 12. Plasma

_____ 13. Serum

_____ 14. Venipuncture

_____ 15. Venous reflux

_____ 16. Venous stasis

A. The liquid part of blood, consisting of a clear, straw-colored fluid that makes up approximately 55% of the blood volume
B. A substance that inhibits blood clotting
C. Health professional trained in the collection of blood specimens
D. The breakdown of blood cells
E. A closed glass or plastic tube that contains a premeasured vacuum
F. The temporary cessation or slowing of the venous blood flow
G. A thin, light-colored layer of white blood cells and platelets that lies between a top layer of plasma and a bottom layer of red blood cells when an anticoagulant has been added to a blood specimen
H. The surface of the arm in front of the elbow
I. Inflammation of bone and cartilage
J. An increase in the concentration of the nonfilterable blood components
K. Plasma from which the clotting factor fibrinogen has been removed
L. Incision of a vein for the removal of blood
M. Inflammation of the bone or bone marrow as a result of bacterial infection
N. A swelling or mass of coagulated blood caused by a break in a blood vessel
O. Puncturing of a vein
P. The backflow of blood (from an evacuated tube) into the patient's vein

B. Word Parts

Directions: Indicate the meaning of each word part in the space provided. List as many medical terms as possible that incorporate the word part in the space provided.

Word Part	Meaning of Word Part	Medical Terms That Incorporate Word Part
1. ante-		
2. anti-		
3. hemat/o		
4. -oma		
5. hem/o		
6. lysis		
7. oste/o		
8. myel/o		
9. -itis		
10. phleb/o		
11. -otomy		
12. ven/o		
13. -ous		

Directions: Fill in each blank with the correct answer.

1. List the three major areas of blood collection included in phlebotomy.

_____

_____

_____

2. What is the purpose of performing a venipuncture?

_____

_____

3. List the two methods that can be used to perform a venipuncture.

_____

_____

_____

4. What are the advantages of using the vacuum tube method of venipuncture?

_____

_____

5. When would the butterfly method of venipuncture be preferred over the vacuum tube method?

_____

_____

_____

6. What reference source should be consulted for collection and handling requirements in the following situations?

   a. The specimen is being transported to an outside laboratory for testing:

   _____

   b. The specimen is being tested in the medical office:

   _____

7. Why should a patient be identified using two forms of identification?

_____

_____

8. What is a unique identifier?

_____

9. Explain how to prevent venous reflux.

_____

_____

10. What is the purpose of the tourniquet?

_____

_____

11. Why are the antecubital veins preferred for performing a venipuncture?

_____

_____

_____

12. After locating a suitable vein for venipuncture, what three qualities should be determined with respect to the vein?

_____

_____

_____

13. List four techniques that can be used to make veins more prominent.

_____

_____

_____

_____

14. Why should the veins of the hand be used only as a last resort when performing a venipuncture?

_____

_____

_____

15. How is a serum specimen obtained?

_____

_____

16. How is a whole blood specimen obtained?

_____

_____

17. List the three layers into which blood separates when it is mixed with an anticoagulant.

_____

_____

18. List the layers into which blood separates when an anticoagulant is not added to it.

_____

_____

19. List six OSHA safety precautions that must be followed when performing a venipuncture and separating serum or plasma from whole blood.

_____

_____

_____

_____

20. What is the range for the gauge and length of the needle used for the vacuum tube method of venipuncture?

_____

_____

21. What is the purpose of the flange on the plastic holder of the vacuum tube system?

_____

_____

22. What type of additive is present in each of the following evacuated tubes?

Red _____

Red/gray speckled _____

Lavender _____

Light blue _____

Green _____

Gray _____

Royal blue _____

23. What color stopper must be used to collect the blood specimen for each of the tests listed?

Complete blood count _____

Prothrombin time _____

Glucose tolerance test _____

Most blood chemistry tests _____

Blood gas determinations _____

Lead testing _____

24. Why is it important to use the correct order of draw when performing a venipuncture?

_____

_____

25. Why is it important to mix a tube containing an anticoagulant immediately after drawing it?

_____

_____

26. What is the range for the gauge and length of needle used for the butterfly method of venipuncture?

_____

_____

27. How can a vein be prevented from rolling when performing a venipuncture on the cephalic or basic veins?

_____

_____

28. What is typically observed when performing a venipuncture on a vein that collapses?

_____

_____

29. What are three ways in which a hematoma may occur?

_____

_____

_____

30. List four ways to prevent a blood specimen from becoming hemolyzed.

_____

_____

_____

_____

31. List examples of substances dissolved in the serum of blood.

_____

_____

_____

32. What is the purpose of performing laboratory tests on serum?

_____

_____

_____

33. List the proper size tube that must be used to obtain the following serum specimens.

2 mL of serum _____

6 mL of serum _____

4 mL of serum _____

34. What is a fibrin clot, and why should it be avoided in a serum specimen?

_____

_____

_____

35. How does a serum separator tube function in the collection of a serum specimen?

_____

_____

_____

36. List four types of solutes contained in the plasma.

_____

_____

_____

_____

37. What is the preferred site for a skin puncture for the following individuals?
    a. Adult _____
    b. Infant _____

38. Why is it important not to penetrate the skin too deeply when performing a skin puncture?

_____

_____

39. How does the medical assistant determine the blade length to use to perform a skin puncture?

_____

_____

40. What are two examples of microcollection devices?

_____

_____

41. Why should a finger puncture not be performed on the index finger?

_____

_____

42. Why should the first drop of blood be wiped away when performing a finger puncture?

_____

_____

CRITICAL THINKING ACTIVITIES

A. Antecubital Veins

Practice palpating the antecubital veins on at least five classmates. Use a tourniquet applied to each person's arm, and ask the individual to clench his or her fist. Record the individual's name and which vein would be considered the best to use on each person when performing venipuncture.

	NAME	SUITABLE VEIN
1.		
2.		
3.		
4.		
5.		

B. Venipuncture—Vacuum Tube Method

Using the principles outlined in the vacuum tube venipuncture procedure, state what can happen under the following circumstances:

1. An evacuated tube is used that is past its expiration date.

_____

_____

2. The vacuum tube is not labeled.

_____

_____

3. The tourniquet is not applied tightly enough.

_____

_____

4. The tourniquet is left on for more than 1 minute.

_____

_____

5. The area that has just been cleansed with an antiseptic is not allowed to dry before the venipuncture is made.

_____

_____

6. The evacuated tube is inserted past the indentation in the plastic holder before the vein is entered.

_____

_____

7. An angle of less than 15 degrees is used when performing venipuncture.

_____

_____

8. An angle of more than 15 degrees is used when performing venipuncture.

_____

_____

9. The needle is moved after inserting it.

_____

_____

10. Venous reflux occurs when using an EDTA evacuated tube.

_____

_____

11. The vacuum tube is removed before it has filled to the exhaustion of the vacuum.

_____

_____

12. The needle is removed from the arm before the tourniquet has been removed.

_____

_____

13. A gauze pad is not placed slightly above the puncture site before removing the needle.

_____

_____

14. The patient bends the arm at the elbow after the needle is removed.

_____

_____

15. The patient lifts a heavy object after the procedure.

_____

_____

C. Venipuncture Situations

You are responsible for performing the venipunctures in your medical office. In the space provided, explain what you would do in each of the following situations:

1. The patient asks you whether the venipuncture will hurt.

_____

_____

2. On palpating the patient's vein, you find that it feels stiff and hard.

_____

_____

3. You have attempted one venipuncture in a patient with small veins by using the vacuum tube method of venipuncture; however, the vein collapsed, and you were unable to obtain blood.

_____

_____

4. The patient moves during the procedure, thus causing the needle to come out of his or her arm.

_____

_____

5. You have inserted the needle in the vein but notice a sudden swelling around the puncture site.

_____

_____

6. You inadvertently puncture the brachial artery after inserting the needle.

_____

_____

7. The patient begins to sweat and tells you that he or she feels warm and light-headed.

_____

_____

D. Separating Serum
Explain why the following guidelines must be observed while separating serum from whole blood.

1. Label the transfer tube with the word serum.

_____

_____

2. Place the tube in an upright position for 30 to 45 minutes.

_____

_____

3. Do not allow the specimen to stand for more than 1 hour before centrifuging it.

_____

_____

4. Make sure the tube is stoppered during centrifugation.

_____

_____

5. Wear personal protective equipment when transferring serum from whole blood.

_____

_____

6. Do not disturb the cell layer while pipetting the serum.

_____

_____

E. Skin Puncture

The medical assistant is performing a skin puncture on an adult patient to obtain a capillary blood specimen for a hemoglobin test. For each of the following situations, write **C** if the technique is correct and **I** if the technique is incorrect. If the technique is correct, explain the rationale for performing it that way; if incorrect, explain what might happen if the technique were performed in the incorrect manner.

_____ 1. Before making the puncture, the medical assistant asks the patient to rinse his or her hand in warm water.

_____

_____

_____ 2. The puncture is made with the patient in a standing position.

_____

_____

_____ 3. The site is allowed to dry thoroughly after it is cleansed with an antiseptic wipe.

_____

_____

_____ 4. The specimen is collected from the lateral part of the tip of the ring finger.

_____

_____

_____ 5. The puncture is made perpendicular to the lines of the fingerprint.

_____

_____

_____ 6. The depth of the puncture is 4 mm.

_____

_____

_____ 7. The first drop of blood is wiped away.

_____

_____

_____ 8. The puncture site is squeezed to obtain the blood specimen.

_____

_____

F. Crossword Puzzle: Phlebotomy

Directions: Complete the crossword puzzle using the clues provided.

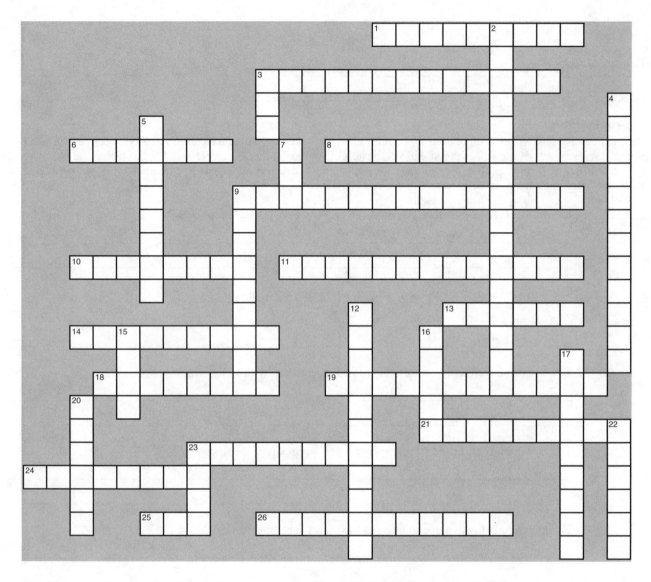

Across

1 What BP does during fainting
3 Makes RBCs clot quicker
6 Rolling vein
8 Best VP vein
9 Inflammation of bone and cartilage
10 Outdated tube problem
11 Inhibits blood clotting
13 Faint position
14 PT tube
18 EDTA tube
19 Back flow of blood
21 For small veins
23 Broken RBCs
24 Bad bruise
25 No additive tube
26 Based on size of pt's finger

Down

2 In front of the elbow
3 Select lavender tube for this test
4 Collects blood
5 First drop of capillary blood?
7 Contains a "separating" gel
9 Time limit for tourniquet
12 Do not use for skin puncture
15 Fluoride/oxalate tube
16 Don't use to palpate vein
17 WBCs and platelets
20 Fainting warning signal
22 Color of serum
23 Last choice veins

Name: _____

Directions:

a. Watch the indicated videos.
b. Mark each true statement with a T and each false statement with an F. For each false statement, change the wording of the question so that it becomes a true statement.

Video: Procedure 17-1: Venipuncture—Vacuum Tube Method

_____ 1. Venipuncture is performed when a large blood specimen is needed for laboratory testing.

_____ 2. The vacuum tube method is the fastest and most convenient venipuncture method.

_____ 3. Identify the patient by asking the patient to state his or her last name and Social Security number.

_____ 4. The patient should be asked whether he or she has prepared properly after performing the venipuncture.

_____ 5. A 25-gauge needle should be used to perform a venipuncture.

_____ 6. A red-stoppered tube should be used to collect a specimen for a CBC.

_____ 7. Outdated evacuated tubes may no longer have a vacuum.

_____ 8. A lavender-stoppered tube should be drawn before a serum separator tube.

_____ 9. The tourniquet should be applied 3 to 4 inches above the bend in the elbow.

_____ 10. The tourniquet should be applied as tightly as possible.

_____ 11. The tourniquet should never be left on for more than 1 minute at a time.

_____ 12. The alcohol should be allowed to dry at the puncture site to provide enough time for it to destroy microorganisms on the skin.

_____ 13. The needle should be positioned at a 30-degree angle to the patient's skin.

_____ 14. As the vein is entered, a sensation of resistance is felt, followed by a "release."

_____ 15. The evacuated tube should be filled to the exhaustion of the vacuum.

_____ 16. The flange should be used to remove the evacuated tube from the holder.

_____ 17. If the tube contains an anticoagulant, it should be vigorously shaken 8 to 10 times.

_____ 18. The needle should be withdrawn at the same angle as that for penetration.

_____ 19. The SST should be allowed to stand in an upright position for 10 to 15 minutes before centrifuging it.

_____ 20. The blood tubes should be placed in a biohazard specimen bag for transport to an outside laboratory.

Video: Procedure 17-2: Venipuncture—Butterfly Method

_____ 1. The butterfly method of venipuncture is also known as the *winged infusion method.*

_____ 2. The butterfly method is used for small or sclerosed veins.

_____ 3. The gauge of the needle for the butterfly method ranges between 18 and 20.

_____ 4. The tubing of the butterfly setup should be stretched slightly to permit a free flow of blood in the tubing.

_____ 5. The vein selected for the venipuncture should be thoroughly palpated with the thumb.

_____ 6. The puncture site should be cleansed using a circular motion.

_____ 7. If the alcohol is not permitted to dry, the patient may experience a stinging sensation when the needle is inserted.

_____ 8. The needle should be positioned so that it points in the same direction as the vein to be entered.

_____ 9. If the butterfly needle is in the vein, a flash of blood will appear at the top of the tubing.

_____ 10. Seating the needle lets you use both hands for changing tubes.

_____ 11. The evacuated tube should be allowed to fill from the top downward.

_____ 12. If the tube is removed before the vacuum is exhausted, the patient will develop a hematoma.

_____ 13. The tube should be gently inverted 5 times if it contains a clot activator.

_____ 14. The needle should be removed before removing the tourniquet.

_____ 15. The patient should be instructed to bend the arm at the elbow after the needle is removed.

Video: Procedures 17-4 and 17-5: Obtaining a Capillary Blood Specimen

_____ 1. The index or little finger should be used when performing a finger puncture.

_____ 2. If the alcohol is not allowed to dry, the blood may leach out and run down the finger.

_____ 3. Wet alcohol should be wiped off the puncture site with a gauze pad.

_____ 4. The puncture should be made in the center of the fingertip.

_____ 5. Moving the lancet too soon after making the puncture can lead to an inadequate puncture and poor blood flow.

_____ 6. The first drop of blood should be wiped away with an antiseptic wipe.

_____ 7. Squeezing or massaging the puncture site excessively causes dilution of the blood sample with tissue fluid leading to inaccurate test results.

PRACTICE FOR COMPETENCY

Procedure 17-1: Venipuncture—Vacuum Tube Method. Practice the procedure for collecting a venous blood specimen with the vacuum tube method. Record the procedure in the chart provided.

Procedure 17-2: Venipuncture—Butterfly Method. Practice the procedure for collecting a venous blood specimen with the butterfly method. Record the procedure in the chart provided.

Procedure 17-3: Separating Serum from Whole Blood. Separate serum from whole blood, and record the procedure in the chart provided.

Procedure 17-4: Disposable Lancet. Obtain a capillary blood specimen using a disposable semiautomatic lancet device.

Procedure 17-5: Reusable Lancet. Obtain a capillary blood specimen using a reusable semiautomatic lancet.

CHART	
Date	

	CHART
Date	

Procedure 17-1: Venipuncture—Vacuum Tube Method

Name: _____   Date: _____

Evaluated by: _____   Score: _____

Performance Objective

Outcome:	Perform a venipuncture using the vacuum tube method.
Conditions:	Given the following: disposable gloves, tourniquet, antiseptic wipe, double-pointed needle, plastic holder, evacuated tubes with labels, gauze pad, adhesive bandage, biohazard sharps container, biohazard specimen bag, and a laboratory request form.
Standards:	Time: 10 minutes. Student completed procedure in _____ minutes.
	Accuracy: Satisfactory score on the Performance Evaluation Checklist.

Performance Evaluation Checklist

Trial 1	Trial 2	Point Value	Performance Standards
		•	Reviewed requirements for collecting and handling the blood specimen.
		•	Sanitized hands.
		•	Greeted the patient and introduced yourself.
		•	Identified the patient.
		•	Asked the patient whether he or she prepared properly.
			Prepared the equipment
		•	Assembled equipment.
		•	Selected the proper evacuated tubes.
		•	Checked the expiration date of the tubes.
		▷	Stated the purpose of checking the expiration date.
		•	Labeled the evacuated tubes.
		•	Completed a laboratory request form, if necessary.
		•	Screwed the plastic holder onto the Luer adapter and tightened securely.
		•	Opened the gauze packet.
		•	Positioned the evacuated tubes in the correct order of draw.
		•	Tapped the evacuated tubes with a powdered additive below the stopper.
		▷	Stated the purpose for tapping the tube.
		•	Placed the first tube loosely in the plastic holder.
			Prepared the patient
		•	Explained the procedure to the patient and reassured the patient.
		•	Performed a preliminary assessment of both arms.
		•	Correctly applied the tourniquet.

Trial 1	Trial 2	Point Value	Performance Standards
		•	Asked the patient to clench fist.
		▷	Stated the purpose of the tourniquet and clenched fist.
		•	Assessed the veins of both arms.
		•	Determined the best vein to use.
		•	Positioned the patient's arm correctly.
		•	Thoroughly palpated the selected vein.
		•	Did not leave the tourniquet on for more than 1 minute.
		▷	Explained why the tourniquet should not be left on for more than 1 minute.
		•	Removed the tourniquet and cleansed the puncture site.
		•	Allowed the puncture site to air dry.
		▷	Explained why the site should be allowed to air dry.
		•	Did not touch the site after cleansing.
		•	Placed supplies within comfortable reach of the nondominant hand.
		•	Reapplied the tourniquet and applied gloves.
			Performed the venipuncture
		•	Correctly positioned the safety shield and removed the cap from the needle.
		•	Properly held the venipuncture setup (bevel up) with the dominant hand.
		•	Positioned the tube with the label facing downward.
		▷	Explained why the label should face downward.
		•	Grasped the patient's arm and anchored the vein correctly.
		•	Positioned the venipuncture setup at a 15-degree angle to the arm, with the needle pointing in the same direction as the vein to be entered.
		•	Positioned the needle approximately $\frac{1}{8}$ inch below the place where the vein is to be entered.
		•	Told the patient that a small stick will be felt.
		•	With one continuous motion, entered the skin and then the vein.
		•	Stabilized the vacuum tube setup.
			Stated why the vacuum tube setup should be stabilized.
		•	Pushed the tube forward slowly to the end of the holder by using the flange.
		•	Allowed evacuated tube to fill to the exhaustion of the vacuum.
		▷	Explained why the tube should be allowed to fill to the exhaustion of the vacuum.
		•	Removed the tube from the plastic holder by using the flange.
		•	Immediately and gently inverted tube 5 times if it contained a clot activator and 8 to 10 times if it contained an anticoagulant.
		•	Inserted the next tube into the holder using the flange.
		•	Continued until the last tube was filled.
		✱	Removed the tourniquet and asked the patient to unclench fist.
		•	Removed the last tube from the holder.
		▷	Stated why the last tube should be removed.

Trial 1	Trial 2	Point Value	Performance Standards
		•	Placed a gauze pad slightly above the puncture site and withdrew the needle slowly and at the same angle as that for penetration.
		•	Immediately moved the gauze over the puncture site and applied pressure.
		•	Pushed the safety shield forward with the thumb until an audible click is heard.
		•	Properly disposed of the holder and needle in a biohazard sharps container.
		•	Instructed the patient to apply pressure with the gauze pad for 1 to 2 minutes.
		▷	Stated why pressure should be applied.
		•	Applied an adhesive bandage to puncture site.
		•	Placed the tube in an upright position in a test tube rack.
		•	Removed gloves and sanitized hands.
		•	Charted the procedure correctly.
		•	Tested the specimen or prepared the specimen for transport according to medical office policy.
		✶	Completed the procedure within 10 minutes.
			Totals

CHART	
Date	

Evaluation of Student Performance

EVALUATION CRITERIA			COMMENTS
Symbol	**Category**	**Point Value**	
✶	Critical Step	16 points	
•	Essential Step	6 points	
▷	Theory Question	2 points	
Score calculation: 100 points			
− _____ points missed			
_____ Score			
Satisfactory score: 85 or above			

CAAHEP Competencies Achieved
Psychomotor (Skills)
☑ I. 2. Perform venipuncture.
Affective (Behavior)
☑ I. 1. Apply critical thinking skills in performing patient assessment and care.
☑ IV. I. Demonstrate empathy in communicating with patients, family, and staff.

ABHES Competencies Achieved
☑ 8. bb. Are impartial and show empathy when dealing with patients.
☑ 10. c. Dispose of biohazardous materials.
☑ 10. d. Collect, label, and process specimens (1) Perform venipuncture.

ⅇ Procedure 17-2: Venipuncture—Butterfly Method

Name: _____   Date: _____

Evaluated by: _____   Score: _____

Performance Objective

Outcome:	Perform a venipuncture using the butterfly method.
Conditions:	Given the following: disposable gloves, tourniquet, antiseptic wipe, winged infusion set, plastic holder, evacuated tubes with labels, gauze pad, adhesive bandage, biohazard sharps container, biohazard specimen bag, and a laboratory request form.
Standards:	Time: 10 minutes. Student completed procedure in _____ minutes.
	Accuracy: Satisfactory score on the Performance Evaluation Checklist.

Performance Evaluation Checklist

Trial 1	Trial 2	Point Value	Performance Standards
		•	Reviewed requirements for collecting and handling the blood specimen.
		•	Sanitized hands.
		•	Greeted the patient and introduced yourself.
		•	Identified the patient.
		▷	Stated why the patient must be correctly identified.
		•	Asked the patient whether he or she prepared properly.
		▷	Explained why it is important for the patient to prepare properly.
			Prepared the equipment
		•	Assembled equipment.
		•	Selected the proper evacuated tubes.
		•	Checked the expiration date of the tubes.
		•	Labeled the evacuated tubes.
		•	Completed a laboratory request form, if necessary.
		•	Removed the winged infusion set from its package.
		•	Extended the tubing to its full length and stretched it.
		▷	Explained why the tubing should be extended and stretched.
		•	Screwed the plastic holder onto the Luer adapter and tightened it securely.
		•	Opened the gauze packet.
		•	Positioned the evacuated tubes in the correct order of draw.
		•	Tapped the evacuated tubes with a powdered additive below the stopper.
		▷	Stated why tubes with powdered additives must be tapped.
		•	Placed the first tube loosely in the plastic holder with the label facing downward.
		•	Explained why the label should be facing downward.

Trial 1	Trial 2	Point Value	Performance Standards
			Prepared the patient
		•	Explained the procedure to the patient and reassured the patient.
		•	Performed a preliminary assessment of both arms.
		•	Correctly applied the tourniquet and asked the patient to clench fist.
		•	Assessed the veins of both arms.
		•	Determined the best vein to use.
		•	Positioned the patient's arm correctly.
		▷	Stated why the arm must be positioned correctly.
		•	Thoroughly palpated the selected vein.
		▷	Stated the purpose of palpating the vein.
		•	Did not leave the tourniquet on for more than 1 minute.
		•	Removed the tourniquet and cleansed the puncture site.
		•	Allowed the puncture site to air dry.
		•	Did not touch the site after cleansing.
		•	Placed supplies within comfortable reach.
		•	Reapplied tourniquet and applied gloves.
			Performed the venipuncture
		•	Grasped the winged infusion set correctly.
		•	Removed the protective shield.
		•	Positioned the needle with the bevel facing upward.
		▷	Explained why the bevel should be facing upward.
		•	Grasped the patient's arm and anchored the vein correctly.
		•	Positioned the needle at a 15-degree angle to arm, with the needle pointing in the same direction as the vein to be entered.
		•	Positioned the needle approximately $\frac{1}{8}$ inch below the place where the vein is to be entered.
		•	Told the patient that a small stick will be felt.
		•	With one continuous motion, entered the skin and then the vein.
		▷	Explained why a continuous motion should be used.
		•	Decreased the angle of the needle to 5 degrees.
		•	Seated the needle.
		▷	Stated the purpose of seating the needle.
		•	Opened the butterfly wings and rested them flat against the skin.
		•	Kept the tube and holder in a downward position.
		•	Slowly pushed the tube forward to the end of the plastic holder.
		•	Allowed the evacuated tube to fill to the exhaustion of the vacuum.
		▷	Explained why the tube should be filled to the exhaustion of the vacuum.
		•	Removed the tube from the plastic holder.
		•	Immediately and gently inverted the evacuated tube 5 times if it contained a clot activator and 8 to 10 times if it contained an anticoagulant.

Trial 1	Trial 2	Point Value	Performance Standards
		▷	Explained why a tube with an anticoagulant must be inverted immediately.
		•	Inserted the next tube into the holder.
		•	Continued until the last tube was filled.
		✻	Removed the tourniquet and asked the patient to unclench fist.
		▷	Stated why the tourniquet must be removed before the needle.
		•	Removed the last tube from the holder.
		•	Placed a gauze pad slightly above the puncture site. Grasped the setup just below the wings and withdrew the needle slowly and at the same angle as that for penetration.
		•	Immediately moved the gauze over the puncture site and applied pressure.
		•	Instructed the patient to apply pressure with the gauze.
		•	Activated the safety shield on the needle.
		•	Properly disposed of the winged infusion set and plastic holder in a biohazard sharps container.
		•	Continued to apply pressure for 1 to 2 minutes.
		•	Applied an adhesive bandage.
		•	Placed the tubes in an upright position in a test tube rack.
		•	Removed gloves and sanitized hands.
		•	Charted the procedure correctly.
		•	Tested the specimen or prepared the specimen for transport according to medical office policy.
		✻	Completed the procedure within 10 minutes.
			Totals

CHART

Date	

Evaluation of Student Performance

EVALUATION CRITERIA			COMMENTS
Symbol	**Category**	**Point Value**	
✻	Critical Step	16 points	
•	Essential Step	6 points	
▷	Theory Question	2 points	

Score calculation: 100 points

− _____ points missed

____ Score

Satisfactory score: 85 or above

Procedure 17-3: Separating Serum from a Blood Specimen

Name: _____ Date: _____

Evaluated by: _____ Score: _____

Performance Objective

Outcome:	Separate serum from whole blood.
Conditions:	Given the following: red evacuated tube venipuncture setup, test tube rack, disposable pipet, transfer tube and label, disposable gloves, face shield or mask and eye protection device, centrifuge, and a biohazard sharps container.
Standards:	Time: 20 minutes. Student completed procedure in _____ minutes.
	Accuracy: Satisfactory score on the Performance Evaluation Checklist.

Performance Evaluation Checklist

Trial 1	Trial 2	Point Value	Performance Standards
		•	Collected the blood specimen by performing a venipuncture.
		▷	Stated why a red-stoppered tube should be used.
		•	Placed the specimen tube in an upright position for 30 to 45 minutes at room temperature while keeping a stopper on the specimen tube.
		▷	Explained why the specimen tube must be placed in an upright position.
		•	Placed the specimen tube in the centrifuge, with stopper end upward.
		▷	Stated why the stopper must remain on the specimen tube.
		•	Balanced the specimen with the same type and weight of tube.
		▷	Stated the purpose for balancing the centrifuge.
		•	Centrifuged the specimen for 10 minutes.
		▷	Explained the purpose of centrifugation.
		•	Put on a face shield or a mask and an eye protection device and applied gloves.
		▷	Stated the purpose of wearing personal protective equipment.
		•	Removed the specimen tube from the centrifuge without disturbing the contents.
		▷	Explained what must be done if the contents of the tube are disturbed.
		•	Carefully removed the stopper from the tube.
		•	Squeezed the bulb of the pipet and placed the tip of the pipet against the side of specimen tube approximately ¼ inch above the cell layer.
		▷	Explained why the bulb should be squeezed before inserting the pipet into serum.
		•	Released the bulb to suction serum into the pipet.
		•	Transferred serum to the transfer tube.
		•	Did not disturb the cell layer.
		•	Continued pipetting until as much serum as possible was removed.

Trial 1	Trial 2	Point Value	Performance Standards
		•	Capped the specimen tube tightly and held it up to the light to examine it for hemolysis.
		▷	Explained what should be done if hemolysis is present in the specimen.
		•	Made sure that the proper amount of serum was obtained.
		•	Properly disposed of equipment.
		•	Removed gloves and sanitized hands.
		•	Tested the specimen or prepared the specimen for transport to an outside laboratory according to medical office policy.
		✶	Completed the procedure within 20 minutes.
			Totals

Evaluation of Student Performance

EVALUATION CRITERIA			COMMENTS
Symbol	**Category**	**Point Value**	
✶	Critical Step	16 points	
•	Essential Step	6 points	
▷	Theory Question	2 points	

Score calculation: 100 points

— _____ points missed

_____ Score

Satisfactory score: 85 or above

CAAHEP Competencies Achieved

Psychomotor (Skills)

☑ III. 2. Practice Standard Precautions.

Affective (Behavior)

☑ III. 1. Display sensitivity to patient rights and feelings in collecting specimens.

ABHES Competencies Achieved

☑ 10. d. Collect, label, and process specimens.

Procedure 17-4: Skin Puncture—Disposable Semiautomatic Lancet Device

Name: _____   Date: _____

Evaluated by: _____   Score: _____

Performance Objective

Outcome:	Obtain a capillary blood specimen.
Conditions:	Given the following: disposable gloves, antiseptic wipe, CoaguChek lancet, gauze pad, and a biohazard sharps container.
Standards:	Time: 5 minutes. Student completed procedure in _____ minutes.
	Accuracy: Satisfactory score on the Performance Evaluation Checklist.

Performance Evaluation Checklist

Trial 1	Trial 2	Point Value	Performance Standards
		•	Sanitized hands.
		•	Greeted the patient and introduced yourself.
		•	Identified the patient.
		•	Asked the patient whether he or she prepared properly.
		•	Assembled equipment.
		•	Opened a sterile gauze packet.
		•	Explained the procedure to the patient and reassured the patient.
		•	Seated the patient in a chair.
		•	Extended the palmar surface of patient's hand facing upward.
		•	Selected a puncture site.
		•	Warmed the site if needed.
		▷	Explained why the site should be warmed.
		•	Cleansed the puncture site and allowed it to air dry.
		▷	Explained why the site should be allowed to air dry.
		•	Did not touch the site after cleansing.
		•	Applied gloves.
		•	Firmly grasped the patient's finger.
		•	Positioned the lancet firmly on the fingertip slightly to the side of center.
		•	Depressed the activation button without moving the lancet or finger.
		▷	Stated why the lancet and finger should not be moved.
		•	Disposed of the lancet in a biohazard sharps container.
		•	Waited a few seconds to allow blood flow to begin.
		•	Wiped away the first drop of blood with a gauze pad.
		▷	Stated why the first drop of blood should be wiped away.

Trial 1	Trial 2	Point Value	Performance Standards
		•	Allowed a second large, well-rounded drop of blood to form.
		•	Did not squeeze finger to obtain blood.
		•	Collected the blood specimen on a test strip or in the appropriate microcollection device.
		•	Instructed the patient to hold a gauze pad over the puncture site with pressure.
		•	Remained with the patient until bleeding stopped.
		•	Applied an adhesive bandage if needed.
		•	Tested the blood specimen following the manufacturer's instructions.
		•	Removed gloves.
		•	Sanitized hands.
		✳	Completed the procedure within 5 minutes.
			Totals

Evaluation of Student Performance

EVALUATION CRITERIA			COMMENTS
Symbol	Category	Point Value	
✳	Critical Step	16 points	
•	Essential Step	6 points	
▷	Theory Question	2 points	

Score calculation: 100 points

      — _____ points missed

      _____ Score

Satisfactory score: 85 or above

CAAHEP Competencies Achieved

Psychomotor (Skills)

☑ I. 3. Perform capillary puncture.

Affective (Behavior)

☑ IV. I. Demonstrate empathy in communicating with patients, family, and staff.

ABHES Competencies Achieved

☑ 8. bb. Are impartial and show empathy when dealing with patients.

☑ 10. d. Collect, label, and process specimens (2) Perform capillary puncture.

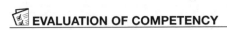 EVALUATION OF COMPETENCY

Procedure 17-5: Skin Puncture—Reusable Semiautomatic Lancet Device

Name: _____   Date: _____

Evaluated by: _____   Score: _____

Performance Objective

Outcome:	Obtain a capillary blood specimen.
Conditions:	Given the following: disposable gloves, antiseptic wipe, Glucolet II lancet device, sterile lancet/endcap, gauze pad, and a biohazard sharps container.
Standards:	Time: 10 minutes. Student completed procedure in _____ minutes.
	Accuracy: Satisfactory score on the Performance Evaluation Checklist.

Performance Evaluation Checklist

Trial 1	Trial 2	Point Value	Performance Standards
		•	Sanitized hands.
		•	Greeted the patient and introduced yourself.
		•	Identified the patient.
		•	Asked the patient whether he or she prepared properly.
		•	Assembled equipment.
		•	Pushed the transparent barrel toward the release button until it clicked into place.
		•	Inserted the lancet/endcap onto the lancet device.
		•	Opened a sterile gauze packet.
		•	Explained the procedure to the patient and reassured the patient.
		•	Seated the patient in a chair.
		•	Extended the palmar surface of patient's hand facing upward.
		•	Selected a puncture site.
		•	Warmed the site if needed.
		▷	Explained how patient's finger can be warmed.
		•	Cleansed the puncture site and allowed it to air dry.
		•	Applied gloves.
		•	Twisted off the plastic post from the endcap.
		•	Firmly grasped the patient's finger.
		•	Placed the endcap firmly on the fingertip slightly to the side of center.
		•	Depressed the activation button without moving the Glucolet or finger.
		•	Wiped away the first drop of blood with a gauze pad.
		•	Allowed a second large, well-rounded drop of blood to form.
		▷	Explained why the finger should not be squeezed.

Trial 1	Trial 2	Point Value	Performance Standards
		•	Collected the blood specimen on a test strip or in the appropriate microcollection device.
		•	Instructed the patient to hold a gauze pad over the puncture site with pressure.
		•	Remained with the patient until bleeding stopped.
		•	Applied an adhesive bandage if needed.
		•	Removed the endcap from the lancet device.
		•	Discarded the endcap in a biohazard waste container.
		•	Tested the blood specimen following the manufacturer's instructions.
		•	Removed gloves.
		•	Sanitized hands.
		•	Sanitized and disinfected the Glucolet.
		•	Stored the Glucolet in its resting position.
		✷	Completed the procedure within 5 minutes.
			Totals

Evaluation of Student Performance

EVALUATION CRITERIA			COMMENTS
Symbol	**Category**	**Point Value**	
✷	Critical Step	16 points	
•	Essential Step	6 points	
▷	Theory Question	2 points	

Score calculation: 100 points

− _____ points missed

_____ Score

Satisfactory score: 85 or above

CAAHEP Competencies Achieved

Psychomotor (Skills)

☑ I. 3. Perform capillary puncture.

Affective (Behavior)

☑ IV. I. Demonstrate empathy in communicating with patients, family, and staff.

ABHES Competencies Achieved

☑ 8. bb. Are impartial and show empathy when dealing with patients.

☑ 10. d. Collect, label, and process specimens (2) Perform capillary puncture.

18 Hematology

CHAPTER ASSIGNMENTS

√ After Completing	Date Due	Textbook Pages	TEXTBOOK ASSIGNMENTS	Possible Points	Points You Earned
		703–725	Read Chapter 18: Hematology		
		709 722	Read Case Study 1 Case Study 1 questions	5	
		715 722	Read Case Study 2 Case Study 2 questions	5	
		716 722	Read Case Study 3 Case Study 3 questions	5	
			Total points		

√ After Completing	Date Due	Study Guide Pages	STUDY GUIDE ASSIGNMENTS (CTA = Critical Thinking Activity)	Possible Points	Points You Earned
		785	Pretest	10	
		786 787	Term Key Term Assessment A. Definitions B. Word Parts (Add 1 point for each medical term)	19 18	
		788–791	Evaluation of Learning questions	42	
		792–794	CTA A: Diseases	40	
		795	CTA B: Hematocrit	5	
		795	CTA C: Iron Content of Food	10	
		796–797	CTA D: Iron-Deficiency Anemia	20	
		798	CTA E: Dear Gabby	10	
		799–802	CTA F: Find It! Game (Record points earned)		
			Evolve Site: Chapter 18: Name That Cell: Identification of Blood Cells (Record points earned)		
		803	CTA G: Crossword Puzzle	23	

√ After Completing	Date Due	Study Guide Pages	STUDY GUIDE ASSIGNMENTS (CTA = Critical Thinking Activity)	Possible Points	Points You Earned
			e Evolve Site: Chapter 18: Time for a Test: Hematologic Tests (Record points earned)		
			e Evolve Site: Chapter 18 Animations (2 points each)	10	
			e Evolve Site: Chapter 18 Nutrition Nugget: Anemias		
			e Evolve Site: Apply Your Knowledge questions	10	
		805–806	*e* Video Evaluation	38	
		785	?▤ Posttest	10	
			ADDITIONAL ASSIGNMENTS		
			Total points		

782

Chapter **18** Hematology

Copyright © 2015, 2012, 2008, 2004, 2000, 1995, 1990 by Saunders, an imprint of Elsevier Inc.
All rights reserved.

√ When Assigned by Your Instructor	Study Guide Pages	Practices Required	LABORATORY ASSIGNMENTS (Procedure Number and Name)	Score*
	807–809	3	Practice for Competency 18-A: Hemoglobin Determination Textbook reference: p. 708	
	811–813		Evaluation of Competency 18-A: Hemoglobin Determination	*
	807–808	3	Practice for Competency 18-1: Hematocrit Textbook reference: pp. 710–712	
	815–817		Evaluation of Competency 18-1: Hematocrit	*
	807–808	10	Practice for Competency 18-2: Preparation of a Blood Smear for a Differential Cell Count Textbook reference: pp. 716–718	
	819–820		Evaluation of Competency 18-2: Preparation of a Blood Smear for a Differential Cell Count	*
			ADDITIONAL ASSIGNMENTS	

Notes

⦅?⦆ PRETEST

True or False

_____ 1. Plasma makes up approximately 55% of the blood volume.

_____ 2. A mature erythrocyte has a biconcave shape and contains a nucleus.

_____ 3. Erythrocytes are responsible for defending the body against infection.

_____ 4. The life span of a red blood cell is 120 days.

_____ 5. The function of hemoglobin is to assist in blood clotting.

_____ 6. Leukocytosis is an abnormal increase in the number of leukocytes.

_____ 7. Another name for a thrombocyte is a platelet.

_____ 8. A low hemoglobin reading occurs with polycythemia.

_____ 9. An increase in neutrophils occurs during an acute infection.

_____ 10. The PT test measures how long it takes for an individual's blood to form a clot.

⦅?⦆ POSTTEST

True or False

_____ 1. A function of the plasma is to transport antibodies, enzymes, and hormones.

_____ 2. The red bone marrow of the sternum produces red blood cells in the adult.

_____ 3. The normal range for a red blood cell count for an adult female is 4 to 5.5 million.

_____ 4. The normal range for hemoglobin for an adult male is 12 to 16 g/dL.

_____ 5. The normal adult range for a white blood cell count is 4500 to 11,000.

_____ 6. Leukocytes do their work in the tissues.

_____ 7. Bilirubin is an orange-colored pigment that is produced through the breakdown of hemoglobin.

_____ 8. An immature form of a neutrophil is known as a seg.

_____ 9. The primary function of a neutrophil is to form antibodies.

_____ 10. The function of warfarin is to inhibit the growth of bacteria in the body.

A. Definitions

Directions: Match each medical term (numbers) with its definition (letters).

_____ 1. Ameboid movement

_____ 2. Anemia

_____ 3. Anisocytosis

_____ 4. Anticoagulant

_____ 5. Bilirubin

_____ 6. Diapedesis

_____ 7. Hematology

_____ 8. Hemoglobin

_____ 9. Hemolysis

_____ 10. Hypochromic

_____ 11. Leukocytosis

_____ 12. Leukopenia

_____ 13. Microcytic

_____ 14. Macrocytic

_____ 15. Normochromic

_____ 16. Normocytic

_____ 17. Oxyhemoglobin

_____ 18. Phagocytosis

_____ 19. Polycythemia

A. An abnormal decrease in the number of white blood cells (less than 4500 per cubic millimeter of blood)

B. The breakdown of erythrocytes with the release of hemoglobin into the plasma

C. Movement used by leukocytes that permits them to propel themselves from the capillaries into the tissues

D. The ameboid movement of blood cells (especially leukocytes) through the wall of a capillary and out into the tissues

E. A disorder in which there is an increase in the red blood cell mass

F. A condition in which there is a decrease in the number of erythrocytes or in the amount of hemoglobin in the blood

G. Hemoglobin that has combined with oxygen

H. The study of blood and blood-forming tissues

I. An abnormal increase in the number of white blood cells (greater than 11,000 per cubic millimeter of blood)

J. An orange-colored bile pigment produced by the breakdown of heme from the hemoglobin molecule

K. The engulfing and destruction of foreign particles, such as bacteria, by special cells called *phagocytes*

L. The protein- and iron-containing pigment of erythrocytes that transports oxygen in the body

M. A substance that inhibits blood clotting

N. A red blood cell with a decreased concentration of hemoglobin

O. An abnormally small red blood cell

P. An abnormally large red blood cell

Q. A red blood cell with a normal concentration of hemoglobin

R. A normal-sized red blood cell

S. A variation in the size of red blood cells

B. Word Parts

Directions: Indicate the meaning of each word part in the space provided. List as many medical terms as possible that incorporate the word part in the space provided.

Word Part	Meaning of Word Part	Medical Terms That Incorporate Word Part
1. anis/o		
2. cyt/o		
3. -ia		
4. -osis		
5. anti-		
6. coagulant		
7. hemato/o		
8. -ology		
9. -lysis		
10. hypo-		
11. chrom/o		
12. -ic		
13. leuk/o		
14. -penia		
15. micro-		
16. norm/o		
17. phag/o		
18. poly-		

Directions: Fill in each blank with the correct answer.

1. List the tests generally included in a complete blood cell count (CBC).

   _____

   _____

2. What is the function of plasma?

   _____

   _____

3. Where are erythrocytes formed in the adult?

   _____

   _____

4. Describe the shape of an erythrocyte, and explain how it acquires this shape.

   _____

   _____

5. Describe the normal appearance of arterial and venous blood.

   _____

   _____

6. What is the average life span of a red blood cell?

   _____

7. What is the function of leukocytes?

   _____

   _____

8. Where do leukocytes do their work?

   _____

9. What is the function of platelets?

   _____

10. What is the normal range for platelets in an adult?

    _____

11. What is the normal hemoglobin range?

    a. Adult female: _____

    b. Adult male: _____

12. List five conditions that cause a decrease in the hemoglobin level.

_____

_____

_____

13. What is the purpose of the hematocrit?

_____

_____

14. What is the normal hematocrit range?

a. Adult female: _____

b. Adult male: _____

15. What is the normal range for the white blood count for an adult?

_____

16. List examples of conditions that may result in leukocytosis.

_____

_____

17. What is the normal range for the red blood count for an adult?

a. Adult female: _____

b. Adult male: _____

18. List the five types of white blood cells and the normal adult range for each.

_____

_____

_____

19. What is measured by each of the following red blood cell indices?

MCV: _____

MCH: _____

MCHC: _____

RDW: _____

20. What is the most common cause of microcytic anemia?

_____

21. What are the most common causes of macrocytic anemia?

_____

22. Hypochromia occurs with what type of conditions?

_____

23. What are the advantages of the following methods for performing a differential cell count?

a. Automatic method: _____

b. Manual: _____

24. Why must the white blood cells be stained when performing a manual differential cell count?

_____

_____

25. The least numerous type of white blood cell is the _____

26. Why are neutrophils also known as "segs"?

_____

_____

27. What is a band?

_____

28. The largest of the white blood cells is the _____

29. What is the function of lymphocytes?

_____

_____

30. List the abbreviation for each of the following tests:

a. Hematocrit _____

b. Hemoglobin _____

c. Differential cell count _____

d. White blood cell count _____

e. Red blood cell count _____

31. What does the PT test measure?

_____

32. What is the PT adult reference range?

_____

33. What is the purpose of performing an INR on a PT test?

_____

_____

Chapter **18** **Hematology**

34. What is the range for a PT/INR result of a healthy individual with a normal clotting ability?

_____

35. What is the function of warfarin?

_____

36. What are the most common conditions for which warfarin is prescribed?

_____

_____

37. What is the usual desired PT/INR range for a patient who is on warfarin therapy for a heart attack or stroke?

_____

38. What is the goal of warfarin therapy?

_____

_____

39. How often should a patient on warfarin therapy have a PT/INR test performed?

_____

40. What color-stoppered tube should be used to collect a specimen for a PT/INR test?

_____

41. Why is it important to fill the blood tube for a PT/INR test to the exhaustion of the vacuum?

_____

_____

42. What are the advantages of PT/INR home testing?

_____

_____

CRITICAL THINKING ACTIVITIES

A. Diseases

1. You and your classmates work at a large clinic. It is National Disease Awareness Week. The physicians at your clinic ask you to develop informative, creative, and colorful brochures for patients about various diseases. Choose a condition from the list, and design a brochure using the blank Frequently Asked Questions (FAQ) brochure provided on the following page. Each student in the class should select a different disease. On a separate sheet of paper, write three true/false questions relating to the information in your brochure.

2. Present your brochure to the class. After all the brochures have been presented, each student should ask three questions to the entire class to see how well the class understands the diseases that were presented. (*Note:* Students can take notes during the presentations and refer to them when answering the questions.)

Conditions
1. Addison's disease
2. Amyotrophic lateral sclerosis
3. Aplastic anemia
4. Bell's palsy
5. Cirrhosis
6. Crohn's disease
7. Cushing's syndrome
8. Cystic fibrosis
9. Degenerative disc disease
10. Epilepsy
11. Hemolytic anemia
12. Hemophilia
13. Hernia
14. Hodgkin's disease
15. Hyperthyroidism
16. Hypothyroidism
17. Leukemia
18. Lupus erythematosus
19. Multiple sclerosis
20. Muscular dystrophy
21. Parkinson's disease
22. Peptic ulcer
23. Pernicious anemia
24. Polycythemia
25. Sickle-cell anemia
26. Ulcerative colitis

FAQ
ON:

Q: A:

Q: A:

Q: A:

Q: A:

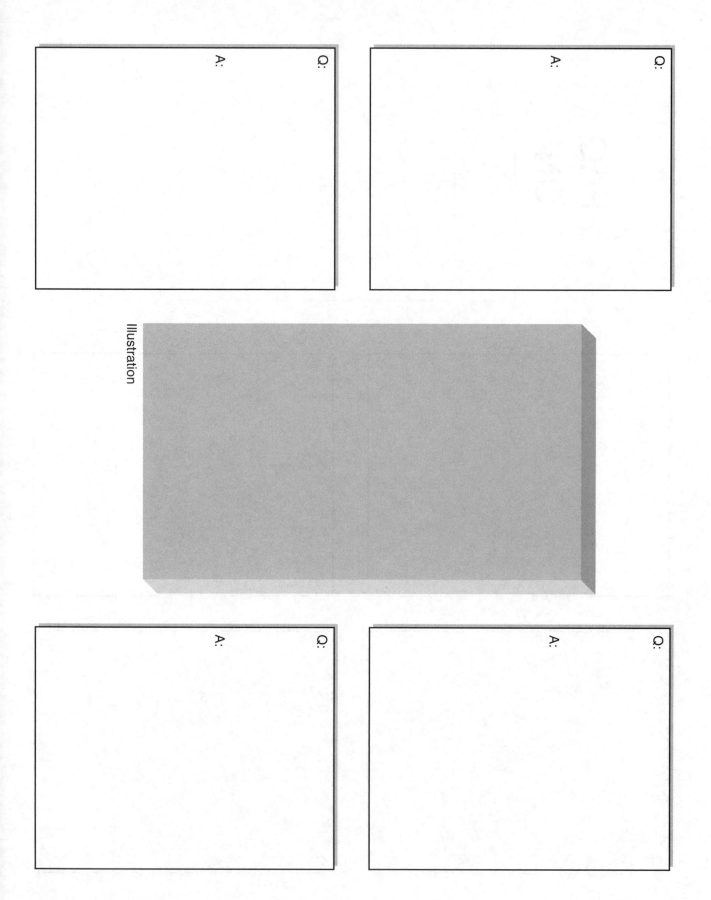

Q:

A:

Q:

A:

Illustration

Q:

A:

Q:

A:

B. Hematocrit

Label the layers of this microhematocrit capillary tube that has been centrifuged. Place an arrow at the point where you would take the hematocrit reading.

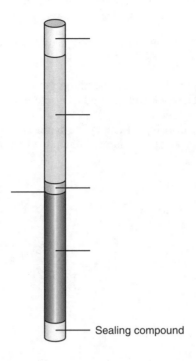

Sealing compound

C. Iron Content of Food

Consuming food that is high in iron helps to prevent iron-deficiency anemia. To become familiar with foods that are high in iron content and foods that contain little or no iron, plan the following two meals. One meal should be as high as possible in iron content, and the other meal should not contain any iron at all.

Meal 1

_____

_____

_____

_____

_____

Meal 2

_____

_____

_____

_____

_____

D. Iron-Deficiency Anemia

Create a profile of an individual who has iron-deficiency anemia following these guidelines:

1. Using colored pencils, crayons, or markers, draw a figure of an individual exhibiting iron-deficiency anemia. Be as creative as possible.

2. Do not use any text on your drawing other than to label items you have drawn in your picture. (A picture is worth a thousand words!)

3. Try to include all of the symptoms of iron-deficiency anemia in your drawing. The Iron-Deficiency Anemia Patient Teaching Box on pp. 709–710 in your textbook can be used as a reference source.

4. In the classroom, find a partner and trade drawings. Identify the symptoms of iron-deficiency anemia in your partner's drawing. With your partner, discuss what treatment is recommended and also what this person could do to prevent iron-deficiency anemia.

IRON-DEFICIENCY ANEMIA

E. Dear Gabby

Gabby is attending her class reunion and wants you to fill in for her. In the space provided, respond to the following letter.

Dear Gabby,

I am a housewife with two adorable children, ages 2 and 4. I have been feeling run down and tired lately, so I bought some vitamin pills at the drugstore. They came individually packaged in foil and plastic. They are hard to open, so I cut each package and transferred the iron pills to a little plastic baggie. When I told my mother about what I thought was a great idea, she got very upset. She told me that I could possibly be putting my children at danger. She said that iron is poisonous to children and that I should not do that. Gabby, my mom has always been overprotective. Is this just another one of her episodes?

Signed,

Curious in Kansas

_____

_____

_____

_____

_____

_____

_____

_____

_____

_____

_____

F. Find It! Game

Object: The object of the game is to identify the different types of blood cells.

Directions:

1. Cut out the game cards on the following page.
2. Refer to Figure 18-5 in your textbook.
3. Using colored pencils, draw the appropriate blood cell types on the blank side of the card.
4. Get into a group of three students.
5. Hold your game cards with the cells facing you.
6. In turn, each player "names" a blood cell. All players should place a blood cell on the table with the cell side facing upward.
7. When all players have placed a card on the table, turn the cards over.
8. Award yourself 5 points if you have correctly determined the proper blood cell. If you have a question regarding the correct answer, consult your instructor.
9. In turn, each player can earn an additional 5 points by stating a fact about that blood cell.
10. Keep track of your points on the score card provided below.
11. Continue the game until all of the game cards have been used.

FIND IT!
SCORE CARD

Name: _____

Recording Points:
Cross off a number each time you properly sequence a game card (starting with 5 and continuing in sequence). Cross off another number if you are able to state a fact about the blood cell. Your points will be equal to the last number you crossed off. Record this number in the space provided, and determine the knowledge level you attained.

Points:	
5	75
10	80
15	85
20	90
25	95
30	100
35	105
40	110
45	115
50	120
55	125
60	130
65	135
70	140

Total points:	_____
LEVEL OF KNOWLEDGE:	_____
☐ 70 to 80 points:	**No Signs of Anemia**
☐ 55 to 65 points:	**A Little Anemic**
☐ 50 points and below:	**Better Take Some Iron**

Notes

Red Blood Cell

Platelets

Neutrophil

Neutrophilic Band

Eosinophil

Basophil

Lymphocyte

Monocyte

G. Crossword Puzzle: Hematology

Directions: Complete the crossword puzzle using the clues provided.

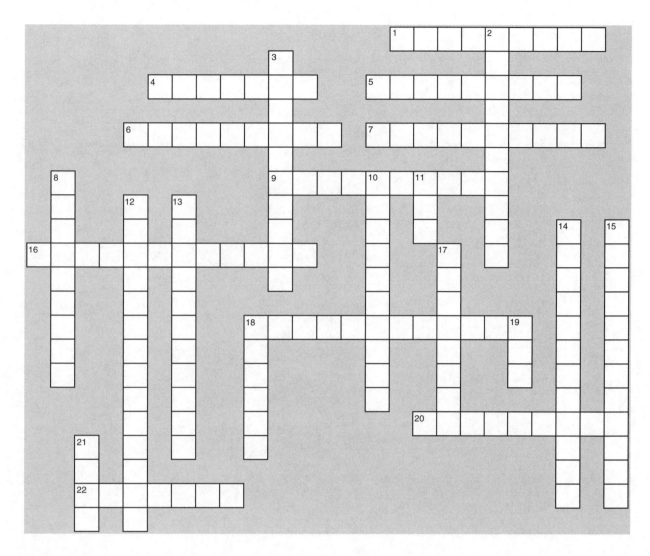

Across
1 Broken RBC
4 WBCs work here
5 Orange bile pigment
6 Platelets and WBCs
7 Study of blood
9 Produces antibodies
16 More than 11,000 WBCs
18 Engulfing pathogens
20 White blood cell
22 Not in an RBC

Down
2 Less than 4500 WBCs
3 Carries oxygen
8 Symptom of anemia
10 To separate blood
11 Common hematology test
12 Common cause of anemia
13 Red blood cell
14 Clots blood
15 Condition of too many RBCs
17 Largest WBC
18 Liquid part of blood
19 Neutrophil's other name
21 Immature neutrophil

Notes

Name: _____

Directions:

a. Watch the indicated videos.
b. Mark each true statement with a T and each false statement with an F. For each false statement, change the wording of the question so that it becomes a true statement.

Video: Procedure 18-A: Hemoglobin Determination

_____ 1. Hemoglobin transports oxygen in the body.

_____ 2. A low hemoglobin level may indicate polycythemia.

_____ 3. The hemoglobin meter must be calibrated each time a new container of test cards is used.

_____ 4. Calibrating the hemoglobin meter compensates for variables that occur in the manufacturing process of the test cards.

_____ 5. Three levels of controls must be run each day before you use the hemoglobin meter for the first time.

_____ 6. If the control result is within the acceptable range, it will fall within the expected control range listed on a reference sheet accompanying the control solution.

_____ 7. The control results should be recorded in the patient's chart.

_____ 8. The puncture site should not be touched after it has been cleansed.

_____ 9. After making the puncture, the first drop of blood should be wiped away with a gauze pad.

_____ 10. To obtain blood for the test, the patient's finger should be vigorously squeezed until a large drop of blood forms.

_____ 11. The hemoglobin test provides a direct reading of the amount of hemoglobin in whole blood in grams per deciliter.

_____ 12. The normal hemoglobin range for a female is 14 to 18 g/dL.

Video: Procedure 18-1: Hematocrit

_____ 1. The hematocrit measures the percentage volume of packed red blood cells in whole blood.

_____ 2. A hematocrit reading that is below normal may indicate anemia.

_____ 3. The patient should be identified by full name and date of birth.

_____ 4. After puncturing the patient's finger, the lancet should be discarded in a biohazard sharps container.

_____ 5. The capillary tube should be filled to the black calibration line.

_____ 6. Air bubbles entering the capillary tube lead to falsely high test results.

_____ 7. The capillary tubes must be sealed to prevent leakage of the blood specimen during centrifugation.

_____ 8. Capillary tubes should be placed in the centrifuge with the sealed ends facing inward.

_____ 9. Centrifuging the capillary tubes causes the red blood cells to become packed and to settle to the bottom of the tube.

_____ 10. When reading the test results, the bottom of the red blood cell column (located just above the sealing compound) should be placed on the zero line.

_____ 11. The hematocrit results should be read at the top of the buffy coat layer.

_____ 12. To be considered valid, the results of the capillary tubes should agree within 2 percentage points.

_____ 13. The normal range for a hematocrit for a female is 37% to 47%.

_____ 14. The capillary tubes should be discarded in a biohazard bag.

Video: Procedure 18-2: Preparation of a Blood Smear for a Differential Cell Count

_____ 1. The purpose of the differential cell count is to identify and count the five types of white blood cells (WBCs).

_____ 2. An increase or decrease in one or more types of WBCs may occur in pathologic conditions.

_____ 3. The normal range for neutrophils is 30% to 50%.

_____ 4. The range for basophils is 0% to 1%.

_____ 5. The frosted edge of the slide should be labeled with the patient's name and date of birth and the date.

_____ 6. The best type of specimen to use for a manual differential cell count is fresh whole blood.

_____ 7. When preparing the slide, the drop of blood should be placed 1 inch from the frosted edge of the slide.

_____ 8. The spreader slide should be placed at a 15-degree angle to the first slide.

_____ 9. The blood smear should be approximately 1½ inches long.

_____ 10. The blood smear should be thickest at the beginning and gradually thin to a very fine, feathered edge.

_____ 11. The spreader slide should be discarded in a biohazard sharps container.

_____ 12. The slides should be placed in a paper envelope for transport to the laboratory.

Procedure 18-A: Hemoglobin Determination.
   a. Run controls on a CLIA-waived hemoglobin analyzer, and record results on the quality control log on p. 809.
   b. Perform a hemoglobin determination on a patient using a CLIA-waived hemoglobin analyzer, and record results in the chart provided. Circle any values that fall outside the normal range.

Procedure 18-1: Hematocrit Determination. Perform a hematocrit determination in duplicate, and record results in the chart provided. Circle any values that fall outside the normal range.

Procedure 18-2: Preparation of a Blood Smear for a Differential Cell Count. Prepare a blood smear for a differential white blood cell count.

CHART	
Date	

CHART	
Date	

QUALITY CONTROL HEMOGLOBIN LOG SHEET

Name of Meter: _____   **Control Lot Number:** _____

Low-Level Range: _____   **Control Exp. Date:** _____

High-Level Range: _____

Date	Test Cards: Lot # and Expiration	Low-Level Value	Accept	Reject	High-Level Value	Accept	Reject	Technician

Procedure 18-A: Hemoglobin Determination

Name: _____   Date: _____

Evaluated by: _____   Score: _____

Performance Objective

Outcome:	Perform a hemoglobin determination.
Conditions:	Using a hemoglobin meter and operating manual and given the following: disposable gloves, antiseptic wipe, lancet, gauze pad, test cards, cod key, control solutions, quality control log, and a biohazard sharps container.
Standards:	Time: 10 minutes. Student completed procedure in _____ minutes.
	Accuracy: Satisfactory score on the Performance Evaluation Checklist.

Performance Evaluation Checklist

Trial 1	Trial 2	Point Value	Performance Standards
		•	Sanitized hands.
		•	Assembled equipment.
		•	Checked the expiration date of the test cards.
		•	Calibrated the hemoglobin meter.
		▷	Stated the purpose of calibrating the meter.
		•	Checked the expiration date of the control solution.
		•	Applied gloves and ran a low and high control.
		▷	Stated the purpose of running controls.
		•	Removed gloves and sanitized hands.
		•	Recorded the control results in the quality control log.
		•	Greeted the patient and introduced yourself.
		•	Identified the patient and explained the procedure.
		•	Turned on the hemoglobin meter and checked the code number.
		•	Inserted a test card into the meter.
		•	Opened gauze packet.
		•	Cleansed the puncture site and allowed it to air dry.
		▷	Stated what happens to the blood drop if the site is not dry.
		•	Applied gloves and performed a finger puncture.
		•	Wiped away the first drop of blood.
		•	Collected the blood specimen.
		•	Placed a gauze pad over the puncture site and applied pressure.
		•	Applied the blood specimen to the test card.
		•	Waited while the hemoglobin meter analyzed the blood specimen.

Trial 1	Trial 2	Point Value	Performance Standards
		•	Read the results on the display screen.
		▷	Stated the normal hemoglobin range for a female (12 to 16 g/dL) and a male (14 to 18 g/dL).
		•	Removed the test card from the meter.
		•	Properly disposed of the test card in a biohazard waste container.
		•	Checked the puncture site and applied an adhesive bandage, if needed.
		•	Removed gloves and sanitized hands.
		•	Charted the test results correctly.
		✶	The hemoglobin recording was identical to the reading on the digital display screen.
		✶	Completed the procedure within 10 minutes.
			Totals
			CHART
Date			

Evaluation of Student Performance

EVALUATION CRITERIA			COMMENTS
Symbol	**Category**	**Point Value**	
✶	Critical Step	16 points	
•	Essential Step	6 points	
▷	Theory Question	2 points	

Score calculation: 100 points

− _____ points missed

_____ Score

Satisfactory score: 85 or above

CAAHEP Competencies Achieved
Psychomotor (Skills)
☑ I. 11. Perform quality control measures.
☑ I. 12. Perform hematology testing.
Affective (Behavior)
☑ II. 2. Distinguish between normal and abnormal test results.

ABHES Competencies Achieved
☑ 10. a. Practice quality control.
☑ 10. b. Perform selected CLIA-waived tests that assist with diagnosis and treatment (2) Hematology testing.

Notes

Procedure 18-1: Hematocrit

Name: _____   Date: _____

Evaluated by: _____   Score: _____

Performance Objective

Outcome:	Perform a hematocrit determination.
Conditions:	Given the following: microhematocrit centrifuge, disposable gloves, lancet, antiseptic wipe, gauze pad, capillary tubes, sealing compound, and a biohazard sharps container.
Standards:	Time: 10 minutes. Student completed procedure in _____ minutes.
	Accuracy: Satisfactory score on the Performance Evaluation Checklist.

Performance Evaluation Checklist

Trial 1	Trial 2	Point Value	Performance Standards
		•	Sanitized hands.
		•	Greeted the patient and introduced yourself.
		•	Identified the patient and explained the procedure.
		•	Assembled equipment.
		•	Opened gauze packet.
		•	Cleansed the site with an antiseptic wipe and allowed it to air dry.
		•	Applied gloves.
		•	Performed a finger puncture and discarded the lancet in a biohazard sharps container.
		•	Wiped away the first drop of blood.
		•	Massaged the finger until a large blood drop formed.
		•	Held one end of the capillary tube horizontally but slightly downward next to the free-flowing puncture.
		•	Kept the tip of the pipet in the blood but did not allow it to press against the skin of the patient's finger.
		▷	Explained why the capillary tube should be kept in the blood specimen.
		•	Filled the capillary tube (calibrated tubes filled to the calibration line; uncalibrated tubes filled approximately three-fourths full).
		▷	Explained why a tube with air bubbles is unacceptable.
		•	Filled a second capillary tube.
		▷	Stated why 2 capillary tubes must be filled.
		•	Placed a gauze pad over the puncture site and applied pressure.
		•	Sealed the dry end of each capillary tube.
		•	Checked the puncture site and applied an adhesive bandage, if needed.
		•	Placed the capillary tubes in the microhematocrit centrifuge with the sealed end facing toward the outside.

Trial 1	Trial 2	Point Value	Performance Standards
		▷	Explained why the sealed end must face toward the outside.
		•	Balanced one tube with the other tube placed opposite it.
		•	Placed the cover over the capillary tubes and locked it securely.
		•	Centrifuged the blood specimen for 3 to 5 minutes.
		▷	Explained the reason for centrifuging the blood specimen.
		•	Allowed the centrifuge to come to a complete stop.
		•	Removed the protective cover from the capillary tubes.
		•	Read the results with the appropriate reading device.
		•	Determined whether the results agreed within 4 percentage points.
		▷	Explained what to do if the results are not within 4 percentage points.
		•	Averaged the values of the two tubes together to derive the test results.
		✶	Results were within ±1% of the evaluator's results.
		▷	Stated the normal hematocrit range for a female (37% to 47%) and a male (40% to 54%).
		•	Properly disposed of the capillary tubes in a biohazard sharps container.
		•	Removed gloves and sanitized hands.
		•	Charted the test results correctly.
		•	Returned equipment.
		✶	Completed the procedure within 10 minutes.
			Totals

CHART

Date	

Evaluation of Student Performance

EVALUATION CRITERIA			COMMENTS
Symbol	**Category**	**Point Value**	
✶	Critical Step	16 points	
•	Essential Step	6 points	
▷	Theory Question	2 points	

Score calculation: 100 points

− _____ points missed

_____ Score

Satisfactory score: 85 or above

CAAHEP Competencies Achieved

Psychomotor (Skills)

☑ I. 11. Perform quality control measures.

☑ I. 12. Perform hematology testing.

Affective (Behavior)

☑ II. 2. Distinguish between normal and abnormal test results.

ABHES Competencies Achieved

☑ 10. a. Practice quality control.

☑ 10. b. Perform selected CLIA-waived tests that assist with diagnosis and treatment (2) Hematology testing.

☑ 10. c. Dispose of biohazardous materials.

Notes

Procedure 18-2: Preparation of a Blood Smear for a Differential Cell Count

Name: _____ Date: _____

Evaluated by: _____ Score: _____

Performance Objective

Outcome:	Prepare a blood smear for a differential white blood cell count.
Conditions:	Given the following: disposable gloves, supplies to perform a finger puncture or venipuncture, slides with a frosted edge, slide container, biohazard specimen bag, laboratory request form, and a biohazard sharps container.
Standards:	Time: 10 minutes. Student completed procedure in _____ minutes.
	Accuracy: Satisfactory score on the Performance Evaluation Checklist.

Performance Evaluation Checklist

Trial 1	Trial 2	Point Value	Performance Standards
		•	Sanitized hands.
		•	Greeted the patient and introduced yourself.
		•	Identified the patient and explained the procedure.
		•	Assembled equipment.
		•	Labeled the slides.
		•	Opened the gauze packet.
		•	Cleansed the puncture site.
		•	Applied gloves.
		•	Performed a venipuncture or finger puncture.
		•	Placed a drop of blood in the middle of each slide approximately ¼ inch from the frosted edge of the slide.
		•	Held a spreader slide at a 30-degree angle to first slide in front of the drop of blood.
		▷	Stated what occurs if the angle is more than 30 degrees or less than 30 degrees.
		•	Moved the spreader slide until it touched the drop of blood.
		•	Spread the blood thinly and evenly across slide using the spreader slide.
		•	Prepared the second blood smear.
		•	Disposed of the spreader slide in a biohazard sharps container.
		•	Laid the blood smears on a flat surface and allowed them to dry.
		▷	Explained why the blood smears should be dried immediately.
		•	The length of the smear was approximately 1½ inches.
		•	The smear was smooth and even, with no ridges, holes, lines, streaks, or clumps.
		•	The smear was not too thick or too thin.
		•	There was a feathered edge at the thin end of the smear.
		•	There was a margin on all sides of the smear.

Trial 1	Trial 2	Point Value	Performance Standards
		•	Placed the slides in a protective slide container.
		•	Placed lavender-stoppered tube and slide container in a biohazard specimen bag.
		•	Removed gloves and sanitized hands.
		•	Completed a laboratory request form.
		•	Placed the lab request in the outside pocket of the specimen bag.
		•	Charted the procedure correctly.
		•	Filed a copy of the lab request in the patient's chart.
		•	Placed the specimen bag in the appropriate location for pickup by the lab courier.
		•	Charted the procedure correctly.
		✷	Completed the procedure within 10 minutes.
			Totals

<table>
<thead>
<tr><th colspan="2">CHART</th></tr>
</thead>
<tbody>
<tr><td>Date</td><td></td></tr>
<tr><td></td><td></td></tr>
<tr><td></td><td></td></tr>
<tr><td></td><td></td></tr>
<tr><td></td><td></td></tr>
</tbody>
</table>

Evaluation of Student Performance

EVALUATION CRITERIA			COMMENTS
Symbol	**Category**	**Point Value**	
✷	Critical Step	16 points	
•	Essential Step	6 points	
▷	Theory Question	2 points	

Score calculation: 100 points

− _____ points missed

_____ Score

Satisfactory score: 85 or above

CAAHEP Competencies Achieved

Psychomotor (Skills)

☑ I. 11. Perform quality control measures.

Affective (Behavior)

☑ I. 1. Apply critical thinking skills in performing patient assessment and care.

ABHES Competencies Achieved

☑ 10. a. Practice quality control

☑ 10. d. Collect, label, and process specimens.

---

19 Blood Chemistry and Immunology

Blood Chemistry and Immunology

CHAPTER ASSIGNMENTS

√ After Completing	Date Due	Textbook Pages	TEXTBOOK ASSIGNMENTS	Possible Points	Points You Earned
		726–757	Read Chapter 19: Blood Chemistry and Immunology		
		734 754	Read Case Study 1 Case Study 1 questions	5	
		735 754	Read Case Study 2 Case Study 2 questions	5	
		746 755	Read Case Study 3 Case Study 3 questions	5	
			Total points		

√ After Completing	Date Due	Study Guide Pages	STUDY GUIDE ASSIGNMENTS (CTA = Critical Thinking Activity)	Possible Points	Points You Earned
		825	Pretest	10	
		826	Term Key Term Assessment	17	
		827–832	Evaluation of Learning questions	55	
		832–834	CTA A: Type 2 Diabetes	40	
		835	CTA B: Oral Glucose Tolerance Test (2 points each)	10	
		835–836	CTA C: Coronary Artery Disease	20	
		837	CTA D: Cholesterol and Saturated Fat (5 points each)	15	
			Evolve Site: Chapter 19 The Right Chemistry: Blood Chemistry Tests (Record points earned)		
		837–838	CTA E: Rh Incompatibility (2 points each)	20	
		838	CTA F: Crossword Puzzle	25	

√ After Completing	Date Due	Study Guide Pages	STUDY GUIDE ASSIGNMENTS (CTA = Critical Thinking Activity)	Possible Points	Points You Earned
			e Evolve Site: Chapter 19 Immunologic Tests (Record points earned)		
			e Evolve Site: Chapter 19 Animations (2 points each)	6	
			e Evolve Site: Chapter 19 Nutrition Nugget: Nutrition and Cardiovascular Disease	10	
			e Evolve Site: Apply Your Knowledge questions	20	
		839	*e* Video Evaluation	16	
		825	[?] Posttest	10	
			ADDITIONAL ASSIGNMENTS		
			Total points		

√ When Assigned by Your Instructor	Study Guide Pages	Practices Required	LABORATORY ASSIGNMENTS (Procedure Number and Name)	Score*
	841–842	3	Practice for Competency 19-A: Performing a Blood Chemistry Test Textbook reference: pp. 727–733	
	847–848		Evaluation of Competency 19-A: Performing a Blood Chemistry Test	*
	841–843	3	Practice for Competency 19-1: Blood Glucose Measurement Using the Accu-Chek Advantage Glucose Meter Textbook reference: pp. 741–744	
	849–851		Evaluation of Competency 19-1: Blood Glucose Measurement Using the Accu-Chek Advantage Glucose Meter	*
	841–845	3	Practice for Competency 19-B: Rapid Mononucleosis Testing (Quick Vue + Mono Test) Textbook reference: pp. 749–750	
	853–854		Evaluation of Competency 19-B: Rapid Mononucleosis Testing (Quick Vue + Mono Test)	*
			ADDITIONAL ASSIGNMENTS	

Notes

Name: _____ Date:_____

True or False

_____ 1. The function of glucose in the body is to build and repair tissue.

_____ 2. Insulin is required for normal use of glucose in the body.

_____ 3. An abnormally low level of glucose in the body is known as *hypoglycemia.*

_____ 4. The hemoglobin A_{1C} test measures the average amount of blood glucose over a 3-month period.

_____ 5. Most of the cholesterol found in the blood comes from the intake of dietary cholesterol.

_____ 6. The primary use of the cholesterol test is to screen for the presence of coronary artery disease.

_____ 7. LDL picks up cholesterol from ingested fats and the liver and carries it to the cells.

_____ 8. An antibody is a substance that is capable of combining with an antigen.

_____ 9. Mononucleosis is transmitted through coughing and sneezing.

_____ 10. Blood antigens (A, B, Rh) are located on the surface of red blood cells.

? POSTTEST

True or False

_____ 1. Serum is required for most blood chemistry tests.

_____ 2. The normal range for a fasting blood glucose level is 120 to 160 mg/dL.

_____ 3. The oral glucose tolerance test is used to assist in the diagnosis of diabetes mellitus.

_____ 4. Before meals, it is recommended that the blood glucose level for a diabetic patient be 60 to 80 mg/dL.

_____ 5. The recommended hemoglobin A_{1C} level for a patient with diabetes is 4% to 6%.

_____ 6. The buildup of plaque (resulting from high cholesterol) on the walls of arteries is known as thrombophlebitis.

_____ 7. An HDL cholesterol level greater than 50 mg/dL is a risk factor for coronary artery disease.

_____ 8. The triglyceride test requires that the patient not eat or drink for 12 hours before the test.

_____ 9. The RPR test is a screening test for syphilis.

_____ 10. The varicella virus causes infectious mononucleosis.

Directions: Match each medical term (numbers) with its definition (letters).

_____ 1. Agglutination

_____ 2. Antibody

_____ 3. Antigen

_____ 4. Antiserum

_____ 5. Blood antibody

_____ 6. Blood antigen

_____ 7. Donor

_____ 8. Gene

_____ 9. Glycogen

_____ 10. HDL cholesterol

_____ 11. Hyperglycemia

_____ 12. Hypoglycemia

_____ 13. In vitro

_____ 14. In vivo

_____ 15. LDL cholesterol

_____ 16. Lipoprotein

_____ 17. Recipient

A. An abnormally high level of glucose in the blood
B. A complex molecule consisting of protein and a lipid fraction such as cholesterol
C. The form in which carbohydrate is stored in the body
D. A lipoprotein consisting of protein and cholesterol that removes excess cholesterol from the cells
E. An abnormally low level of glucose in the blood
F. A lipoprotein, consisting of protein and cholesterol, that picks up cholesterol and delivers it to the cells
G. A substance that is capable of combining with an antigen resulting in an antigen-antibody reaction
H. Substance capable of stimulating the formation of antibodies
I. One who receives something, such as a blood transfusion, from a donor
J. Clumping of blood cells
K. A protein present on the surface of red blood cells that determines a person's blood type
L. Occurring in the living body or organism
M. A unit of heredity
N. A serum that contains antibodies
O. One who furnishes something, such as blood, tissue, or organs to be used in another individual
P. Occurring in glass; refers to tests performed under artificial conditions, as in the laboratory
Q. A protein present in the blood plasma that is capable of combining with its corresponding blood antigen to produce an antigen-antibody reaction

EVALUATION OF LEARNING

Directions: Fill in each blank with the correct answer.

1. What type of specimen is required for most blood chemistry tests?

_____

2. What is the purpose of quality control?

_____

_____

3. What is the purpose of calibrating a blood chemistry analyzer?

_____

_____

4. At a minimum, when should a calibration check be performed on a blood chemistry analyzer?

_____

5. What is the purpose of running a control on a blood chemistry analyzer?

_____

_____

6. List three reasons why a control may not produce expected results.

_____

_____

7. When running controls on a blood chemistry analyzer, what should be done if the controls do not perform as expected?

_____

8. What is the function of glucose in the body?

_____

_____

9. Explain the function of insulin in the body.

_____

_____

10. List the abbreviation for each of the following tests:

   a. Fasting blood glucose _____

   b. Two-hour postprandial blood glucose _____

   c. Oral glucose tolerance test _____

11. What type of patient preparation is required for a fasting blood glucose test?

_____

_____

12. List two reasons for performing a fasting blood glucose test.

_____

13. What is prediabetes?

_____

_____

14. What are the values recommended by the American Diabetes Association for interpreting fasting blood glucose results?

a. Normal _____

b. Prediabetes _____

c. Diabetes _____

15. What type of patient preparation is required for a 2-hour postprandial blood glucose test?

_____

_____

16. Describe the procedure for performing a 2-hour postprandial blood glucose test.

_____

_____

17. What is the purpose of an oral glucose tolerance test?

_____

_____

18. What type of patient preparation is required for an oral glucose tolerance test?

_____

_____

19. Describe the procedure for an oral glucose tolerance test.

_____

_____

20. Define hypoglycemia and list three conditions that may cause it to occur.

_____

_____

21. Why is it important for a patient with insulin-dependent diabetes to perform self-monitoring of blood glucose (SMBG)?

_____

_____

22. What is the ideal insulin testing schedule for SMBG?

_____

_____

23. What type of damage can occur to the body from prolonged high blood glucose levels?

_____

_____

24. List three advantages of blood glucose monitoring at home.

_____

_____

_____

25. What is the recommended blood glucose level for a diabetic patient during the following times of the day?

    a. Before meals _____

    b. One to 2 hours after meals _____

    c. At bedtime _____

26. What information is provided by a hemoglobin A_{1C} test?

_____

_____

27. What is the normal A_{1C} range for an individual without diabetes?

_____

28. What is the recommended A_{1C} percentage for an individual with diabetes?

_____

_____

29. What are the storage requirements for blood glucose reagent test strips?

_____

_____

30. When should the calibration (coding) procedure be performed on a glucose meter?

_____

31. What is cholesterol?

_____

_____

32. List the two main sources of cholesterol in the blood.

_____

_____

33. What is atherosclerosis, and why is it a health risk?

_____

_____

34. Why is LDL cholesterol referred to as *bad cholesterol* and HDL referred to as *good cholesterol*?

_____

_____

_____

_____

35. What does a total cholesterol test measure?

_____

_____

36. List the ranges for each of the following cholesterol categories:

   a. Desirable cholesterol level _____

   b. Borderline cholesterol level _____

   c. High cholesterol level _____

37. At what level is HDL cholesterol considered a risk factor for coronary heart disease?

_____

_____

38. What is the primary use of the cholesterol test?

_____

_____

39. What type of patient preparation is required for a triglyceride test?

_____

_____

40. List the ranges for each of the following triglyceride categories:

   a. Normal _____

   b. Borderline high _____

   c. High _____

   d. Very high _____

41. What conditions result in elevated blood triglycerides?

_____

_____

_____

42. What is the purpose of performing a BUN?

_____

_____

43. What is the definition of immunology?

_____

_____

_____

44. List three examples of antigens.

_____

_____

45. What is the purpose of performing each of the following serologic tests?

   a. Rheumatoid factor

_____

_____

   b. Antistreptolysin test

_____

_____

   c. C-reactive protein

_____

_____

   d. ABO and Rh blood typing

_____

_____

46. How is infectious mononucleosis transmitted?

_____

_____

47. What are the symptoms of infectious mononucleosis?

_____

_____

48. What happens when a blood antigen and antibody combine?

_____

_____

49. Where are the A, B, and Rh antigens located?

_____

50. Why is agglutination of blood in vivo a threat to life?

_____

_____

51. If a person has type A blood, what antigens and antibodies are present?

_____

_____

_____

52. If a person has type B blood, what antigens and antibodies are present?

_____

_____

53. If a person has type AB blood, what antigens and antibodies are present?

_____

54. If a person has type O blood, what antigens and antibodies are present?

_____

55. What is the difference between Rh-positive and Rh-negative blood?

_____

_____

CRITICAL THINKING ACTIVITIES

A. Type 2 Diabetes

You are working for a physician specializing in internal medicine. The physician is concerned about the increased numbers of patients developing type 2 diabetes mellitus. He asks you to design a colorful, creative, and informative brochure on type 2 diabetes using the brochure format provided on the next page. This brochure will be published and placed in the waiting room to provide patients with education on type 2 diabetes. The diabetes Internet sites listed under On the Web at the end of Chapter 19 in your textbook can be used to complete this activity.

Chapter **19** **Blood Chemistry and Immunology**

FAQ
ON:

Q: A:

Q: A:

Q: A:

Q: A:

Q:

A:

Q:

A:

Illustration

Q:

A:

Q:

A:

B. Oral Glucose Tolerance Test

Marty Wolf has arrived at your office for an oral glucose tolerance test. What should you tell her regarding the following subjects? Explain the reason for each answer.

1. Consumption of food and fluid

   _____

   _____

2. Water consumption

   _____

   _____

3. Smoking

   _____

   _____

4. Leaving the test site

   _____

   _____

5. Activity

   _____

   _____

C. Coronary Artery Disease

Create a profile of an individual who is at risk for coronary artery disease (CAD) following these guidelines:

1. Using colored pencils, crayons, or markers, draw a figure of an individual exhibiting risk factors for CAD. Be as creative as possible.

2. Do not use any text on your drawing other than to label items you have drawn in your picture. (A picture is worth a thousand words!)

3. Try to include at least eight risk factors for CAD in your drawing. The *Highlight on Heart Disease* box on p. 745 in your textbook can be used as a reference source.

4. In the classroom, find a partner and trade drawings. Identify the risk factors for CAD in your partner's drawing. With your partner, discuss what this person could do to lower his or her chances of developing coronary heart disease.

AT RISK FOR CAD

D. Cholesterol and Saturated Fat

Using a reference source, complete the following activities:

1. Create a dinner meal that is as high as possible in saturated fat and cholesterol.

_____

_____

_____

_____

_____

2. Create a dinner meal that is as low as possible in saturated fat and cholesterol.

_____

_____

_____

_____

_____

3. Choose a fast-food restaurant, and plan a meal that is as low as possible in saturated fat and cholesterol.

_____

_____

_____

_____

_____

E. Rh Incompatibility

Erythroblastosis fetalis is a blood disorder of the newborn. It usually is caused by incompatibility between the infant's blood and the mother's blood. Using a reference source, answer the following questions regarding this condition in the space provided.

1. Explain how Rh incompatibility between the mother and infant can cause this condition to occur.

_____

_____

_____

_____

2. Describe the symptoms associated with erythroblastosis fetalis.

_____

_____

_____

_____

3. Explain the treatment used for this condition.

_____

_____

_____

4. How can this condition be prevented?

_____

_____

_____

F. Crossword Puzzle: Blood Chemistry and Immunology

Directions: Complete the crossword puzzle using the clues provided.

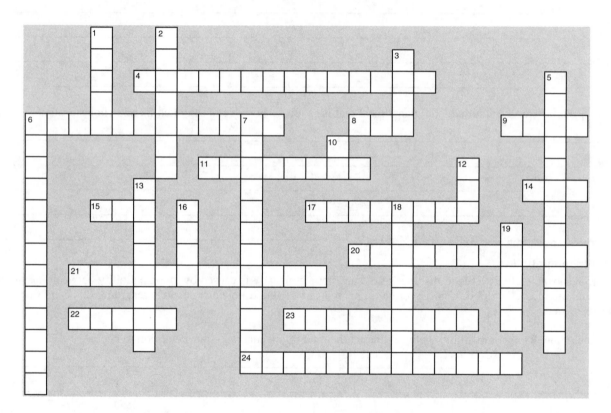

Across
4 Cholesterol: 200-239
6 #1 killer in the U.S.
8 Detects liver disease
9 Unit of heredity
11 Combines with an antigen
14 Detects renal disease
15 Bad cholesterol
17 Unsaturated fat (ex)
20 FBG: 100-125 mg/dL
21 Low BG
22 Makes cholesterol
23 Blood donor disqualifier
24 Normal: Less than150 mg/dL

Down
1 Thyroid function test
2 Risk factor for CAD
3 Series of glucose tests
5 Kissing disease
6 High BG
7 Raises cholesterol level
10 Assists in confirming an MI
12 Good cholesterol
13 Stored glucose
16 Syphilis test
18 Increases HDL cholesterol
19 Keep diabetic A_1C below this

VIDEO EVALUATION FOR CHAPTER 19: BLOOD CHEMISTRY AND IMMUNOLOGY

Name: _____

Directions:

a. Watch the indicated videos.
b. Mark each true statement with a T and each false statement with an F. For each false statement, change the wording of the question so that it becomes a true statement.

Video: Procedure 19-1: Blood Glucose Measurement Using the Accu-Chek Advantage Glucose Meter

_____ 1. Blood glucose test results are used to detect diabetes mellitus.

_____ 2. Blood glucose is usually measured when the patient is in a fasting state.

_____ 3. Calibrating the glucose meter with a code key compensates for variations that occur in the manufacturing of the test strips.

_____ 4. The 3-digit code number displayed on the glucose meter must match the code number that is indicated on the control solution container.

_____ 5. Two levels of controls must be run each day before you use the meter for the first time.

_____ 6. Replacing the lid of the test strip container as soon as possible protects the strips from being exposed to insects.

_____ 7. After making the puncture, the first drop of blood should be wiped away with a gauze pad.

_____ 8. The yellow target area of the test strip must be completely covered with blood.

Video: Procedure 19-B: Performing a Rapid Mononucleosis Test

_____ 1. Mononucleosis is caused by bacteria.

_____ 2. Mononucleosis is transmitted through saliva by direct oral contact.

_____ 3. Controls should be run when a patient has a positive test result.

_____ 4. If the puncture site is touched after it is cleansed with alcohol, the cleansing process needs to be repeated.

_____ 5. The first drop of blood should be wiped away with a gauze pad.

_____ 6. The puncture site should be gently massaged until a large drop of blood forms.

_____ 7. If the "test complete" line is not visible after 10 minutes, the test is considered valid.

_____ 8. A negative result is indicated by a horizontal blue line.

Notes

PRACTICE FOR COMPETENCY

Procedure 19-A: Blood Chemistry Test. Perform a blood chemistry test, and record results in the chart provided. Examples of blood chemistry tests: cholesterol, triglycerides, and BUN.

Procedure 19-1: Blood Glucose Measurement.
a. Run controls on a CLIA-waived glucose meter, and record results on the quality control log on page 843.
b. Perform a fasting blood glucose test, and record results in the chart provided.

Procedure 19-B: Rapid Mononucleosis Test.
a. Run controls on a CLIA-waived mono, and record results on the quality control log on page 845.
b. Perform a rapid mononucleosis test, and record results in the chart provided.

CHART	
Date	

CHART	
Date	

QUALITY CONTROL LOG

BLOOD GLUCOSE

NAME OF METER		CONTROLS
Test Strips: Lot Number: _____ Exp Date: _____ Code Number: _____		**Low-Level Control:** Lot Number: _____ Exp Date: _____ Expected Range: _____ **High-Level Control:** Lot Number: _____ Exp Date: _____ Expected Range: _____

Date	Low-Level Control	Accept	Reject	High-Level Control	Accept	Reject	Technician

Notes

QUALITY CONTROL LOG

MONONUCLEOSIS TEST

Date	Name of Test	Control Lot #	Control Expiration Date	External Positive Control	External Negative Control	Technician

Notes

EVALUATION OF COMPETENCY

Procedure 19-A: Performing a Blood Chemistry Test

Name: _____   Date: _____

Evaluated by: _____   Score: _____

Performance Objective

Outcome:	Perform a fasting blood glucose test.
Conditions:	Given the following: disposable gloves, an antiseptic wipe, a lancet, gauze pad, quality control log, and a biohazard sharps container. Using an automated blood chemistry analyzer and operating manual.
Standards:	Time: 10 minutes. Student completed procedure in _____ minutes.
	Accuracy: Satisfactory score on the Performance Evaluation Checklist.

Performance Evaluation Checklist

Trial 1	Trial 2	Point Value	Performance Standards
		•	Sanitized hands.
		•	Assembled equipment.
		•	Calibrated the blood chemistry analyzer.
		•	Applied gloves and ran controls.
		•	Recorded the results in the quality control log.
		•	Sanitized hands.
		•	Greeted the patient and introduced yourself.
		•	Identified the patient and explained the procedure.
		•	Applied gloves.
		•	Performed a finger puncture.
		•	Collected the specimen according to the manufacturer's instructions.
		•	Placed a gauze pad over the puncture site and applied pressure.
		•	Inserted the specimen into the blood chemistry analyzer according to the manufacturer's instructions.
		•	Operated the blood chemistry analyzer according to the manufacturer's instructions.
		•	Read the results on the digital display screen.
		•	Properly disposed of used materials.
		•	Checked the puncture site and applied an adhesive bandage if needed.
		•	Removed gloves.
		•	Sanitized hands.
		•	Charted the test results correctly.
		✱	The recording was identical to the reading on the digital display screen.
		✱	Completed the procedure within 10 minutes.
			Totals

Chapter **19 Blood Chemistry and Immunology**

CHART	
Date	

Evaluation of Student Performance

EVALUATION CRITERIA			COMMENTS
Symbol	**Category**	**Point Value**	
✶	Critical Step	16 points	
•	Essential Step	6 points	
▷	Theory Question	2 points	

Score calculation: 100 points

− _____ points missed

_____ Score

Satisfactory score: 85 or above

CAAHEP Competencies Achieved

Psychomotor (Skills)

☑ I. 11. Perform quality control measures.

☑ I. 13. Perform chemistry testing.

☑ II. 2. Maintain laboratory test results using flow sheets.

Affective (Behavior)

☑ II. 2. Distinguish between normal and abnormal test results.

ABHES Competencies Achieved

☑ 10. a. Practice quality control.

☑ 10. b. Perform selected CLIA-waived tests that assist with diagnosis and treatment (3) Chemistry testing.

Procedure 19-1: Blood Glucose Measurement Using the Accu-Chek Advantage Glucose Meter

Name: _____   Date: _____

Evaluated by: _____   Score: _____

Performance Objective

Outcome:	Perform a fasting blood glucose test.
Conditions:	Given the following: disposable gloves, Accu-Chek Advantage glucose meter, reagent test strips, check strip, code key, control solutions, lancet, antiseptic wipe, gauze pad, quality control log, and a biohazard sharps container.
Standards:	Time: 10 minutes. Student completed procedure in _____ minutes.
	Accuracy: Satisfactory score on the Performance Evaluation Checklist.

Performance Evaluation Checklist

Trial 1	Trial 2	Point Value	Performance Standards
		•	Sanitized hands.
		•	Assembled equipment.
		•	Checked the expiration date on the container of test strips.
		•	Calibrated the meter using the code key.
		▷	Stated the purpose of calibrating the meter.
		•	Ran a low and high control.
		▷	Stated the purpose for running controls.
		•	Recorded the results in the quality control log.
		•	Sanitized hands.
		•	Greeted the patient and introduced yourself.
		•	Identified the patient and explained the procedure.
		•	Asked the patient whether he or she prepared properly.
		▷	Stated the preparation required for a fasting blood glucose test.
		•	Removed a test strip from the container.
		•	Immediately replaced the lid of the container.
		▷	Explained why the lid should be replaced immediately.
		•	Gently inserted the test strip into the test strip guide.
		•	Checked that the code number matches the code number on the test strip container.
		•	Opened a gauze packet.
		•	Cleansed the puncture site with an antiseptic wipe and allowed it to dry.
		•	Applied gloves.
		•	Performed a finger puncture.
		•	Disposed of the lancet in the biohazard sharps container.

		•	Wiped away the first drop of blood with a gauze pad.
		▷	Explained why the first drop of blood should be wiped away.
		•	Placed the patient's hand in a dependent position and gently massaged the finger until a large drop of blood formed.
		•	Applied the drop of blood to the yellow target area of the test strip.
		•	Completely filled the yellow target area with blood.
		▷	Explained what to do if the yellow area is not completely covered with blood.
		•	Placed a gauze pad over puncture site and applied pressure.
		•	Observed the digital display of the test results.
		▷	Stated the reference range for a fasting blood glucose level (70 to 99 mg/dL), prediabetes (100 to 125 mg/dL), and diabetes (above 126 mg/dL).
		•	Removed the test strip from the meter and discarded it in a biohazard waste container.
		•	Turned off the meter.
		•	Checked the puncture site and applied an adhesive bandage, if needed.
		•	Removed gloves and sanitized hands.
		•	Charted the test results correctly.
		✶	The recording was identical to the reading on the digital display screen.
		•	Properly stored the glucose meter.
		✶	Completed the procedure within 10 minutes.
			Totals

Evaluation of Student Performance

EVALUATION CRITERIA			COMMENTS
Symbol	**Category**	**Point Value**	
✶	Critical Step	16 points	
•	Essential Step	6 points	
▷	Theory Question	2 points	

Score calculation: 100 points

            −_____ points missed
            _____ Score

Satisfactory score: 85 or above

CAAHEP Competencies Achieved

Psychomotor (Skills)

☑ I. 11. Perform quality control measures.

☑ I. 13. Perform chemistry testing.

☑ II. 2. Maintain laboratory test results using flow sheets.

Affective (Behavior)

☑ II. 2. Distinguish between normal and abnormal test results.

ABHES Competencies Achieved

☑ 10. a. Practice quality control.

☑ 10. b. Perform selected CLIA-waived tests that assist with diagnosis and treatment (3) Chemistry testing.

Notes

Procedure 19-B: Rapid Mononucleosis Testing (Quick Vue + Mono Test)

Name: _____   Date: _____

Evaluated by: _____   Score: _____

Performance Objective

Outcome:	Perform a rapid mononucleosis test.
Conditions:	Given the following: disposable gloves, the supplies needed to perform a finger puncture, a mononucleosis testing kit, and a biohazard container.
Standards:	Time: 10 minutes. Student completed procedure in _____ minutes.
	Accuracy: Satisfactory score on the Performance Evaluation Checklist.

Performance Evaluation Checklist

Trial 1	Trial 2	Point Value	Performance Standards
		•	Sanitized hands.
		•	Assembled equipment.
		•	Checked the expiration date on the testing kit.
		•	Applied gloves and ran a positive and a negative control, if necessary.
		•	Removed gloves and recorded the results in the quality control log.
		•	Greeted the patient and introduced yourself.
		•	Identified the patient and explained the procedure.
		•	Cleansed the puncture site and allowed it to air dry.
		•	Applied gloves.
		•	Performed a finger puncture.
		•	Disposed of the lancet in a biohazard sharps container.
		•	Wiped away the first drop of blood.
		•	Collected the blood specimen with a capillary tube.
		•	Placed a gauze pad over puncture site and applied pressure.
		•	Dispensed the blood specimen into the add well on the test cassette.
		•	Added 5 drops of developing solution to the add well.
		•	Waited 5 minutes and read the results.
		▷	Described the appearance of a positive and negative test result.
		•	Disposed of the test cassette in a biohazard waste container.
		•	Checked the puncture site and applied an adhesive bandage, if needed.
		•	Removed gloves.
		•	Sanitized hands.
		•	Charted the results correctly.

Trial 1	Trial 2	Point Value	Performance Standards
		•	The results were identical to the evaluator's results.
		•	Completed the procedure within 10 minutes.
			Totals
			**CHART**
Date			

Evaluation of Student Performance

EVALUATION CRITERIA			COMMENTS
Symbol	**Category**	**Point Value**	
✱	Critical Step	16 points	
•	Essential Step	6 points	
▷	Theory Question	2 points	

Score calculation: 100 points

− _____ points missed

_____ Score

Satisfactory score: 85 or above

CAAHEP Competencies Achieved

Psychomotor (Skills)

☑ I. 11. Perform quality control measures.

☑ I. 13. Perform immunology testing.

Affective (Behavior)

☑ II. 2. Distinguish between normal and abnormal test results.

ABHES Competencies Achieved

☑ 10. a. Practice quality control.

☑ 10. b. Perform selected CLIA-waived tests that assist with diagnosis and treatment (4) Immunology testing.

20 Medical Microbiology

√ After Completing	Date Due	Textbook Pages	TEXTBOOK ASSIGNMENTS	Possible Points	Points You Earned
		758–780	Read Chapter 20: Medical Microbiology		
		761 777	Read Case Study 1 Case Study 1 questions	5	
		769 777	Read Case Study 2 Case Study 2 questions	5	
		774 777	Read Case Study 3 Case Study 3 questions	5	
			Total points		

√ After Completing	Date Due	Study Guide Pages	STUDY GUIDE ASSIGNMENTS (CTA = Critical Thinking Activity)	Possible Points	Points You Earned
		859	Pretest	10	
		860	Term Key Term Assessment	15	
		860–863	Evaluation of Learning questions	31	
		864	CTA A: Stages of an Infectious Disease	20	
			Evolve Site: Chapter 20 Microscope Identification (Record points earned)		
		865–870	CTA B: Choose-a-Clue (Record points earned)		
		871	CTA C: Disease and Infection Control	10	
		871	CTA D: Sensitivity Testing	12	
		872	CTA E: Crossword Puzzle	21	
			Evolve Site: Chapter 20 Animations (2 points each)	14	
			Evolve Site: Chapter 20 Nutrition Nugget: Vegetarianism	10	

√ After Completing	Date Due	Study Guide Pages	STUDY GUIDE ASSIGNMENTS (CTA = Critical Thinking Activity)	Possible Points	Points You Earned
			Evolve Site: Apply Your Knowledge questions	10	
		873	Video Evaluation	15	
		859	Posttest	10	
			ADDITIONAL ASSIGNMENTS		
			Total points		

Chapter **20** **Medical Microbiology**

√ When Assigned by Your Instructor	Study Guide Pages	Practices Required	LABORATORY ASSIGNMENTS (Procedure Number and Name)	Score*
	875–876	3	Practice for Competency 20-1: Using the Microscope Textbook reference: pp. 765–767	
	877–879		Evaluation of Competency 20-1: Using the Microscope	*
	875–876	3	Practice for Competency 20-2: Collecting a Throat Specimen Textbook reference: pp. 769–770	
	881–883		Evaluation of Competency 20-2: Collecting a Throat Specimen	*
	875–876	3	Practice for Competency 20-A: Rapid Strep Testing Textbook reference: pp. 771–773	
	885–887		Evaluation of Competency 20-A: Rapid Strep Testing	*
	875–876	3	Practice for Competency 20-3: Preparing a Smear Textbook reference: p. 776	
	889–890		Evaluation of Competency 20-3: Preparing a Smear	*
			ADDITIONAL ASSIGNMENTS	

Notes

Name: _____ Date: _____

True or False

_____ 1. Microbiology is the scientific study of microorganisms and their activities.

_____ 2. A disease that can be spread from one person to another is known as an *infectious disease.*

_____ 3. Droplet infection is the transfer of pathogens from a fine spray emitted from a person already infected with the disease.

_____ 4. Streptococci are round bacteria that grow in pairs.

_____ 5. Chickenpox is caused by a virus.

_____ 6. The course adjustment on a microscope is used to obtain precise focusing of an object.

_____ 7. The purpose of transport media is to provide nutrients for the multiplication of the specimen.

_____ 8. A throat specimen should be collected from the tonsillar area and posterior pharynx.

_____ 9. A wet mount is used to examine microorganisms in the living state.

_____ 10. A smear is material spread on a slide for microscopic examination.

?≣ **POSTTEST**

True or False

_____ 1. Microorganisms that reside in the body but do not cause disease are known as *transient flora.*

_____ 2. The invasion of the body by a pathogenic microorganism is known as *infection.*

_____ 3. The interval of time between the invasion by a pathogen and the first symptoms of disease is known as the *prodromal period.*

_____ 4. Staphylococcal infections usually result in pus formation.

_____ 5. *Escherichia coli* normally reside in the urinary tract.

_____ 6. The high-power objective has a magnification of 40×.

_____ 7. Examination of urine sediment requires the use of the oil immersion objective.

_____ 8. A mixed culture contains two or more types of microorganisms.

_____ 9. The purpose of sensitivity testing is to identify the type of microorganism present.

_____ 10. When viewed under a microscope, gram-positive bacteria appear pink or red.

Directions: Match each medical term (numbers) with its definition (letters).

_____ 1. Bacilli

_____ 2. Cocci

_____ 3. Contagious

_____ 4. Culture

_____ 5. Culture medium

_____ 6. Incubate

_____ 7. Incubation period

_____ 8. Infectious disease

_____ 9. Inoculate

_____ 10. Microbiology

_____ 11. Normal flora

_____ 12. Sequelae

_____ 13. Smear

_____ 14. Specimen

_____ 15. Spirilla

A. A disease caused by a pathogen that produces harmful effects on its host
B. Capable of being transmitted directly or indirectly from one person to another
C. To introduce microorganisms into a culture medium for growth and multiplication
D. Bacteria that have a round shape
E. The scientific study of microorganisms and their activities
F. Material spread on a slide for microscopic examination
G. Morbid (secondary) condition occurring as a result of a less serious primary infection
H. A mixture of nutrients in which microorganisms are grown in the laboratory
I. The interval of time between invasion by a pathogenic microorganism and the appearance of the first symptoms of the disease
J. Bacteria that have a spiral or curved shape
K. Harmless, nonpathogenic microorganisms that normally reside in many parts of the body but do not cause disease
L. Bacteria that have a rod shape
M. The propagation of a mass of microorganisms in a laboratory culture medium
N. In microbiology, the act of placing a culture in a chamber that provides optimal growth requirements for the multiplication of the organisms, such as the proper temperature, humidity, and darkness
O. A small sample or part taken from the body to show the nature of the whole

EVALUATION OF LEARNING

Directions: Fill in each blank with the correct answer.

1. What occurs when pathogens invade the body, and what is the response of the body to the invasion?

_____

_____

2. What is droplet infection?

_____

_____

3. What is the prodromal period of an infectious disease?

_____

_____

4. List three infectious diseases caused by *Staphylococcus aureus*.

_____

_____

5. List three infectious diseases caused by different types of streptococci.

_____

_____

6. List three infectious diseases caused by different types of bacilli.

_____

_____

7. In what part of the body do *E. coli* bacteria normally reside?

_____

8. List four infectious diseases caused by different viruses.

_____

_____

9. Explain the purpose of each of the following parts of a microscope:

Stage

_____

_____

Substage condenser

_____

_____

Iris diaphragm

_____

_____

Coarse adjustment

_____

_____

Fine adjustment

_____

_____

Ocular lens

_____

_____

10. Describe the function of each of the following objective lenses:

Low power

_____

_____

High power

_____

_____

Oil immersion

_____

_____

11. What is the purpose of using oil with the oil-immersion objective?

_____

_____

12. List five guidelines that should be followed for proper care of the microscope.

_____

_____

_____

_____

13. List five common areas of the body from which a microbiologic specimen may be obtained.

_____

_____

14. List two ways to prevent contamination of a specimen with extraneous microorganisms.

_____

_____

15. List two precautions a medical assistant should take to prevent infecting herself or himself with a microbiologic specimen.

_____

_____

16. Why should a specimen be processed as soon as possible after it is collected?

_____

_____

17. What is the purpose of a transport medium?

_____

_____

18. How should a collection and transport system be stored?

_____

_____

19. Describe the procedure for collecting a wound specimen.

_____

_____

20. A throat specimen is used to perform tests that assist in the diagnosis of what conditions?

_____

_____

21. What is the purpose of culturing a microbiologic specimen?

_____

_____

22. What is the purpose of adding sheep's blood to an agar culture medium?

_____

_____

23. What is the name given to the type of culture that contains two or more types of microorganisms?

_____

24. Why is it important to diagnose and treat streptococcal pharyngitis as early as possible?

_____

_____

25. What type of reaction is used to identify streptococci with the direct antigen identification test?

_____

26. What is the advantage of using the direct antigen identification test to diagnose streptococci compared with a culture test?

_____

_____

27. When performing a hemolytic reaction and bacitracin susceptibility test, what is observed on the blood agar medium if a patient has streptococcal pharyngitis?

_____

_____

28. What is the purpose of performing a sensitivity test on a bacterial culture?

_____

29. List two reasons for examining a microorganism in the living state.

_____

_____

30. What is the purpose of staining a smear?

_____

_____

31. What color do the following bacteria exhibit in a Gram-stained smear?

Gram-positive bacteria: _____

Gram-negative bacteria:_____

CRITICAL THINKING ACTIVITIES

A. Stages of an Infectious Disease

Your physician wants you to design a poster to hang in the office that outlines the stages of an infectious disease. Complete this project using the following diagram in your study guide.

STAGES OF INFECTIOUS DISEASE

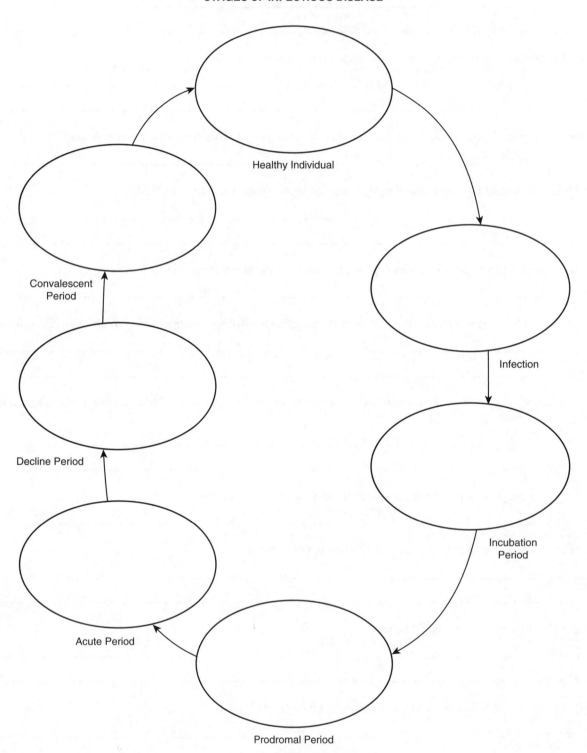

B. Choose-a-Clue

Object: The object of the game is to become familiar with infectious diseases.

Directions:

1. Cut out the game cards on the following pages.

2. List three clues for each condition specified on the reverse of the card. Your clues should include information about symptoms, prevention, and treatment. The name of the disease must not be written on this side of the card.

3. Use the game cards as flash cards to study the diseases.

4. Get into a group of three students.

5. Place your game cards on the table in front of you with the clues facing up.

6. One of the players should name the first disease on the list provided.

7. Each player places the appropriate game card in the middle of the table with the clues facing upward.

8. When all players have placed a card on the table, turn the cards over.

9. Award yourself 5 points if you have correctly determined the disease.

10. Review the information each player listed on his or her game card.

11. Keep track of your points on the score card provided on the next page.

12. Internet reference sources (www.merck.com, www.kidshealth.org) can help you find clues.

Conditions

1. Botulism

2. Common cold

3. Diphtheria

4. Gonorrhea

5. H1N1 influenza

6. Infectious mononucleosis

7. Meningitis

8. Poliomyelitis

9. Rabies

10. Rheumatic fever

11. Rubella

12. Rubeola

13. *Salmonella* food poisoning

14. Staphylococcal food poisoning

15. Syphilis

16. Tetanus

CHOOSE-A-CLUE SCORE CARD

Name: _____

Recording Points:

Cross off a number each time you properly identify a disease (starting with 5 and continuing in sequence). Your total points will be equal to the last number you crossed off. Record this number in the space provided, and determine the knowledge level you attained.

Points:	
5	75
10	80
15	85
20	90
25	95
30	100
35	105
40	110
45	115
50	120
55	125
60	130
65	135
70	140

Total points: _____

LEVEL: _____

☐ 75 points and above: **Free from Infection**

☐ 65 to 70 points: **Putting Up a Good Fight**

☐ 55 to 60 points: **Susceptible**

☐ 50 points and under: **Infected**

Botulism	**Common cold**
Diphtheria	**Gonorrhea**
H1N1 influenza	**Infectious mononucleosis**
Meningitis	**Poliomyelitis**

Sym:

_____

_____

Prev:

_____

_____

Tx:

_____

_____

Sym:

_____

_____

Prev:

_____

_____

Tx:

_____

_____

Sym:

_____

_____

Prev:

_____

_____

Tx:

_____

_____

Sym:

_____

_____

Prev:

_____

_____

Tx:

_____

_____

Sym:

_____

_____

Prev:

_____

_____

Tx:

_____

_____

Sym:

_____

_____

Prev:

_____

_____

Tx:

_____

_____

Sym:

_____

_____

Prev:

_____

_____

Tx:

_____

_____

Sym:

_____

_____

Prev:

_____

_____

Tx:

_____

_____

Rabies

Rheumatic fever

Rubella

Rubeola

Salmonella food poisoning

Staphylococcal food poisoning

Syphilis

Tetanus

Sym:

_____

_____

Prev:

_____

Tx:

_____

_____

Sym:

_____

_____

Prev:

_____

Tx:

_____

_____

Sym:

_____

_____

Prev:

_____

Tx:

_____

_____

Sym:

_____

_____

Prev:

_____

Tx:

_____

_____

Sym:

_____

_____

Prev:

_____

Tx:

_____

_____

Sym:

_____

_____

Prev:

_____

Tx:

_____

_____

Sym:

_____

_____

Prev:

_____

Tx:

_____

_____

Sym:

_____

_____

Prev:

_____

Tx:

_____

_____

C. Disease and Infection Control

Obtain a current journal article on disease and infection control. The Internet sites listed under On the Web at the end of Chapter 20 in your textbook can be used to locate an article. List the important parts of your article below.

_____

_____

_____

_____

_____

_____

_____

_____

D. Sensitivity Testing

Refer to Figure 20-9 in your textbook on p. 773. Place a check mark next to each antibiotic that is effective against the pathogen growing on the culture medium in the Petri plate.

_____ 1. azithromycin

_____ 2. cephalothin

_____ 3. ciprofloxacin

_____ 4. cefprozil

_____ 5. clarithromycin

_____ 6. doxycycline

_____ 7. erythromycin

_____ 8. nitrofurantoin

_____ 9. norfloxacin

_____ 10. penicillin

_____ 11. sulfisoxazole

_____ 12. tetracycline

E. Crossword Puzzle: Medical Microbiology

Directions: Complete the crossword puzzle using the clues provided.

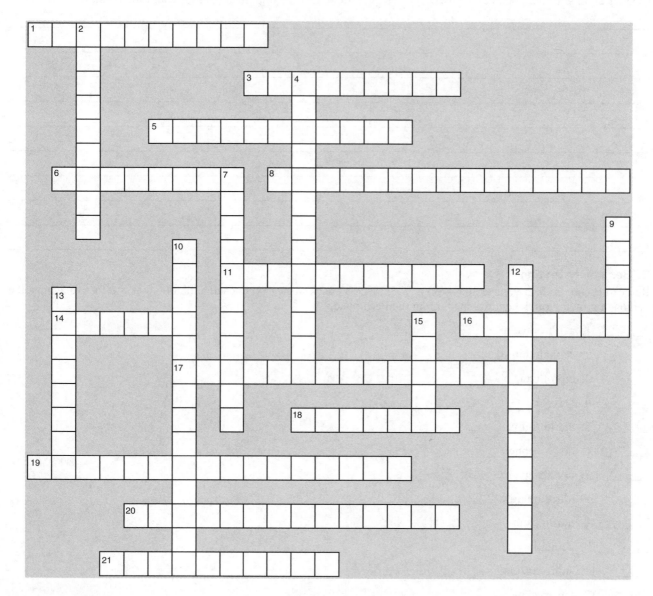

Across
1 It is everywhere!
3 Invasion by pathogens
5 Only 1 MO growing
6 Disease producing MO
8 Which antibiotic?
11 Tx for strep throat
14 Color of gram+ bacteria
16 Rod-shaped bacteria
17 Way to transmit pathogens
18 Mass of MOs on a medium
19 Between invasion and first sym
20 Sequela to strep throat
21 Can catch it!

Down
2 Introduce MOs to a culture
4 Not really present
7 Harmless MOs residing in body
9 Round bacteria
10 For precise focusing
12 Study of MOs
13 Sample of the body
15 Material spread on a slide

VIDEO EVALUATION FOR CHAPTER 20: MEDICAL MICROBIOLOGY

Name: _____

Directions:

a. Watch the indicated videos.

b. Mark each true statement with a T and each false statement with an F. For each false statement, change the wording of the question so that it becomes a true statement.

Video: Procedure 20-2: Collecting a Throat Specimen

_____ 1. A specimen is a mass of microorganisms growing on a culture medium.

_____ 2. If a specimen is contaminated with extraneous microorganisms, it may not be possible to identify pathogens that may be present.

_____ 3. The purpose of a transport medium is to preserve a specimen in its original state until it reaches its destination.

_____ 4. The swab should be firmly rubbed over any lesions or white or inflamed areas of the throat.

_____ 5. A rotating motion should be used when collecting a specimen to prevent contamination of the swab with normal flora.

_____ 6. The tonsillar area and the uvula should be swabbed when obtaining a throat specimen.

_____ 7. The swab should be completely immersed in the transport medium in the collection tube.

_____ 8. The specimen should be transported to the laboratory within 60 minutes after collection.

Video: Procedure 20-A: Rapid Strep Testing

_____ 1. Strep throat primarily affects children and young adults.

_____ 2. In some patients, strep throat can develop into tuberculosis.

_____ 3. Controls should be run when a new testing kit is opened.

_____ 4. The blue internal control line indicates that the proper volume of fluid entered the test cassette.

_____ 5. If the blue control line does not appear, the results are recorded as negative.

_____ 6. When collecting a throat specimen, the swab should not be allowed to touch the patient's tongue or mouth.

_____ 7. If the test results are invalid, the test should be repeated.

Notes

PRACTICE FOR COMPETENCY

Procedure 20-1: Using the Microscope. Practice using a microscope.

Procedure 20-2: Collecting a Throat Specimen. Obtain a throat specimen by using a sterile cotton swab or a collection and transport system. Record the procedure in the chart provided.

Procedure 20-A: Rapid Strep Testing. Perform a strep test using a rapid strep testing kit, and record the results in the chart provided.

Procedure 20-3: Preparing a Smear. Prepare a microbiologic smear.

CHART	
Date	

CHART	
Date	

Procedure 20-1: Using the Microscope

Name: _____   Date: _____

Evaluated by: _____   Score: _____

Performance Objective

Outcome:	Use a microscope.
Conditions:	Given a microscope, lens paper, specimen slide, tissue or gauze, immersion oil, xylene, and a soft cloth.
Standards:	Time: 15 minutes. Student completed procedure in _____ minutes.
	Accuracy: Satisfactory score on the Performance Evaluation Checklist.

Performance Evaluation Checklist

Trial 1	Trial 2	Point Value	Performance Standards
		•	Cleaned the ocular and objective lenses with lens paper.
		•	Turned on the light source.
		•	Rotated the nosepiece to the low-power objective.
		•	Used the coarse adjustment to provide sufficient working space for placing the slide on the stage.
		•	Placed the slide on the stage, specimen side up, and secured it.
		•	Positioned the low-power objective until it almost touched the slide using the coarse adjustment.
		•	Observed this step.
		▷	Explained why this step should be observed.
		•	Looked through the ocular lens.
		•	Brought the specimen into coarse focus using the coarse adjustment knob.
		•	Observed the specimen until it came into coarse focus.
		•	Used the fine-adjustment knob to bring the specimen into sharp, clear focus.
		•	Adjusted the light as needed using the iris diaphragm.
		•	Rotated the nosepiece to the high-power objective.
		•	Used the fine-adjustment knob to bring the specimen into a precise focus.
		•	Did not use the coarse-adjustment knob to focus the high-power objective.
		▷	Explained why the coarse-adjustment knob should not be used for focusing at this point.
		•	Examined the specimen as required by the test or procedure being performed.
		•	Turned off the light after use.
		•	Removed the slide from the stage.
		•	Cleaned the stage with a tissue or gauze.

Trial 1	Trial 2	Point Value	Performance Standards
		•	Properly cared for and stored the microscope.
			Using the oil-immersion objective:
		•	Rotated the nosepiece to the oil-immersion objective.
		•	Placed the objective to one side.
		•	Placed a drop of immersion oil on the slide directly over the center opening in the stage.
		•	Moved the oil-immersion objective into place.
		•	Made sure the objective did not touch the stage or slide.
		•	Used the coarse adjustment to position the oil-immersion objective.
		•	Brought the objective down until the lens touched the oil but did not come in contact with the slide.
		•	Looked through the eyepiece.
		•	Focused slowly using the coarse objective until the object was visible.
		•	Used the fine adjustment to bring the object into sharp focus.
		•	Adjusted the light as needed using the iris diaphragm.
		•	Examined the specimen as required by the test or procedure being performed.
		•	Turned off the light after use.
		•	Removed the slide from the stage.
		•	Cleaned the oil-immersion objective with lens paper.
		▷	Explained why the lens must be cleaned immediately.
		•	Cleaned the oil from the slide by immersing it in xylene and wiping it with a soft cloth.
		✶	Completed the procedure within 15 minutes.
			Totals

Evaluation of Student Performance

EVALUATION CRITERIA			COMMENTS
Symbol	**Category**	**Point Value**	
✶	Critical Step	16 points	
•	Essential Step	6 points	
▷	Theory Question	2 points	

Score calculation: 100 points

−_____ points missed

_____ Score

Satisfactory score: 85 or above

Notes

e **Procedure 20-2: Collecting a Throat Specimen**

Name: _____ Date: _____

Evaluated by: _____ Score: _____

Performance Objective

Outcome:	Collect a throat specimen.
Conditions:	Given the following: disposable gloves, tongue depressor, sterile swab, collection and transport system, laboratory request form, and a biohazard specimen bag.
Standards:	Time: 15 minutes. Student completed procedure in _____ minutes.
	Accuracy: Satisfactory score on the Performance Evaluation Checklist.

Performance Evaluation Checklist

Trial 1	Trial 2	Point Value	Performance Standards
			Throat specimen—sterile swab for strep testing in medical office
		•	Sanitized hands.
		•	Assembled equipment.
		•	Greeted the patient and introduced yourself.
		•	Identified the patient and explained the procedure.
		•	Positioned the patient and adjusted the light.
		•	Applied gloves.
		•	Removed the sterile swab from its peel-apart package and took care not to contaminate it.
		•	Depressed the patient's tongue with a tongue depressor.
		•	Placed a swab at the back of patient's throat and firmly rubbed it over lesions or white or inflamed areas of the tonsillar area and posterior pharynx.
		▷	Explained why the swab should be rubbed over suspicious-looking areas.
		•	Constantly rotated the swab as the specimen was being obtained.
		▷	Described why a rotating motion should be used.
		•	Did not allow the swab to touch any area other than the throat.
		▷	Explained why the swab should not be allowed to touch any areas other than the throat.
		•	Kept the patient's tongue depressed and withdrew the swab and removed the tongue depressor.
		•	Disposed of the tongue depressor.
		•	Performed the rapid strep test according to the directions accompanying the rapid strep testing kit.
		•	Removed gloves and sanitized hands.
		•	Charted the test results correctly.
		✶	Completed the procedure within 5 minutes.

Trial 1	Trial 2	Point Value	Performance Standards
			Throat specimen—collection and transport system
		•	Sanitized hands.
		•	Greeted the patient and introduced yourself.
		•	Identified the patient and explained the procedure.
		•	Positioned the patient and adjusted the light.
		•	Applied gloves.
		•	Checked the expiration date on the peel-apart package.
		•	Peeled open the package and removed the cap from the collection tube.
		•	Removed the cap/swab unit from the peel-apart package.
		•	Depressed the patient's tongue with a tongue depressor.
		•	Placed the swab at the back of the patient's throat and firmly rubbed it over lesions or white or inflamed areas of the tonsillar area and posterior pharynx.
		•	Constantly rotated the swab as the specimen was being obtained.
		•	Did not allow the swab to touch any area other than the collection site.
		•	Kept the patient's tongue depressed and withdrew the swab and removed the tongue depressor.
		•	Disposed of the tongue depressor.
		•	Inserted the swab into the collection tube.
		•	Pushed the cap or swab in as far as it would go.
		•	Made sure the cap was tightly in place.
		•	Removed gloves and sanitized hands.
		•	Labeled the tube.
		•	Completed a laboratory request form.
		•	Placed the tube in a biohazard specimen transport bag.
		•	Placed the laboratory request in the outside pocket of the bag.
		•	Charted the procedure.
		•	Transported the specimen to the laboratory within 24 hours.
		▷	Explained why the specimen must be transported within 24 hours.
		✳	Completed the procedure within 5 minutes.
			Totals
		CHART	
Date			

Evaluation of Student Performance

EVALUATION CRITERIA			COMMENTS
Symbol	**Category**	**Point Value**	
✱	Critical Step	16 points	
•	Essential Step	6 points	
▷	Theory Question	2 points	

Score calculation: 100 points

        − _____ points missed

           _____ Score

Satisfactory score: 85 or above

CAAHEP Competencies Achieved

Psychomotor (Skills)

☑ III. 7. Obtain specimens for microbiological testing.

Affective (Behavior)

☑ III. 1. Display sensitivity to patient rights and feelings in collecting specimens.

☑ III. 2. Explain the rationale for performance of a procedure to the patient.

☑ III. 3. Show awareness of patients' concerns regarding their perceptions related to the procedures being performed.

ABHES Competencies Achieved

☑ 8. cc. Communicate on the recipient's level of comprehension.

☑ 10. d. Collect, label, and process specimens (4) Obtain throat specimens for microbiologic testing.

Notes

Procedure 20-A: Rapid Strep Testing

Name: _____   Date: _____

Evaluated by: _____   Score: _____

Performance Objective

Outcome:	Perform a rapid strep test.
Conditions:	Given the following: disposable gloves, tongue blade, a Quick Vue rapid strep testing kit, controls, manufacturer's instructions, quality control log, and a biohazard sharps container.
Standards:	Time: 10 minutes. Student completed procedure in _____ minutes.
	Accuracy: Satisfactory score on the Performance Evaluation Checklist.

Performance Evaluation Checklist

Trial 1	Trial 2	Point Value	Performance Standards
		•	Sanitized hands.
		•	Assembled equipment.
		•	Checked the expiration date on the testing kit.
		•	Applied gloves and ran a positive and negative control, if needed.
		▷	Stated when controls should be run.
		•	Disposed of the test cassettes and swabs in a biohazard waste container.
		•	Removed gloves and sanitized hands.
		•	Recorded the results in the quality control log.
		•	Greeted the patient and introduced yourself.
		•	Identified the patient and explained the procedure.
		•	Positioned the patient and adjusted the light.
		•	Sanitized hands and applied gloves.
		•	Removed the test cassette from its foil pouch, and placed it on a clean, dry, level surface.
		•	Removed the sterile swab from its peel-apart package.
		•	Depressed the patient's tongue with a tongue depressor.
		•	Placed the swab at the back of the patient's throat and firmly rubbed it over lesions or white or inflamed areas of the tonsillar area and posterior pharynx.
		•	Constantly rotated the swab as the specimen was being obtained.
		▷	Stated why the swab should be rotated.
		•	Did not allow the swab to touch any area other than the throat.
		•	Kept the patient's tongue depressed and withdrew the swab.
		•	Removed the tongue depressor and discarded it.
		•	Inserted the swab completely into the swab chamber.

Trial 1	Trial 2	Point Value	Performance Standards
		•	Squeezed the extraction bottle once to break the glass ampule.
		•	Vigorously shook the extraction bottle five times.
		•	Filled the swab chamber to the rim.
		•	Started the timer.
		•	Waited 5 minutes and read the results.
		▷	Described the appearance of a positive and negative result.
		▷	Described the appearance of an invalid result.
		▷	Explained what to do if an invalid result occurs.
		✱	The results were identical to the evaluator's results.
		•	Disposed of the test cassette and swab in a biohazard waste container.
		•	Removed gloves and sanitized hands.
		•	Recorded the results in patient's chart.
		✱	Completed the procedure within 10 minutes.
			Totals

CHART	
Date	

Evaluation of Student Performance

EVALUATION CRITERIA			COMMENTS
Symbol	**Category**	**Point Value**	
✱	Critical Step	16 points	
•	Essential Step	6 points	
▷	Theory Question	2 points	

Score calculation: 100 points

− _____ points missed

_____ Score

Satisfactory score: 85 or above

CAAHEP Competencies Achieved

Psychomotor (Skills)

☑ I. 11. Perform quality control measures.

☑ III. 7. Obtain specimens for microbiological testing.

☑ III. 8. Perform CLIA-waived microbiology testing.

Affective (Behavior)

☑ II. 2. Distinguish between normal and abnormal test results.

☑ III. 1. Display sensitivity to patient rights and feelings in collecting specimens.

☑ III. 3. Show awareness of patients' concerns regarding their perceptions related to the procedures being performed.

ABHES Competencies Achieved

☑ 10. a. Practice quality control.

☑ 10. b. Perform selected CLIA-waived tests that assist with diagnosis and treatment (2) Microbiology testing (6) Kit testing (b) Quick strep.

☑ 10. c. Dispose of biohazardous materials.

Notes

Procedure 20-3: Preparing a Smear

Name: _____   Date: _____

Evaluated by: _____   Score: _____

Performance Objective

Outcome:	Prepare a microbiologic smear.
Conditions:	Given the following: disposable gloves, Bunsen burner, clean glass slide, microbiologic specimen, slide forceps, sterile swab, and a biohazard waste container.
Standards:	Time: 15 minutes. Student completed procedure in _____ minutes. Accuracy: Satisfactory score on the Performance Evaluation Checklist.

Performance Evaluation Checklist

Trial 1	Trial 2	Point Value	Performance Standards
		•	Sanitized hands.
		•	Assembled equipment.
		•	Labeled the slide.
		•	Applied gloves and held the edge of slide between the thumb and index finger.
		•	Started at the right side of slide, used a rolling motion, and gently and evenly spread the material from the specimen over the slide.
		▷	Explained why the material should not be rubbed over the slide.
		•	Allowed the smear to air dry.
		▷	Explained why heat should not be applied at this point.
		•	Held the slide with slide forceps and heat-fixed the smear.
		•	Stated the purpose of heat-fixing the smear.
		•	Allowed the slide to cool completely.
		•	Prepared the slide for examination under the microscope by the physician.
		✻	Completed the procedure within 15 minutes.
			Totals

EVALUATION CRITERIA			COMMENTS
Symbol	**Category**	**Point Value**	
✱	Critical Step	16 points	
•	Essential Step	6 points	
▷	Theory Question	2 points	

Score calculation: 100 points

−   _____ points missed

_____ Score

Satisfactory score: 85 or above

CAAHEP Competencies Achieved

Psychomotor (Skills)

☑ III. 7. Obtain specimens for microbiological testing.

ABHES Competencies Achieved

☑ 10. d. Collect, label, and process specimens.

21 Emergency Medical Procedures

CHAPTER ASSIGNMENTS

√ After Completing	Date Due	Textbook Pages	TEXTBOOK ASSIGNMENTS	Possible Points	Points You Earned
		781–807	Read Chapter 21: Emergency Medical Procedures		
		798 804	Read Case Study 1 Case Study 1 questions	5	
		799 804	Read Case Study 2 Case Study 2 questions	5	
		802 804–805	Read Case Study 3 Case Study 3 questions	5	
			Total points		

√ After Completing	Date Due	Study Guide Pages	STUDY GUIDE ASSIGNMENTS (CTA = Critical Thinking Activity)	Possible Points	Points You Earned
		893	Pretest	10	
		894	Term Key Term Assessment	16	
		895–899	Evaluation of Learning questions	27	
		900	CTA A: First Aid Kit	10	
		900	CTA B: EMD Information	5	
		900	CTA C: Emergency Care	6	
		901–902	CTA D: Emergency Situations	55	
			Evolve Site: Chapter 21 Nutrition Nugget: Nutrition and Burns	10	
			Evolve Site: Apply Your Knowledge questions	10	
		893	Posttest	10	
			ADDITIONAL ASSIGNMENTS		
			Total points		

Notes

Name: _____   Date: _____

True or False

_____ 1. A specially equipped cart for holding and transporting medications, equipment, and supplies needed in an emergency is known as a *crash cart*.

_____ 2. Symptoms of an asthmatic attack include dyspnea and wheezing.

_____ 3. Symptoms of a heart attack include sudden weakness on one side of the body.

_____ 4. Another name for a stroke is a coronary occlusion.

_____ 5. Arterial bleeding is characterized by a slow and steady flow of blood that is dark red.

_____ 6. A laceration is an example of a closed wound.

_____ 7. Symptoms of a fracture include pain, swelling, deformity, and loss of function.

_____ 8. A sprain is a tearing of ligaments at a joint.

_____ 9. Heatstroke is a life-threatening emergency.

_____ 10. Insulin enables glucose to enter the body's cells and be converted to energy.

?📄 POSTTEST

True or False

_____ 1. When providing emergency care, you should obtain information about what happened from bystanders.

_____ 2. Emphysema is a progressive lung disorder in which there is a loss of elasticity of the alveoli of the lungs.

_____ 3. Symptoms that may occur with hyperventilation include rapid and deep respirations and tachycardia.

_____ 4. The first priority for hypovolemic shock is to control bleeding.

_____ 5. Status asthmaticus is the type of shock caused by a reaction of the body to a substance to which an individual is highly allergic.

_____ 6. Another name for a nosebleed is epistaxis.

_____ 7. The type of fracture in which the broken ends of the bone are forcefully jammed together is a greenstick fracture.

_____ 8. The type of seizure in which the abnormal electrical activity is localized into very specific areas of the brain is a tonic-clonic seizure.

_____ 9. Chipmunks have a high incidence of rabies.

_____ 10. Emergency care for insulin shock is to give the patient sugar immediately.

Directions: Match each medical term (numbers) with its definition (letters).

_____ 1. Burn

_____ 2. Crash cart

_____ 3. Crepitus

_____ 4. Dislocation

_____ 5. Emergency medical services

_____ 6. First aid

_____ 7. Fracture

_____ 8. Hypothermia

_____ 9. Poison

_____ 10. Pressure point

_____ 11. Seizure

_____ 12. Shock

_____ 13. Splint

_____ 14. Sprain

_____ 15. Strain

_____ 16. Wound

A. A network of community resources, equipment, and personnel that provides care to victims of injury or sudden illness

B. Any substance that causes illness, injury, or death if it enters the body

C. An injury to the tissues caused by exposure to thermal, chemical, electrical, or radioactive agents

D. Any device that immobilizes a body part

E. A grating sensation caused by fractured bone fragments rubbing against each other

F. A sudden episode of involuntary muscular contractions and relaxation, often accompanied by a change in sensation, behavior, and level of consciousness

G. A stretching or tearing of muscles or tendons caused by trauma

H. The immediate care that is administered to an individual who is injured or suddenly becomes ill before complete medical care can be obtained

I. A break in the continuity of an external or internal surface caused by physical means

J. A specially equipped cart for holding and transporting medications, equipment, and supplies needed for performing lifesaving procedures in an emergency

K. Any break in a bone

L. The failure of the cardiovascular system to deliver enough blood to all the vital organs of the body

M. An injury in which one end of a bone making up a joint is separated or displaced from its normal anatomic position

N. A life-threatening condition in which the temperature of the entire body falls to a dangerously low level

O. A site on the body where an artery lies close to the surface of the skin and can be compressed against an underlying bone to control bleeding

P. Trauma to a joint that causes tearing of ligaments

Directions: Fill in each blank with the correct answer.

1. What is the purpose of first aid?

   _____

   _____

   _____

   _____

2. What is the purpose of the office crash cart?

   _____

   _____

   _____

   _____

3. What is the difference between an EMT-basic and an EMT-paramedic?

   _____

   _____

   _____

4. What are the responsibilities of an emergency medical dispatcher?

   _____

   _____

   _____

5. List five OSHA Standards that should be followed when administering first aid.

   _____

   _____

   _____

   _____

6. What is the reason for performing each of the following during an emergency situation?

   a. Remaining calm and speaking in a normal tone of voice

   _____

   _____

   b. Making sure it is safe before approaching the patient

   _____

   _____

c. Following OSHA Standards when providing emergency care

_____

_____

d. Activating the emergency medical services

_____

_____

e. Not moving the patient unnecessarily

_____

_____

f. Checking the patient for a medical alert tag

_____

_____

7. What are the symptoms of asthma?

_____

_____

8. What is emphysema?

_____

_____

9. What are the symptoms of hyperventilation?

_____

_____

10. What are the symptoms of a heart attack?

_____

_____

11. What are the symptoms of a stroke?

_____

_____

12. What is the cause of the following types of shock?

a. Hypovolemic

_____

_____

b. Cardiogenic

_____

_____

c. Neurogenic

_____

_____

d. Anaphylactic

_____

_____

e. Psychogenic

_____

_____

13. What are the characteristics of each of the following types of external bleeding?
    a. Capillary

_____

_____

    b. Venous

_____

_____

    c. Arterial

_____

_____

14. What is the difference between an open wound and a closed wound?

_____

_____

15. What are the signs and symptoms of a fracture?

_____

_____

16. What are the characteristics of each of the following types of fractures?
    a. Impacted

_____

_____

    b. Greenstick

_____

_____

c. Transverse

_____

_____

d. Oblique

_____

_____

e. Comminuted

_____

_____

f. Spiral

_____

_____

17. What are the characteristics of each of the following types of burns?
   a. Superficial

_____

_____

   b. Partial thickness

_____

_____

   c. Full thickness

_____

_____

18. What is the difference between a partial seizure and a generalized seizure?

_____

_____

19. List two examples of each of the following types of poisoning:
   a. Ingested

_____

_____

   b. Inhaled

_____

_____

c. Absorbed

_____

_____

d. Injected

_____

_____

20. What spiders (found in the United States) have bites that can result in serious or life-threatening reactions?

_____

_____

21. What species of snakes (found in the United States) are poisonous?

_____

_____

22. What animals tend to have a high incidence of rabies?

_____

_____

23. What factors place an individual at higher risk for developing heat- and cold-related injuries?

_____

_____

24. What areas of the body are most susceptible to frostbite?

_____

_____

25. What is the difference between type 1 diabetes and type 2 diabetes?

_____

_____

26. What is insulin shock, and what causes it to occur?

_____

_____

27. What is diabetic coma, and what causes it to occur?

_____

_____

CRITICAL THINKING ACTIVITIES

A. First Aid Kit

You are assembling a first aid kit. What supplies should be included in your kit? Identify one use for each of the supplies you list.

_____

_____

_____

_____

_____

_____

_____

_____

_____

B. EMD Information

Jeff Stickler suddenly develops weakness in his left arm and leg, has difficulty speaking, and has a severe headache and dizziness. You immediately call the Emergency Medical Services (EMS). What information should you be prepared to relay to the emergency medical dispatcher (EMD)?

_____

_____

_____

C. Emergency Care

In which of the following emergency situations would you be legally permitted to administer first aid? Explain your answers.

1. A patient is unconscious and bleeding profusely.

_____

_____

2. You identify yourself and state your level of training and what you plan to do. You ask the patient if it is all right to administer emergency care. The patient responds by saying, "Yes, please help me."

_____

_____

3. You ask the patient whether you can administer emergency care, but the patient refuses your help.

_____

_____

900

Chapter **21** **Emergency Medical Procedures**

D. Emergency Situations

Explain what you would do in each of the following situations.

1. Holly Murphy falls while roller skating. She comes down hard on her left arm, which begins to swell and discolor. Holly guards her arm and complains of intense pain.

_____

_____

_____

_____

2. John Phillips is mowing the grass and mows over a yellow jacket nest. He is stung twice and soon starts complaining of intense itching and exhibits erythema and hives on his arms, torso, and face.

_____

_____

_____

_____

3. Steve Williams complains of severe indigestion and squeezing pain in the chest. He is short of breath and perspiring profusely.

_____

_____

_____

_____

4. Clara Miller is playing basketball and is accidentally hit in the face with the ball. Her nose begins bleeding profusely.

_____

_____

_____

_____

5. Debbie Carter, age 4 years, finds some children's chewable vitamins that have been left open on a table. She eats about 10 of them.

_____

_____

_____

_____

6. Rita Preston accidentally cuts her finger with a knife while preparing dinner. Her finger begins bleeding profusely.

_____

_____

_____

_____

7. Jose Perez is jogging on a cinder track. He falls and scrapes his left knee on the cinders.

_____

_____

_____

_____

8. Charlotte Lambert is getting ready to perform a piano recital for her entire church congregation. Suddenly she starts breathing very rapidly and deeply and complains that she feels light-headed and dizzy.

_____

_____

_____

_____

9. Bruce Jones has diabetes. He is in a hurry and forgets to eat breakfast. He begins exhibiting behavior similar to that of someone who is intoxicated.

_____

_____

_____

_____

10. Debra Murray is delivering newspapers and is bitten by a strange dog. The bite causes several puncture marks and slight bleeding.

_____

_____

_____

_____

11. Tanya Howe is playing tennis on a hot and humid day and begins to feel weak and nauseous. Her skin feels cold and clammy, and she is sweating profusely and complains of dizziness.

_____

_____

_____

_____

Notes

Notes

Notes

Notes

Notes

Notes